VOLUME 615   JANUARY 2008

THE ANNALS

of The American Academy of Political
and Social Science

PHYLLIS KANISS, *Executive Editor*

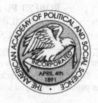

Overweight and Obesity in America's Children: Causes, Consequences, Solutions

Special Editor of this Volume

AMY B. JORDAN
The Annenberg Public Policy Center, University of Pennsylvania

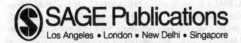

SAGE Publications
Los Angeles • London • New Delhi • Singapore

The American Academy of Political and Social Science

3814 Walnut Street, Fels Institute of Government, University of Pennsylvania,
Philadelphia, PA 19104-6197; (215) 746-6500; (215) 573-3003 (fax); www.aapss.org

Origin and Purpose. The Academy was organized December 14, 1889, to promote the progress of political and social science, especially through publications and meetings. The Academy does not take sides in controverted questions, but seeks to gather and present reliable information to assist the public in forming an intelligent and accurate judgment.

Meetings. The Academy occasionally holds a meeting in the spring extending over two days.

Publications. THE ANNALS of The American Academy of Political and Social Science is the bimonthly publication of the Academy. Each issue contains articles on some prominent social or political problem, written at the invitation of the editors. Also, monographs are published from time to time, numbers of which are distributed to pertinent professional organizations. These volumes constitute important reference works on the topics with which they deal, and they are extensively cited by authorities throughout the United States and abroad. The papers presented at the meetings of the Academy are included in THE ANNALS.

Membership. Each member of the Academy receives THE ANNALS and may attend the meetings of the Academy. Membership is open only to individuals. Annual dues: $94.00 for the regular paperbound edition (clothbound, $134.00). Members may also purchase single issues of THE ANNALS for $18.00 each (clothbound, $27.00). Student memberships are available for $52.00.

Subscriptions. THE ANNALS of The American Academy of Political and Social Science (ISSN 0002-7162) (J295) is published six times annually—in January, March, May, July, September, and November—by Sage Publications, 2455 Teller Road, Thousand Oaks, CA 91320. Telephone: (800) 818-SAGE (7243) and (805) 499-0721; Fax/Order line: (805) 375-1700; e-mail: journals@sagepub.com. Copyright © 2008 by The American Academy of Political and Social Science. Institutions may subscribe to THE ANNALS at the annual rate: $661.00 (clothbound, $747.00). Single issues of THE ANNALS may be obtained by individuals who are not members of the Academy for $34.00 each (clothbound, $47.00). Single issues of THE ANNALS have proven to be excellent supplementary texts for classroom use. Direct inquiries regarding adoptions to THE ANNALS c/o Sage Publications (address below). Periodicals postage paid at Thousand Oaks, California, and at additional mailing offices. POSTMASTER: Send address changes to The Annals of The American Academy of Political and Social Science, c/o Sage Publications, 2455 Teller Road, Thousand Oaks, CA 91320.

All correspondence concerning membership in the Academy, dues renewals, inquiries about membership status, and/or purchase of single issues of THE ANNALS should be sent to THE ANNALS c/o Sage Publications, 2455 Teller Road, Thousand Oaks, CA 91320. Telephone: (800) 818-SAGE (7243) and (805) 499-0721; Fax/Order line: (805) 375-1700; e-mail: journals@sagepub.com. *Please note that orders under $30 must be prepaid.* Sage affiliates in London and India will assist institutional subscribers abroad with regard to orders, claims, and inquiries for both subscriptions and single issues.

Printed on acid-free paper

THE ANNALS

© 2008 by The American Academy of Political and Social Science

Editorial Office: 3814 Walnut Street, Fels Institute for Government, University of Pennsylvania, Philadelphia, PA 19104-6197.
For information about membership* (individuals only) and subscriptions (institutions), address:
Sage Publications
2455 Teller Road
Thousand Oaks, CA 91320

For Sage Publications: Dan Wollrich (Production) and Sandra Hopps (Marketing)

From India and South Asia, write to:
SAGE PUBLICATIONS INDIA Pvt Ltd
B-42 Panchsheel Enclave, P.O. Box 4109
New Delhi 110 017
INDIA

From Europe, the Middle East, and Africa, write to:
SAGE PUBLICATIONS LTD
1 Oliver's Yard, 55 City Road
London EC1Y 1SP
UNITED KINGDOM

*Please note that members of the Academy receive THE ANNALS with their membership.
International Standard Serial Number ISSN 0002-7162
International Standard Book Number ISBN 978-1-4129-6684-9 (Vol. 615, 2008) paper

The articles appearing in *The Annals* are abstracted or indexed in Academic Abstracts, Academic Search, America: History and Life, Asia Pacific Database, Book Review Index,CABAbstracts Database, Central Asia: Abstracts &Index, Communication Abstracts, Corporate ResourceNET, Criminal Justice Abstracts, Current Citations Express, Current Contents: Social & Behavioral Sciences, Documentation in Public Administration, e-JEL, EconLit, Expanded Academic Index, Guide to Social Science & Religion in Periodical Literature, Health Business FullTEXT, HealthSTAR FullTEXT, Historical Abstracts, International Bibliography of the Social Sciences, International Political Science Abstracts, ISI Basic Social Sciences Index, Journal of Economic Literature on CD, LEXIS-NEXIS, MasterFILE FullTEXT, Middle East: Abstracts&Index, North Africa: Abstracts&Index, PAIS International, Periodical Abstracts, Political Science Abstracts, Psychological Abstracts, PsycINFO, Sage Public Administration Abstracts, Scopus, Social Science Source, Social Sciences Citation Index, Social Sciences Index Full Text, Social Services Abstracts, SocialWork Abstracts, Sociological Abstracts, Southeast Asia: Abstracts& Index, Standard Periodical Directory (SPD), TOPICsearch, Wilson OmniFileV, and Wilson Social Sciences Index/Abstracts, and are available on microfilm from ProQuest, Ann Arbor, Michigan.

Information about membership rates, institutional subscriptions, and back issue prices may be found on the facing page.

Advertising. Current rates and specifications may be obtained by writing to The Annals Advertising and Promotion Manager at the Thousand Oaks office (address above).

Claims. Claims for undelivered copies must be made no later than six months following month of publication. The publisher will supply missing copies when losses have been sustained in transit and when the reserve stock will permit.

Change of Address. Six weeks' advance notice must be given when notifying of change of address to ensure proper identification. Please specify name of journal.

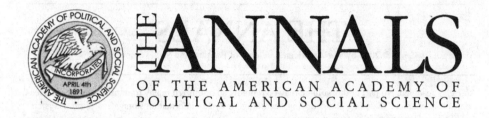

THE ANNALS

OF THE AMERICAN ACADEMY OF POLITICAL AND SOCIAL SCIENCE

Volume 615   January 2008

IN THIS ISSUE:

Overweight and Obesity in America's Children: Causes, Consequences, Solutions

Special Editor: AMY B. JORDAN

FORTHCOMING

Public Diplomacy in a Changing World
Special Editors: GEOFFREY COWAN and NICHOLAS CULL
Volume 616, March 2008

The Politics of History in Comparative Perspective
Special Editor: MARTIN O. HEISLER
Volume 617, May 2008

Preface

By
AMY B. JORDAN

This special issue of *The Annals* is dedicated to exploring the topic of childhood overweight and obesity. It brings together researchers, practitioners, and policy makers in a forum designed to identify the contexts of a child's life that help to determine weight status, including the home, the community, and the school, as well as the larger contexts of children's development influenced by media and culture. The approach we take in this forum reflects the great tradition of *The Annals*—we have the unique opportunity to bring to bear numerous disciplinary perspectives to inform the causes and consequences of childhood overweight, and collectively we are inspired to use our expertise to make empirically based, creative suggestions for strategies to overcome the problem. Our authors are health care practitioners, social scientists, philanthropists, advocates, and policy makers. Where else but in *The Annals* could such a group of distinguished influentials come together?

As the authors who have written for this volume argue, the problem of childhood overweight has reached near-epidemic proportions in the United States. The Centers for Disease Control and Prevention (CDC)—a federal agency that has tracked the prevalence of overweight across the decades—finds that the number of children who are obese (at or above the 95th percentile for age- and gender-adjusted height and weight) has tripled since the 1970s.

Amy B. Jordan is director of the Media and the Developing Child sector of the Annenberg Public Policy Center at the University of Pennsylvania. She is the coauthor (with Victor Strasburger and Barbara Wilson) of Children, Adolescents and the Media *(Sage Publications, forthcoming in 2008) and coeditor (with Sandra Calvert) of* Children in the Digital Age *(Greenwood Press, 2002). She received the International Communications Association award for Most Important Applied/Policy Research (2001) for her work on the implementation and impact of federal children's television regulations.*

DOI: 10.1177/0002716207309670

Equally concerning is the steep trajectory of increase in the number of America's children that have a clinical and significant weight problem (at or above the 85th percentile) (Ogden et al. 2006). Pediatricians William H. Dietz and Thomas N. Robinson write that being overweight as a child makes one significantly more likely to be overweight as an adult. It also puts the child at risk for a host of associated medical problems. Family physician Laure DeMattia and her coauthor Shannon Lee Denney present the reader with the long list of complicating diseases associated with childhood overweight, including diabetes, hyperinsulinemia, dyslipidemia, joint abnormalities, polycystic ovarian syndrome, nonalcoholic fatty liver disease, and sleep disturbances. Recently released studies have also pointed out the social and psychological problems that overweight children face: overweight children are stigmatized, ostracized, and bullied in ways that their normal-weight peers are not (Puhl and Latner 2007). Clearly, we need to help the 9 million children in this country who are overweight, and we need to do it now. Moreover, we need to find ways to effectively prevent future generations from falling into the same unhealthy lifestyles that led to this problem in the first place.

Clearly, we need to help the 9 million children in this country who are overweight, and we need to do it now.

Tackling this problem begins with finding the right words to talk about it. You may notice that contributors to this special issue use various words to describe weight status: "at risk for overweight," "overweight," and "obese." An explanation may be in order, as experts are still debating whether it is accurate or fair to label children "obese." As recently as a year ago, a committee with representatives from the CDC, the American Medical Association, and the American Academy of Pediatrics considered changing the language we use to describe children with weight problems. Currently, parents with a child whose a body mass index (BMI) is between the 85th and 94th percentile are told by their pediatricians that their child is "at risk for overweight." Parents with a child whose BMI is 95th percentile or higher are told that their child is "overweight." (By contrast, adults in the same percentiles are told simply that they are "overweight" or "obese.")

Softer words were chosen almost two decades ago, before the problem of childhood obesity reached epidemic proportions. But the time has come to use the correct words. Because parents often see their children as having "baby fat" or being "big-boned" (Baughcum et al. 2000), labeling a child as "at risk for overweight" is probably not going to catalyze parents to take action. Beyond the pediatrician's office, the public also deserves a less obscure view of the extent and causes of the problem. The current terminology would lead us to believe that only 18 percent of children are overweight and that no child is, strictly speaking, obese. But the more accurate picture—which includes all children who are too heavy—shows that nearly one-third of America's children are afflicted. For this reason, we have decided to title this special issue of *The Annals* "Overweight and Obesity in America's Children: Causes, Consequences, Solutions."

The time has come to ask ourselves the hard question: "How did this happen?" So much has changed over the past two decades that it is virtually impossible to isolate a single or even most important catalyst for the epidemic. In this volume, we have identified distinct contexts that shape weight status—for example, home, school, media—but all of our authors recognize that the environments of the developing child overlap in their influence, exacerbating or alleviating the conditions that put children at risk for developing weight problems. For example, children who grow up in homes where parents socialize children to perceive food as nourishment rather than comfort will have more strategies to resist the ubiquitous junk food marketing that bombards them in schools and through media.

Brown University pediatrician Kyung Rhee writes that parents profoundly shape children's relationship with food and patterns of physical activity through their general approaches to child rearing. The parenting strategies they use—authoritative, authoritarian, permissive, and neglectful—mold specific eating practices, but also influence children's attitudes and beliefs about food. Rhee believes understanding the impact of parenting practices on childhood overweight—and developing interventions that leverage this knowledge—may provide health care professionals and parent educators with new strategies for addressing childhood overweight.

Although parents may be the earliest and most consistent influence on children's beliefs and behaviors, they are not the only influence. Children grow up, go to school, play outside the home, and have access to a host of media and marketing messages. City and regional planning expert Amy Hillier, whose academic home is in the School of Design at the University of Pennsylvania, writes that children are engaging much less with the world outside their homes in terms of physical activity and much more in terms of eating. By exploring the "built environment" of the child, she writes, we can obtain a clearer picture of the opportunities children have to exercise (or not) and the access they have to healthy food choices (or not). Her concern about the increasingly sedentary nature of childhood that has resulted from passive media technology is translated into hope that in the near future these same technologies can be transformed into more active leisure pursuits for children and even tools for researchers (as they use handheld computers to map the built environment). Milwaukee-based family physician Laure DeMattia and law and communications expert Shannon Lee Denney write about the significance of the physical community, including the ways in which the modern restructuring of "neighborhood" often renders safe outdoor play spaces obsolete and walking to school unthinkable. Moreover, they write, children most at risk for overweight (low-income minority youth) are more likely to have access to fast-food restaurants and corner stores stocked with convenience foods than produce stands or grocery stores. Their concern about the negative impact of unhealthful communities is mitigated by the hope they have for changes that could occur at the local, state, and national level. For example, they highlight successful community-based programs that have brought back walking to school in some cities, that teach healthful nutrition and cooking through peer modeling, and that protect the rights of mothers who choose breastfeeding (which has been shown to be a protective factor against childhood obesity).

The school environment has also changed dramatically over the decades. Laura C. Leviton of the Robert Wood Johnson Foundation describes the increasing presence of "competitive foods" in schools (including snack bars and vending machines) which "compete" with the healthier but perhaps less tasty meals offered in the cafeteria. She also notes the decreasing opportunities children have to exercise during the school day. While schools are certainly limited in what they can do to mitigate childhood obesity, Leviton—a senior program officer at a philanthropic organization that has pledged hundreds of millions of dollars to this cause—says there are also many opportunities for action including holding schools accountable to meeting federal dietary guidelines, supporting schools with financial and technical assistance to maximize students' exposure to healthy foods and physical activities, and developing a research base from the many evaluations of school-based efforts under way across the nation.

Media, in particular television, are often blamed for exacerbating the problem of childhood obesity. Stanford pediatrician Thomas N. Robinson and I recently chaired an expert panel on children, television, and weight status. The panel was made up of experts from nutrition, psychology, public health, and a host of other disciplines and examined the relevant literature to determine just why screen media might be implicated. In addition to creating more sedentary children who burn fewer calories than they would otherwise, as well as encouraging the consumption of more calories, media may be persuading children to eat foods that are filled with sugar, salt, and fat and are devoid of nutritional value.

Ariel Chernin, a communications researcher at Harvard University's Center on Media and Child Health, conducted a clever experiment with five- to eleven-year-olds and found that food advertising does indeed increase children's preferences for the advertised foods. Intriguingly, her data show that children's age did not moderate this effect. Susan Linn and Courtney L. Novosat, of the national coalition Campaign for a Commercial-Free Environment, would not be surprised by Chernin's findings. They lay out the massive and somewhat dizzying ways in which food marketers reach children of all ages—from television commercials to product tie-ins to school-based promotionals to cell-phone spam. While each of the authors who write about media and marketing would argue that some degree of "media literacy" is helpful (in which children and families are taught to be more deliberate about their media consumption and more critical of media messages), they also recommend policy initiatives as a necessary and complementary approach to what families and educators can teach.

This issue of *The Annals* concludes with some careful thinking about the public policy options that are available to redress this problem. Samantha Kate Graff, an attorney with the California-based Public Health Institute, weighs the First Amendment implications of restricting food and beverage marketing in schools and concludes that districts do have a legal leg to stand on if they decide to take action in a survey they conducted with experts in nutrition, psychology, and medicine, Victoria L. Brescoll, Kelly D. Brownell (of the Rudd Center at Yale University) and Rogan Kersh (of the New York University Wagner School of Public Health), examine the perceived health efficacy and political feasibility of fifty-one federal policy options for addressing childhood obesity. Their results are fascinating and show a clear path for moving forward. Laura M. Segal and Emily A. Gadola, of Trust for America's Health, persuade us that successes can be found—at the community, state, and federal levels—and that childhood obesity intervention and prevention efforts can work.

The final section of the volume consists of thoughtful comments from leaders at the front lines in the fight against childhood obesity—Senator Sam Brownback, Senator Tom Harkin, and CDC Division Director William Dietz and Stanford's Thomas N. Robinson. Each offers a series of persuasive arguments that it is *not* too late to mobilize and that there *are* clear steps we can take as a nation that cares about the health of its children. Across the volume, our authors provide a research agenda that, if implemented, will continue the interdisciplinary approach we have taken to understanding the problem of childhood overweight and obesity and the collective effort we will need to solve it.

References

Baughcum, Amy E., Leigh A. Chamberlin, C. M. Deeks, Scott W. Powers, and Robert C. Whitaker. 2000. Maternal perceptions of overweight preschool children. *Pediatrics* 106:1380-86.

Ogden, C. L., M. D. Carroll, L. R. Curtin, M. A. McDowell, C. J. Tabak, and K. M. Flegal. 2006. Prevalence of overweight and obesity in the United States, 1999-2004. *Journal of the American Medical Association* 295:1549-55.

Puhl, Rebecca M., and Janet D. Latner. 2007. Stigma, obesity and the health of the nation's children. *Psychological Bulletin* 133 (4): 557-80.

SECTION ONE

Home, School,
and Community

Childhood Overweight and the Relationship between Parent Behaviors, Parenting Style, and Family Functioning

By
KYUNG RHEE

This article discusses the relationship between parent behaviors, parenting style, and how a family functions with respect to the development of childhood overweight. Parents can influence a child's weight through specific feeding and activity practices and perhaps more broadly through their parenting style and management of family functioning. These more global influences of parenting style and family functioning provide a framework in which specific parent behaviors can be interpreted by the child. Therefore, understanding the impact of specific parent behaviors within the context of parenting style and family functioning needs to be explored. This article highlights the pervasive influence of parents around the development of dietary habits, and suggests that additional efforts to examine the interaction between specific feeding behaviors and parenting style/family functioning should be promoted to better inform the development of interventions that may help stem the growing prevalence of obesity among our children.

Keywords: childhood overweight; feeding practices; parenting style; family functioning

The prevalence of childhood overweight has more than tripled in the past several decades and, according to data from the 2003–2004 National Health and Nutrition Examination Surveys (NHANES), continues to rise (Ogden, Carroll, et al. 2006; Ogden, Flegal, et al. 2002). Currently 17 percent of U.S. children aged two to nineteen years are overweight (body mass index [BMI] for age and gender ≥ 95th percentile by the Centers for Disease Control National Center for Health Statistics norms) (Kuczmarski et al. 2002), and nearly another 17 percent are at risk for overweight (BMI for age and gender ≥ 85th but < 95th percentile)

Kyung Rhee, MD, MS, is an assistant professor of pediatrics at the Warren Alpert Medical School of Brown University and conducts pediatric obesity research at the Weight Control and Diabetes Research Center at the Centers for Behavioral and Preventive Medicine. Her interest is in the impact of parenting style on the development of childhood overweight and the role of parental warmth and involvement in the success of pediatric weight control interventions.

DOI: 10.1177/0002716207308400

(Ogden et al. 2006). Looking more closely at these trends, a significant jump in the prevalence of children at risk for overweight and overweight children occurs between preschool (ages two to five) and grade school (ages six to eleven) years (26 to 37 percent) (Ogden et al. 2006). Early interventions that promote the development of healthy habits may help to reduce this rise in prevalence. Given the wide range of influence parents have over children in this early time period, it makes sense to target parents in childhood obesity prevention efforts.

Many factors have been attributed to the overall rise in obesity, including changes in dietary habits, the availability of high-calorie nutrient-poor foods, increasing portion sizes, frequent patronage of fast-food establishments, increasing time in front of the TV or computer, and the lack of physical activity at school and at home (Hill and Peters 1998). But something closer to the child can potentially mediate or buffer the impact of many of these factors: the parent. Parents play an important role in the growth, development, and socialization of children (Darling and Steinberg 1993). Parents influence their children through the use of specific parenting practices, modeling specific behaviors and attitudes, and more broadly through their interpersonal interactions within the family. They also create a home environment that promotes certain behaviors, expectations, beliefs, and social norms. Because of this overarching influence, parents play an important role in the prevention and treatment of childhood overweight. Not only can parents influence the development of eating and activity behaviors through the use of specific feeding techniques and the modeling of healthy dietary and leisure-time activity habits, but they also have direct control over the home environment and what foods or activities are available in the house.

Parenting goes beyond just shaping and reinforcing specific behaviors. The socioemotional environment created in the home through specific parenting styles and attitudes toward food and sedentary behaviors can assist in the development of a healthier approach toward weight-related domains with presumably lifelong impacts. Research examining the influence of parents on childhood overweight has expanded in recent years to include the area of parenting style and family functioning (Moens, Braet, and Soetens 2007; Rhee et al. 2006; van der Horst et al. 2007; Zeller et al. 2007). Through this work, we have begun to understand the potential scope of parental influence on the development and treatment of childhood overweight. However, the relationship between specific parent behaviors and more global influences like parenting style or family functioning has not been examined. Through the exploration of this interaction, the relationship between parents and children with regards to the development and treatment of obesity may be more clearly defined.

This article will explore the relationship between three levels of parental influence as it impacts dietary behaviors and the development of childhood overweight: (1) specific parent feeding practices that are targeted toward the child with the intent to shape eating behaviors and intake; (2) general parent behaviors which are not necessarily targeted at the child, such as food availability and parent modeling, but also influence the development of child behaviors; and (3) global influences like parenting style and family functioning that shape the socioemotional environment at home. This article will highlight the complex interactions between parents and children and how these interactions can affect a child's weight. Furthermore, we will address possible interactions between these parent-level influences and future areas of work that may improve our understanding of how parents affect their child's weight-related behaviors. Despite this focus on parents, the intent of this article is not to place sole responsibility or blame on the parent. Parents are not parenting in isolation, but in response to inherent child traits and perceived risks unique to the child, as well as other environmental and social factors. However, parents can have an enormous influence on child behaviors; understanding the scope of this influence may help to improve our efforts to prevent and treat childhood obesity.

The socioemotional environment created in the home through specific parenting styles and attitudes toward food and sedentary behaviors can assist in the development of a healthier approach toward weight-related domains with presumably lifelong impacts.

Targeted Parent Feeding Practices

The greatest focus to date has been on specific parent feeding practices that target child intake. Common behaviors such as limiting access to desired foods, promising a child dessert if she eats her vegetables, or encouraging a child to clean his plate can have unintended consequences that may contribute to the development of unhealthy eating practices among children (Birch et al. 1982, 1987; Birch, Zimmerman, and Hind 1980; Fisher and Birch 1999). These practices often stem from parental concern with the quality and quantity of a child's intake, especially during the toddler and early preschool years when child energy consumption and growth are substantially decreased or slower than what occurred in the first year of life (Leung and Robson 1994). However, these concerns and subsequent feeding behaviors regarding quantity of intake may be unwarranted. Infants and young children appear to be sensitive to internal hunger and satiety cues and have the ability to regulate their energy intake. In an experimental study, preschool children given a high-energy-density snack (preload) before lunch were able to adjust their caloric intake and eat less at lunch time (Birch and Deysher 1986). This regulation also occurred across a series of meals in a twenty-four-hour period, indicating that young children are able to make caloric compensations over time resulting in a stable daily energy consumption (Birch et al. 1991). However, as children age, this ability to adjust their intake according to satiety cues appears to dissipate (Cecil et al. 2005; Johnson and Taylor-Holloway 2006). Many studies among adults also demonstrate this lack of sensitivity to internal satiety cues (Rolls, Morris, and Row 2002; Rolls, Row, Kral, et al. 2004; Rolls, Row, and Meengs 2006). Recognizing factors in a child's environment that may undermine this ability and identifying parental behaviors that will help a child make healthier or more appropriate choices regarding intake will be important in our efforts to prevent and treat obesity.

Prompting to Eat

One feeding behavior that has been evaluated is the use of prompts or encouragements to eat. This behavior can be used to alter the quality and quantity of a child's intake, particularly in the preschool and early grade school years. However, some observational studies have found that simply offering food to a child in an open-ended manner (i.e., "would you like more soup?") or directly prompting or encouraging the child to eat (i.e. "eat your chicken") has been associated with elevated child weight and increased total eating time (Klesges et al. 1983, 1986). This relationship seems to be stronger with direct prompts, a behavior that may leave less room for child autonomy and option for refusal. The rate of prompts has also been related to child caloric intake and meal time such that a higher frequency of prompting by the mother was associated with faster eating by the child (Drucker et al. 1999). Despite these findings, other studies similar in design have found no association (Koivisto, Fellenius, and Sjödén 1994) or a modest negative association (McKenzie et al. 1991) between prompts/offers and child BMI. The variability in these results suggests that the relationship between parental prompting and child BMI may be more complicated than it appears. Lumeng and Burke (2006) demonstrated that three- to six-year-old children of obese mothers were more compliant with prompts to eat, particularly if the food was novel, while children of nonobese mothers were not. Interestingly, obese mothers also prompted their child more often when the food was novel than when it was familiar. Further examination of the child's response to prompts, stratified by weight category, and differences in prompting behaviors based on parental weight status may help us further understand the impact of maternal prompting to eat on child weight status. As we will see with other parenting behaviors, certain feeding behaviors may be a response to the child's perceived weight risk, the parent's own weight, or have a differential effect depending on the child's current weight status. Including these factors when examining specific feeding behaviors will help to further clarify the relationship between parent behaviors and child overweight risk.

Use of Rewards

Another commonly used feeding practice is the promise of a reward if the child cleans his plate. In this case, parents are using an external factor or reward to encourage eating, whether or not the child is full, rather than relying on the child's self-regulatory ability to determine when to stop eating. Birch et al. (1987) demonstrated in an experimental study that rewarding four-year-old children if they "cleaned their plate" resulted in less responsiveness to the energy density of the food, and thereby greater calorie consumption, than if children were allowed to focus on more internal cues of how full their stomachs felt. Using the promise of a reward to encourage a child to eat seemed to override the child's ability to self-regulate his intake and resulted in the child eating more regardless of whether or not he was full. This sort of parenting practice, if used continuously, may have long-term detrimental effects on a child's ability to self-regulate calorie consumption and result in an increased reliance on external cues that dictate how much to eat.

Use of external rewards can also have an effect on the development of food preferences. Parents often use another food item, like dessert, as a reward if the child eats her vegetables. The first food, or food that is being required to eat (e.g., vegetables) then becomes a "means to an end" (eating dessert), and the second food (e.g., dessert) becomes the reward. This behavior seems to increase the value or liking of the dessert item and decrease the preference for the required item (Birch et al. 1982; Birch, Zimmerman, and Hind 1980; Newman and Taylor 1992). Newman and Taylor (1992) demonstrated this effect among four- to seven-year-old children using snack foods that were neither strongly liked nor disliked. Although both snack items were initially ranked equally prior to the manipulation, snacks that were given as a reward increased in preference after the manipulation, while the initial snack, or snack that was required to eat before getting the reward, decreased in preference (see Figure 1). While this practice of using rewards to encourage eating may get a child to increase consumption of the initial food that he or she is being required to eat (which is often a vegetable), it also appears to affect the intrinsic value of this food. Thus, while a child may finish eating her vegetables when promised a reward, she may also learn to devalue or dislike the vegetable and therefore not prefer this food in the future when given a choice.

Restricting Access to Food

The act of restricting access to foods can vary tremendously from telling a child she cannot have a second serving of mashed potatoes at dinner, to storing desired foods in the cupboard and informing the child that these foods are off-limits or only allowed under particular circumstances, to not having specific foods in the home. Certain restrictive feeding practices have been associated with an altered sensitivity to internal satiety cues. In lab-based experimental studies where targeted food items were left on the table in full view of preschool and early-grade-school children, restricting access to the desired foods resulted in

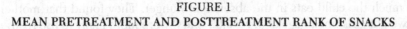

FIGURE 1
MEAN PRETREATMENT AND POSTTREATMENT RANK OF SNACKS

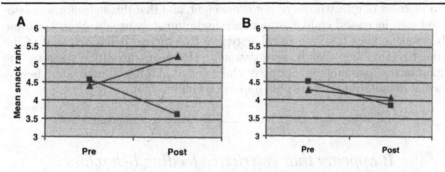

NOTE: Pretreatment and posttreatment snack rankings in the "means to an end" contingency manipulation (Fig. 1a) and the mere exposure condition (Fig. 1b). In the "means to an end" contingency manipulation, children were told that they would be able to "win a chance to eat the second snack" if they ate some of the first snack. Therefore, the second snack was the reward for eating the first snack. In the mere exposure condition, children were shown both snacks and allowed to eat them both, without any contingencies. Ranking range is 1 to 8, with lower scores indicating greater preference. ▲ = first snack or "means" snack; ■ = second snack or "reward" snack (Newman and Taylor 1992).

greater intake of the food when it was no longer being restricted (Fisher and Birch 1999), learning to eat the food in the absence of hunger (Fisher and Birch 2000), and having an increased risk of overweight (Fisher and Birch 2002). Interestingly, many of these findings were found only among girls, not boys. Similar forms of restrictive feeding practices may be used by parents to limit access to palatable foods, like snacks or dessert, in which parents bring these foods into the house but tell the child that they are not available for consumption. While these practices are intended to improve the child's nutritional intake, they may have detrimental effects on his or her overall approach to healthy eating. It is hypothesized that in these situations children learn to place a higher value on the restricted items and consequently eat them whenever they are available or unrestricted, whether or not they are hungry. External cues of availability therefore may become stronger determinants of food consumption than internal cues of hunger and satiety.

In many of these studies, it is assumed that parental restriction is causing increased child intake and overweight. However, because of the predominantly cross-sectional design of these studies, it is difficult to determine whether restriction is causing the increased consumption or whether parents are restricting in response to the child's increased calorie intake or weight status. A few studies have begun to look more closely at this reflective or bidirectional relationship. Birch and Fisher (2000) first demonstrated this phenomenon while performing structural equation modeling on data from an experimental study. This study used questionnaires to assess maternal feeding behaviors and concerns regarding child weight and the "free access procedure" to determine child energy consumption. This procedure involves leaving desired foods in full view of the child while experimenters measure how much the child eats in the absence of hunger. They found that mothers of overweight girls (mean age of 5.4 ± 0.02 years) were more likely to use restriction than mothers of girls who were not overweight, and that this behavior was associated with increased child energy intake and ultimately weight. Whether these lab-based findings translate to other types of restrictive behaviors used in the home has not been clearly demonstrated. However, this study suggests the importance of parental perception of child weight in influencing feeding behaviors and demonstrates its possible impact on child weight.

It appears that restrictive feeding behaviors can have a differential effect on a child's weight depending on the child's overweight risk or current weight status, resulting in more harm among those who are genetically or biologically at risk and those who are already overweight.

Using a longitudinal design, Faith and colleagues (2004) also demonstrated greater parental concern for child weight if the child was born to a mother with a prepregnancy weight > 66th percentile (mean BMI = 30.3 ± 4.2) (high-risk family). This concern predicted increased BMI z-scores for children from high-risk families but not low-risk families (children born to mothers with a prepregnancy weight < 33rd percentile, mean BMI = 19.5 ± 1.1). While they did not demonstrate significant differences in the use of restriction based on this concern or family risk status, they did reveal that among high-risk families, parent's self-report of restrictive behavior predicted increased child BMI z-scores two years later at the age of seven, even after controlling for child weight status at age three. The impact of restrictive behavior on children of low-risk families was not significant. Birch, Fisher, and Davison (2003) demonstrated a similar relationship among girls and energy intake using a longitudinal study design. They found that the use of parent-reported restrictive feeding practices among overweight five-year-old girls was related to greater increases in energy consumption over time (followed until age nine) compared to that of nonoverweight five-year-olds (see Figure 2). Therefore, it appears that restrictive feeding behaviors can have a differential effect on a child's weight depending on the child's overweight risk or current weight status, resulting in more harm among those who are genetically or biologically at risk and those who are already overweight. Additional consideration of these factors in future analyses will help to better delineate the impact of specific behaviors and inform the recommendations that can be made for children who are overweight or at risk for overweight.

FIGURE 2
MATERNAL RESTRICTION AND CHILD OVERWEIGHT STATUS
AT FIVE YEARS OF AGE PREDICT THE DEVELOPMENT
OF CHILD EATING IN THE ABSENCE OF HUNGER (EAH)
AT CHILD AGES FIVE TO NINE YEARS

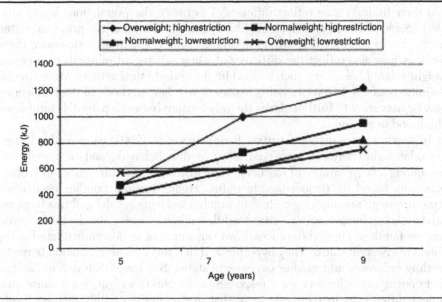

NOTE: The figure presents four-year trajectories for changes in eating in the absence of hunger levels, which are expressed as total energy intake (kJ) during laboratory protocol meals. Trajectories are displayed for the following four groups of daughters, based on daughter overweight status and degree of maternal feeding restriction at 5 years of age: overweight + high restriction (♦); overweight + low restriction (×); normal weight + high restriction (■); normal weight + low restriction (▲). EAH levels increased between five and nine years of age for all groups; however, this increase was most pronounced for girls who were overweight and whose eating was restricted at age five years (Faith and Kerns 2005).

SOURCE: Reproduced with permission from *Maternal and Child Nutrition* 1, no. 3 (2005): 164-68. Copyright © 2005 by Blackwell Publishing Ltd.

Control over Child Intake

The impact of parental control over a child's intake and weight status has had mixed results. This may in part be due to the wide range of behaviors that this construct incorporates, including some restrictive behaviors, and the meaning these questions have for participants (Jain et al. 2004). While Saelens, Ernst, and Epstein (2000) did not find an association between controlling behaviors and child weight status within families, Robinson et al. (2001) found a small inverse relationship such that greater parental control over child dietary intake was associated with lower BMIs among girls. Both of these studies defined control as parents making sure their child finishes his or her plate, has enough to eat, eats healthy food items, only eats at mealtimes, and is reprimanded for playing with his or her food. Robinson and colleagues conducted their cross-sectional survey in a large, ethnically and socioeconomically diverse population of third-graders, and their findings may reflect differences between the populations being sampled. (Saelens, Ernst, and Epstein's [2000] study and most of the previously cited research was conducted in white, middle-income populations.) However, these findings may also reflect the difficulty of using self-report methods to measure weight-related behaviors, such as food intake and physical activity. More precise definitions of the behaviors being assessed or other methods of data collection may be necessary to further clarify the relationship between parental control and childhood overweight.

In another cross-sectional survey, Baughcum et al. (2001) were unable to find any relationship between more controlling feeding behaviors and overweight status among a large sample of toddlers. They instead found differences in feeding behaviors based on socioeconomic status. Higher-income families used more structure (e.g., not allowing a child to watch TV during meals) and less inappropriate feeding behaviors (e.g., giving toddlers a bottle during the day) than lower-income families. These differences, however, were not significantly related to the child's overweight status. They hypothesized that this lack of association between feeding behaviors and toddler overweight status may have been due to the fact that controlling behaviors are a response to the child's weight, not a cause, and reflect differences in parenting style that are related to family income levels. They also postulated that these feeding practices might be related to child weight status in the future, as the child ages. Unfortunately, since they did not follow these families over time, they were unable to determine the true nature of the relationship.

General Parent Behaviors

Exposure to and Availability of Foods

Parents can also shape their child's food preferences by exposing him or her to healthy foods at home and making them more easily accessible. Frequent exposure to an unfamiliar food can result in increased consumption, liking, and preference for that food (Wardle, Cooke, et al. 2003; Wardle, Herrera, et al. 2003). Children are also more likely to eat these foods when they are made available to them in the home (Reinaerts et al. 2007). Since high preference for healthy foods such as fruits and vegetables is a significant factor in a child's consumption of these foods (Nicklas et al. 2001), shaping these preferences via frequent exposure and increasing availability may be an important tool early in a child's life.

Besides exposure and availability, behavioral theories suggest that making fruits and vegetables more easily accessible by putting them in a place where the child can easily reach them (e.g., in a bowl on the table or on a lower shelf in the refrigerator) and preparing them into sizes that are easy to eat (e.g., fruit cut into bite-size pieces) may increase the child's intake of these foods (Baranowski, Cullen, and Baranowski 1999). Knowing this, it is easy to see why snack foods are more readily consumed. Not only are they flavorful, they are packaged in easily accessible containers and prepared for immediate consumption. However, since parents are responsible for buying food for the house and deciding what is available to the children, they can play a large role in shaping child food preferences and consumption patterns. Going one step further and increasing the accessibility of fruits and vegetables can be helpful in increasing the consumption of these foods, particularly among children with low initial preferences for these foods (Cullen et al. 2003). Therefore, helping parents increase availability and accessibility of targeted foods is important since it appears to increase the likelihood that children will eat these foods and can be one of the strongest predictors of future consumption (Reinaerts et al. 2007).

Portion Size

In addition to availability and accessibility, portion size plays an important role in the amount of food a child consumes. While portion size is often thought of as an environmental factor that is predetermined by industry, parents have some influence over this as well. In studies assessing child intake at a single time point, preschool and grade school children have been found to eat a greater amount (in grams and calories) when given larger portion sizes (Fisher 2007; Orlet Fisher, Rolls, and Birch 2003; Rolls, Engell, and Birch 2000). Thus, it appears that large portion sizes can easily overwhelm a child's ability to self-regulate caloric intake. While there has been some suggestion of a developmental shift in this ability such that younger children (age three) can self-regulate their intake when presented with large portions while older children (age five) cannot (Rolls, Engell, and Birch 2000), other studies have not shown this to be the case. Fisher (2007) demonstrated that children as young as two would also eat more when given larger portion sizes. This study, as well as research with adult samples (Rolls, Morris, and Row 2002; Rolls, Row, Kral, et al. 2004; Rolls, Row, and Meengs 2006; Rolls, Row, Meengs, et al. 2004), highlights the pervasive effect of larger portions on an individual's consumption, no matter what the age. However, the long-term effect of large portions on a child's ability to regulate caloric intake has not been demonstrated. It may be that children learn to rely solely on these external cues regarding consumption rather than their internal ones regarding calorie density. On the other hand, we may find that older children are still able to make caloric compensations between meals over a twenty-four-hour period, as Birch found among preschool children. Whatever the case may be, determining methods to maintain a child's ability to make caloric compensations is needed.

One means of circumventing the impact of large portion sizes may be to allow children to chose their own portion size, or serve themselves. In one study, children (mean age of 4 ± 0.5 years) who were presented with a large amount of food (double the standard amount) but given the opportunity to determine their own portion size ate 24 percent less of the entrée than when given the same large portion, but this time on their plate (Orlet Fisher, Rolls, and Birch 2003). This simple technique of encouraging children to make their own decisions regarding intake may allow them to take advantage of their own self-regulatory ability and avoid overeating. Whether this technique is as effective in older or overweight children, whose ability to self-regulate intake may already be compromised, is unknown. Teaching parents to serve age-appropriate portions for these children may be more beneficial and help children adjust their intake. Further studies examining different methods of encouraging portion control for overweight and normal weight children are needed to help inform future recommendations.

Modeling

Parents can indirectly influence their children's eating habits by modeling good eating behaviors (Brown and Ogden 2004). When children were asked to describe their eating patterns at home, they reported more healthy eating habits if their parents reported eating fruits and vegetables (Fisher et al. 2002) and had low dietary fat intake (Tibbs et al. 2001). Addessi et al. (2005) demonstrated in a laboratory setting that two- to five-year-old children accepted a novel food more quickly and ingested more of that food when the adult was eating a similar food (of the same color) rather than when the adult was eating a food of a different color or just sitting together but not eating anything. The impact of modeling may also be enhanced by positive social responses that are tied to the food. Hendy and Raudenbush (2000) demonstrated that enthusiastic comments made by a teacher about the targeted food were associated with greater acceptance and consumption of the new food by preschool children. Thus, this combination of modeling with positive comments and social affect toward the food may provide an additional means for adults to help promote healthy eating behaviors among children. Unfortunately, modeling of negative behaviors can have an equally strong, but opposite effect and has been associated with the development of emotional eating, snacking, and body dissatisfaction (Brown and Ogden 2004). Nevertheless, the importance of parent modeling is supported by the success of child weight control programs where parents are the primary agent of change (Epstein, McCurley, et al. 1990; Epstein, Valoski, et al. 1990; Golan and Crow 2004; Golan et al. 1998). Not only are parents taught behavioral modification and parenting skills to help make changes in the home, but they are also encouraged to adopt these behaviors themselves and therefore model healthy eating and activity behaviors for their child. Through these studies it is clear that parents can indirectly shape child behaviors through modeling and that encouraging parents to adopt healthy behaviors themselves may aid in our efforts to curb childhood obesity.

It is clear that parents can indirectly shape child behaviors through modeling and that encouraging parents to adopt healthy behaviors themselves may aid in our efforts to curb childhood obesity.

Global Parenting Influences

Parenting Style

While quite a bit of research examines specific parenting behaviors and practices, less research examines the impact of more global domains such as parenting style. Parenting style is thought of as the general pattern of parenting that provides the emotional background in which parent behaviors are expressed and interpreted by the child. Parenting behaviors or practices have been described as what parents do (e.g., reprimand or praise), while parenting style describes how parents do it (e.g., with warmth or hostility). It has also been suggested that parenting style modifies or impacts the relationship between parent practices and child outcomes such that a behavior delivered within the context of a more positive parenting style will have a different impact on the child than one delivered in a more negative parenting style.

Maccoby and Martin (1983) operationalized Baumrind's (1971) original definition of parenting style into two dimensions—demandingness (expectations for displays of maturity by their children, parental control, and discipline) and responsiveness (parental displays of warmth, sensitivity, affection, and involvement with their children)—to allow for the creation of a fourfold classification of parenting style (see Figure 3). A positive parenting style, namely, the authoritative parenting style, is classified by high displays of sensitivity, emotional warmth, and involvement by the parent as well as high expectations and demands for maturity and self-control from the child. This parenting style has been associated with positive childhood outcomes such as higher academic achievement, increased self-regulatory ability, more frequent use of adaptive strategies, fewer depressive symptoms, and fewer risk-taking behaviors (Aunola, Stattin, and Nurmi 2000; Glasgow et al. 1997; Radziszewska et al. 1996; Steinberg et al. 1994,

FIGURE 3
PARENTING STYLE

	High Demandingness	Low Demandingness
High Responsiveness	Authoritative: Respectful of child's opinions, but maintains clear boundaries	Permissive: Indulgent, without discipline
Low Responsiveness	Authoritarian: Strict disciplinarian	Neglectful: Emotionally uninvolved and does not set rules

SOURCE: Reproduced with permission from *Pediatrics* 117 (2006): 2047-54. Copyright ©
2006 by the AAP.

1992). In contrast, the other parenting styles have been associated with one of
several child outcomes like lower academic grades, lower levels of self-control,
and poorer psychosocial and emotional development (Dornbusch et al. 1987;
Lamborn et al. 1991; Radziszewska et al. 1996). Given these findings, one could
hypothesize that parent behaviors around weight control delivered within the
context of an authoritative parenting style would have better outcomes than if
delivered within the context of one of the other parenting styles.

While one study examining the effect of parenting style on child weight status
showed no association (Agras et al. 2004), our own work demonstrated that children of authoritarian parents (strict disciplinarians) had almost a fivefold increase
in odds of having overweight children in first grade than authoritative parents
(firm but warm and accepting) (Rhee et al. 2006). A critical dimension of parenting style may be parental warmth and sensitivity toward the child. It was this
dimension of maternal sensitivity that we found to be independently associated
with a lower risk of child overweight by first grade. Parental warmth and sensitivity has also been shown to be related to greater fruit and vegetable intake and
physical activity behaviors (Kremers et al. 2003; Schmitz et al. 2002). Finally, the
importance of this dimension was further demonstrated in a study where overweight adolescents identified maternal support as a key factor in reducing psychological risk (Valtolina and Marta 1998).

Examination of parenting style in pediatric weight management may therefore
be important because it provides the environmental and emotional context for
child rearing and socialization as well as the context in which specific parenting
behaviors are interpreted by the child (Darling and Steinberg 1993). Recently, in
a paper by van der Horst and colleagues (2007), an interaction between parenting
practices and parenting style was demonstrated such that the practice of limiting

consumption of sugar-sweetened beverages (via verbal regulation of how much and which types of beverages to consume as well as regulating availability in the house) was most effective in decreasing adolescent consumption if parents displayed high levels of involvement and moderate levels of strictness or demandingness. This study lends evidence to support the idea that the use of specific behavior modification strategies may be more effective when the child perceives greater involvement or warmth from the parent. Adjustments in parenting style, or how the parent interacts with the child on an emotional level, may therefore be an important factor in the success of weight management for children.

The use of specific behavior modification strategies may be more effective when the child perceives greater involvement or warmth from the parent.

Given these data, it appears that targeting parenting style, or how a parent interacts with his or her child, in an intervention may be important to its success. However, this dimension is rarely examined and it is unclear whether family-based weight control programs effectively change parenting style. Stein et al. (2005) tried to examine the role of parenting style in an intervention by asking eight- to twelve-year-old children in a family-based weight control program to assess their parents' levels of acceptance, psychological autonomy, and control. These children reported that both mothers and fathers became more accepting during the program, suggesting that the program modified this aspect of their parenting. However, it was the father's increase in acceptance that was significantly correlated with child weight loss. This factor accounted for nearly 21 percent of the variance in weight loss. Further study on the impact of parent behavior training to modify parenting style will help inform the development of more effective interventions for childhood weight loss.

Family Functioning

A broader dimension that may impact the ability of parents to control their child's weight is family functioning. How members of a family function, that is, how they manage daily routines, fulfill parenting roles, and communicate and connect emotionally with each other, provides another context in which parenting behaviors are interpreted by the child and may impact child development and behaviors. While poor family functioning has been related to poorer adherence to treatment in families with cystic fibrosis and diabetes (DeLambo et al. 2004; Lewin et al. 2006), its role in pediatric overweight management has not been thoroughly explored. It is often argued that childhood obesity is a chronic illness that adds additional stress and management needs to the lives of families (Barlow and Dietz 1998; Rippe, Crossley, and Ringer 1998). Some studies suggest that families of obese children are more conflicted and less cohesive (Beck and Terry 1985; Mendelson, White, and Schliecker 1995; Wilkins et al. 1998; Zeller et al. 2007). Zeller et al. (2007) found greater maternal reports of family conflict and mealtime challenges among overweight families in a pediatric weight management clinic. Moens, Braet, and Soetens (2007) found that parents with overweight children used more maladaptive control or management strategies regarding food than parents with nonoverweight children. Finally, an analysis of normal and overweight children with asthma revealed that while all families scored in the "unhealthy" range of family functioning, those families with overweight children had statistically significantly increased difficulty managing family meals, affect, and fulfilling role assignments than families with normal weight asthmatics (Jacobs and Fiese 2007). Dysfunction in many aspects of family functioning, like managing daily routines, accomplishing tasks, fulfilling parenting roles that assist in pediatric weight control efforts, communicating with family members, and controlling child behaviors, may contribute to the poor energy regulation capabilities of overweight children. Family dysfunction may also undermine efforts to control a child's weight by creating greater levels of stress and an environment less capable of supporting healthier lifestyles.

Family meals are often used as a proxy for family functioning since many aspects of how a family functions are represented during the planning, carrying out, and eating of a family meal. Given their complexity, family meals are often considered mildly stressful events in themselves. The stress of a meal can be magnified for families of children with chronic diseases, such as diabetes mellitus, where compliance with dietary recommendations is an important component of management and is related to health outcomes (Powers et al. 2002; Wysocki et al. 1989). Despite this level of stress, in cross-sectional analyses, consistent family meals were associated with a lower prevalence of child overweight (Sen 2006; Taveras et al. 2005). Eating meals as a family has also been associated with greater intake of fruits and vegetables, dairy products, and basic vitamins and minerals along with decreased soft drink consumption (Gillman et al. 2000; Neumark-Sztainer et al. 2003; Videon and Manning 2003). There are many possible explanations for these findings. With regards to specific dietary behaviors, it has been suggested that parent modeling may be involved. However, Klesges et al. (1991) found that when children were told that parents would be inspecting their food selection for lunch, children also chose fewer unhealthy items. There was a tenfold decrease in the sugar content of the foods chosen, a decrease in total calories, and a decrease in the percentage of saturated fat. Thus, it appears that parents may be better able to enforce eating rules that encourage healthy choices when eating a meal together as well as allow for the positive effects of modeling to pervade.

On the other hand, families who function more efficiently and cohesively may be able to have more family meals, and it is this improved family functioning that is influencing the child's healthier dietary habits. As with parenting style, positive family functioning may provide a context within which specific feeding behaviors are delivered and interpreted by the child. Positive family interactions and order in the household may create an atmosphere that allows for greater acceptance by children of particular parent behaviors regarding overweight management. Furthermore, as we saw in the modeling literature, the influence of positive social interactions and comments about food during a meal may enhance the adoption of healthy eating behaviors (Hendy and Raudenbush 2000).

Positive family interactions and order in the household may create an atmosphere that allows for greater acceptance by children of particular parent behaviors regarding overweight management.

Despite the positive association between family meals and child weight status, the impact may vary by ethnic group. Sen (2006) examined this relationship over a three-year period using a large ethnically diverse sample from the National Longitudinal Survey of Youth, 1997. Among non-Hispanic white teens, he found that those who ate at least three meals per week with their family had decreased odds of becoming overweight ($OR = 0.20$ to 0.34), and those who were overweight initially and ate seven meals per week with their family had increased odds of losing weight ($OR = 2.74$). The odds of becoming overweight among black and Hispanic youth were not significantly affected by family meals; however, they had lower odds of losing weight if they were initially overweight and took part in frequent family meals ($OR = 0.23$ to 0.50). Cultural differences regarding the types of foods consumed at family meals as well as other social and environmental influences from peers, school, or mass media may influence the eating behaviors of minority youth and attenuate or alter the effect of family meals. Overall, additional longitudinal studies that incorporate better family measurements regarding frequency of family meals, family functioning, and other cultural and environmental factors may help to clarify the role of family meals across ethnic groups. Despite these findings, family meals are generally considered important for adolescent health and well-being (Eisenberg et al. 2004; Fulkerson et al. 2006) as well as BMI (Sen 2006; Taveras et al. 2005), and have therefore been identified as an important tool in the management of pediatric overweight (Barlow and Dietz 1998).

As we have seen in the other parenting dimensions, the causal relationship between overweight and family functioning has not been clearly defined. One could argue that it is poor family functioning that creates a level of chaos or stress in the household, which then contributes to the poor development and control of dietary habits in a child. This level of chaos or stress may even impact a child's food preferences and the development of obesity on a biological level. Among lab animals tested in stressful conditions, elevated levels of corticosteroids were associated with the development of central obesity (Björntorp 1996) and, in the presence of insulin, appeared to influence the consumption of comfort foods or high-fat foods (la Fleur et al. 2004). The ingestion of these foods has also been linked to a reduction in the neuroendocrine stress response, which further reinforces these behaviors (Bell et al. 2002; Nanni et al. 2003; Pecoraro et al. 2004). On the other hand, the relationship between family functioning and childhood obesity may not be unidirectional. Poor family functioning may contribute to a child's overweight risk, and this increased risk may lead to parents responding with additional maladaptive family interactions and poor management of weight-related behaviors. Longitudinal studies that assess these global factors as well as account for the child's and parent's overweight risk/status will help us better understand the relationship between family functioning and child overweight.

Interaction of Parent-Level Factors

This article has reviewed several different levels of parent influence that are associated with childhood obesity (see Table 1). Similar to the social ecological model (Bronfenbrenner 1979), a model of parent-level influences can be created that depicts the interdependence between these factors and how as a whole it impacts child energy consumption and ultimately weight status (see Figure 4). As suggested by the model, global influences of parenting style and family functioning may provide a context and influence the delivery and impact of specific parent behaviors. These specific behaviors may also impact and reflect on one's parenting style and how the family functions. As a whole, these parent-level factors can influence child energy consumption and ultimately overweight status. As mentioned in the discussion of specific parent behaviors and family functioning, child weight can also influence the use of specific feeding behaviors and likely contribute to the socioemotional functioning of the household. While the potential interdependence of these different levels has been discussed, studies that include assessments of parental influences at all these levels are lacking. In addition, most of the evidence in this article has focused on the relationship between

TABLE 1
ASSOCIATIONS BETWEEN PARENT-LEVEL FACTORS AND CHILD OUTCOMES

	Increased Food Intake (Calories or Quantity)	Increased Child Body Mass Index (BMI) or Weight	Additional Comments
Negative factors			
Prompting to eat	+	+/–	(1) Also associated with increased total eating time; (2) Children of obese mothers may be more compliant with prompts
Use of rewards	+		(1) Also affects the preference or intrinsic value of foods
Restricting access to food	+	+	(1) Most associations are only among girls; (2) Also results in eating in the absence of hunger; (3) Seems to have a greater impact on those who are already overweight or have risk factors for becoming overweight; (4) Seems to be used more in overweight children and may be a response to a child's weight
Control over intake	+	+/–	(1) May also be a response to a child's weight status rather than a cause
Large portion sizes	+		(1) Also increases preference for the food; (2) Effective in the context of exposure to or availability of healthy foods
Positive factors			
Exposure and/or availability of specific foods	+		(1) Effective in the context of accessibility to healthy foods
Accessibility of specific foods	+		
Self-regulation or portion control	(–)		(1) Some children may need the assistance of parents to determine appropriate portion sizes; (2) No studies have assessed the effect of true portion control on child intake
Parent modeling of food consumption	+		(1) Most studies describe increased intake of healthy foods when parents model healthy eating
Parental warmth or sensitivity		–	(1) Also associated with greater fruit and vegetable intake and decreased sugar sweetened beverage consumption
Family meals		–	(1) Also associated with greater fruit, vegetable, dairy, vitamins, and mineral intake as well as decreased soft-drink consumption

NOTE: + indicates positive association with child outcome; – indicates negative association with child outcome.

FIGURE 4
RELATIONSHIP BETWEEN PARENT (FEEDING) BEHAVIOR,
PARENTING STYLE, AND FAMILY FUNCTIONING IN
CHILD WEIGHT MANAGEMENT

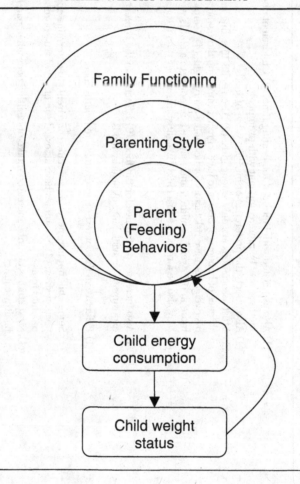

parents and young children. While this relationship most likely exists with older children and adolescents, it may be modified due to the difference in the developmental stages of these children. Nevertheless, modifications in more global areas like family functioning and parenting style may have an effect on how specific parent behaviors regarding feeding will be delivered and interpreted by the child. Because of this interdependence, addressing these larger parent-driven influences may aid in the treatment and prevention of childhood overweight.

To date, few studies have examined the relationship between more global aspects of parenting and child overweight outcomes. As mentioned previously,

Stein and colleagues (2005) demonstrated that child report of increasing levels of acceptance from parents, particularly fathers, during a family-based weight control intervention was correlated with increased child weight loss. They suggested that this increased acceptance may have motivated children to change their behaviors. This change in behavior may have also reflected an improved family functioning where fathers were more involved and assisted in the management of daily routines. Finally, they proposed that children may have felt better toward their parents as a result of their own success and rated their parent's acceptance more positively than was actually the case. It is clear from this study that there is a need for additional research that includes more detailed and objective measures of parenting style and family functioning, particularly before and after an intervention. Studies will also need to measure specific parent behaviors regarding overweight management in conjunction with these more global parenting influences to better understand the possible interdependence between these factors. Finally, longitudinal prospective studies will greatly assist in defining the relationship and relative importance of these factors over time.

It is important to note that many of the previous studies have involved surveys or self-report measures to assess behaviors. How a participant interprets a question can be difficult to determine (Jain et al. 2004) and could affect the results of the study. To bypass these issues, home observational studies can be conducted to determine what behaviors are truly being used in the home and help create a more accurate definition of the behaviors of interest and their impact. These studies, however, are often costly and time-consuming to conduct. Observational studies conducted in the laboratory setting are another alternative, but again, there is a question of validity regarding the behaviors being evaluated and whether these findings can be applied to real-world situations. Given these challenges, future studies need to consider the implication of their study design and how it will add to or clarify the existing body of literature in this area.

Another aspect to consider when conducting these studies is the role of genetically determined overweight risk, current weight status, and parental concern for future overweight in the development of childhood overweight. These factors may influence the specific feeding practices and how a family implements overweight management skills. Large studies with diverse samples will be needed to determine the relative impact of and interaction between biological factors, parental perceptions, specific parent feeding behaviors, and more global parent-level influences on childhood overweight, particularly as it varies between different racial and ethnic groups.

Despite the paucity of information regarding the relationship between parenting style, family functioning, and childhood overweight, facilitators are interested in modifying current weight control programs to address these more global parent level factors. Recently, Golley and colleagues (2007) examined the effectiveness of a parenting skills training program (Positive Parenting Program, Triple P [Sanders 1999]) with or without obesity-related lifestyle education on childhood overweight. Parenting skills training programs typically focus on changing parent reinforcement strategies, problem-solving abilities, and parent–child interactions. Using play therapy and videotapes of parent–child interactions, these interventions address the socioemotional aspects of parenting and help parents develop new strategies to relate to their child while increasing the use of such techniques as positive reinforcement. These types of programs have demonstrated improved parenting skills (Scott et al. 2001; Webster-Stratton and Hammond 1998; Webster-Stratton, Reid, and Hammond 2001, 2004) as well as improvements in parental affect, involvement with the child, and use of praise (Forgatch and DeGarmo 1999; Webster-Stratton and Hammond 1997). In the intervention conducted by Golley and colleagues (2007), six- to nine-year-old children were able to significantly reduce BMI z-scores over the twelve-month period in both the parenting intervention and the Parenting + Lifestyle intervention (by 6 percent and 9 percent, respectively). Unfortunately, since they did not compare their interventions to a standard family-based lifestyle intervention alone, they were unable to determine the incremental effect of parenting skills training on a traditional family-based weight control program, the current state-of-the-art intervention for childhood overweight management (Jelalian and Saelens 1999). Studies examining whether a traditional family-based intervention changes parenting style and the benefit of adding parenting skills training to a family-based intervention are needed to assess the relevance of this dimension on overweight management.

Conclusion

The role of parents in helping to control childhood overweight is multifaceted and complex. Parents not only help mold and shape specific behaviors in a child but also influence children's attitudes and beliefs about food and eating practices. Traditionally, we have examined the impact of specific feeding practices on child calorie intake and weight. But the socioemotional impact of parenting and the stability provided by effective family functioning can also play a role in the development of healthy eating behaviors. We argue that these larger parent-level influences interact with specific behaviors to modify their impact on childhood overweight. Understanding the impact of these more global parent influences and trying to intervene at this level may provide additional strategies to help curb the growing rate of obesity. As we have seen elsewhere in this volume, the impact of specific behaviors on childhood overweight must be considered within the context of the larger community and culture. It is with further understanding of these complex interactions that a more comprehensive and potentially more effective strategy can be implemented to help reduce the rates of overweight among our children.

References

Addessi, Elsa, Amy T. Galloway, Elisabetta Visalberghi, and Leann L. Birch. 2005. Specific social influences on the acceptance of novel foods in 2-5-year-old children. *Appetite* 45:264-71.

Agras, W. Stewart, Lawrence D. Hammer, Fiona McNicholas, and Helena C. Kraemer. 2004. Risk factors for childhood overweight: A prospective study from birth to 9.5 years. *J Pediatr* 145:20-25.

Aunola, Kaisa, Hakan Stattin, and Jari-Erik Nurmi. 2000. Parenting styles and adolescents' achievement strategies. *J Adolesc* 23:205-22.

Baranowski, Tom, Karen W. Cullen, and Janice Baranowski. 1999. Psychosocial correlates of dietary intake: Advancing dietary intervention. *Annu Rev Nutr* 19:17-40.

Barlow, Sarah E., and William H. Dietz. 1998. Obesity evaluation and treatment: Expert Committee recommendations. The Maternal and Child Health Bureau, Health Resources and Services Administration and the Department of Health and Human Services. *Pediatrics* 102:E29.

Baughcum, Amy E., Scott W. Powers, Suzanne B. Johnson, Leigh A. Chamberlin, Cindy M. Deeks, Anjali Jain, and Robert C. Whitaker. 2001. Maternal feeding practices and beliefs and their relationships to overweight in early childhood. *Developmental and Behavioral Pediatrics* 22:391-408.

Baumrind, Diana. 1971. Current patterns of parental authority. *Developmental Psychology Monograph* 4:101-3.

Beck, Steven, and Karen Terry. 1985. A comparison of obese and normal-weight families' psychological characteristics. *American Journal of Family Therapy* 13:55-59.

Bell, M. Elizabeth, Aditi Bhargava, Liza R. Soriano, Kevin D. Laugero, Susan F. Akana, and Mary F. Dallman. 2002. Sucrose intake and corticosterone interact with cold to modulate ingestive behaviour, energy balance, autonomic outflow and neuroendocrine responses during chronic stress. *J Neuroendocrinol* 14:330-42.

Birch, Leann L., D. Birch, D. W. Marlin, and L. Kramer. 1982. Effects of instrumental consumption on children's food preference. *Appetite* 3:125-34.

Birch, Leann L., and M. Deysher. 1986. Caloric compensation and sensory specific satiety: Evidence for self-regulation of food intake by young children. *Appetite* 7:323-31.

Birch, Leann L., and Jennifer Orlet Fisher. 2000. Mothers' child-feeding practices influence daughters' eating and weight. *Am J Clin Nutr* 71:1054-61.

Birch, Leann L., Jennifer Orlet Fisher, and Kirsten K. Davison. 2003. Learning to overeat: Maternal use of restrictive feeding practices promotes girls' eating in the absence of hunger. *Am J Clin Nutr* 78:215-20.

Birch, Leann L., Susan L. Johnson, G. Andresen, John C. Peters, and M. C. Schulte. 1991. The variability of young children's energy intake. *N Engl J Med* 324:232-5.

Birch, Leann L., Linda McPhee, B. C. Shoba, Lois Steinberg, and Ruth Krehbiel. 1987. "Clean up your plate": Effects of child feeding practices on the conditioning of meal size. *Learn Motiv* 18:301-17.

Birch, Leann L., Sheryl Itkin Zimmerman, and Honey Hind. 1980. The influences of social-affective context on preschool children's food preferences. *Child Development* 51:856-61.

Björntorp, P. 1996. The regulation of adipose tissue distribution in humans. *Int J Obes Relat Metab Disord* 20:291-302.

Bronfenbrenner, Urie. 1979. *The ecology of human development*. Cambridge, MA: Harvard University Press.

Brown, Rachel, and Jane Ogden. 2004. Children's eating attitudes and behaviour: A study of the modelling and control theories of parental influence. *Health Educ Res* 19:261-71.

Cecil, Joanne E., Colin N. A. Palmer, Wendy Wrieden, Inez Murrie, Caroline Bolton-Smith, Pete Watt, Deborah J. Wallis, and Marion M. Hetherington. 2005. Energy intakes of children after preloads: Adjustment, not compensation. *Am J Clin Nutr* 82:302-8.

Cullen, Karen W., Tom Baranowski, Emiel Owens, Tara Marsh, Latroy Rittenberry, and Carl de Moor. 2003. Availability, accessibility, and preferences for fruit, 100% fruit juice, and vegetables influence children's dietary behavior. *Health Educ Behav* 30:615-26.

Darling, Nancy, and Laurence Steinberg. 1993. Parenting style as context: An integrative model. *Psychological Bulletin* 113:487-96.

DeLambo, Kirsten E., Carolyn E. Ievers-Landis, Dennis Drotar, and Alexandra L. Quittner. 2004. Association of observed family relationship quality and problem-solving skills with treatment adherence in older children and adolescents with cystic fibrosis. *J Pediatr Psychol* 29:343-53.

Dornbusch, Sanford M., Philip L. Ritter, P. Herbert Leiderman, Donald F. Roberts, and Michael J Fraleigh. 1987. The relation of parenting style to adolescent school performance. *Child Dev* 58:1244-57.

Drucker, Robin R., Lawrence D. Hammer, W. Stewart Agras, and Susan Bryson. 1999. Can mothers influence their child's eating behavior? *J Dev Behav Pediatr* 20:88-92.

Eisenberg, Marla E., Rachel E. Olson, Dianne Neumark-Sztainer, Mary Story, and Linda H. Bearinger.
   2004. Correlations between family meals and psychosocial well-being among adolescents. *Arch Pediatr
   Adolesc Med* 158:792-96.
Epstein, Leonard H., James McCurley, Rena R. Wing, and Alice M. Valoski. 1990. Five-year follow-up of
   family-based behavioral treatments for childhood obesity. *J Consult Clin Psychol* 58:661-64.
Epstein, Leonard H., Alice M. Valoski, Rena R. Wing, and James McCurley. 1990. Ten-year follow-up of
   behavioral, family-based treatment for obese children. *Jama* 264:2519-23.
Faith, Myles S., Robert I. Berkowitz, Virginia A. Stallings, Julia Kerns, Megan Storey, and Albert J.
   Stunkard. 2004. Parental feeding attitudes and styles and child body mass index: Prospective analysis
   of a gene-environment interaction. *Pediatrics* 114:e429-36.
Faith, Myles S., and Julia Kerns. 2005. Infant and child feeding practices and childhood overweight: The
   role of restriction. *Matern Child Nutr* 1:164-68.
Fisher, Jennifer O. 2007. Effects of age on children's intake of large and self-selected food portions.
   Obesity (Silver Spring) 15:403-12.
Fisher, Jennifer O., and Leann L. Birch. 1999. Restricting access to foods and children's eating. *Appetite*
   32:405-19.
———. 2000. Parents' restrictive feeding practices are associated with young girls' negative self-evaluation
   of eating. *J Am Diet Assoc* 100:1341-46.
———. 2002. Eating in the absence of hunger and overweight in girls from 5 to 7 y of age. *Am J Clin Nutr*
   76:226-31.
Fisher, Jennifer O., Diane C. Mitchell, Helen Smiciklas-Wright, and Leann L. Birch. 2002. Parental influences on young girls' fruit and vegetable, micronutrient, and fat intakes. *J Am Diet Assoc* 102:58-64.
Forgatch, Marion S., and David S. DeGarmo. 1999. Parenting through change: An effective prevention
   program for single mothers. *J Consult Clin Psychol* 67:711-24.
Fulkerson, Jayne A., Mary Story, Alison Mellin, Nancy Leffert, Dianne Neumark-Sztainer, and Simone A.
   French. 2006. Family dinner meal frequency and adolescent development: Relationships with devel-
   opmental assets and high-risk behaviors. *J Adolesc Health* 39:337-45.
Gillman, Matthew W., Sheryl L. Rifas-Shiman, Lindsay Frazier, Helaine R. Rockett, Carlos A. Camargo
   Jr., Alison E. Field, Catherine S. Berkey, and Graham A. Colditz. 2000. Family dinner and diet quality
   among older children and adolescents. *Arch Fam Med* 9:235-40.
Glasgow, Kristan, Sanford M. Dornbusch, Lisa Troyer, Laurence Steinberg, and Philip L. Ritter. 1997.
   Parenting styles, adolescents' attributions, and educational outcomes in nine heterogeneous high
   schools. *Child Development* 68:507-29.
Golan, Moria, and Scott Crow. 2004. Targeting parents exclusively in the treatment of childhood obesity:
   Long-term results. *Obes Res* 12:357-61.
Golan, Moria, Abraham Weizman, Alan Apter, and Menahem Fainaru. 1998. Parents as the exclusive
   agents of change in the treatment of childhood obesity. *Am J Clin Nutr* 67:1130-35.
Golley, Rebecca K., Anthea M. Magarey, Louise A. Baur, Katherine S. Steinbeck, and Lynne A. Daniels.
   2007. Twelve-month effectiveness of a parent-led, family-focused weight-management program for
   prepubertal children: A randomized, controlled trial. *Pediatrics* 119:517-25.
Hendy, H. M., and B. Raudenbush. 2000. Effectiveness of teacher modeling to encourage food acceptance
   in preschool children. *Appetite* 34:61-76.
Hill, James O., and John C. Peters. 1998. Environmental contributions to the obesity epidemic. *Science*
   280:1371-74.
Jacobs, Matthew P., and Barbara H. Fiese. 2007. Family mealtime interactions and overweight children
   with asthma: Potential for compounded risks? *J Pediatr Psychol* 32:64-68.
Jain, Anjali, Susan N. Sherman, Leigh A. Chamberlin, and Robert C. Whitaker. 2004. Mothers misunder-
   stand questions on a feeding questionnaire. *Appetite* 42:249-54.
Jelalian, Elissa, and Brian E. Saelens. 1999. Empirically supported treatments in pediatric psychology:
   Pediatric obesity. *J Pediatr Psychol* 24:223-48.
Johnson, Susan L., and Lisa A. Taylor-Holloway. 2006. Non-Hispanic white and Hispanic elementary
   school children's self-regulation of energy intake. *Am J Clin Nutr* 83:1276-82.
Klesges, Robert C., Thomas J. Coates, Guendoline Brown, Janet Sturgeon-Tillisch, Lisa M. Moldenhauer-
   Klesges, Barbara Holzer, Joan Wollfrey, and Jim Vollmer . 1983. Parental influences on children's
   eating behavior and relative weight. *J Appl Behav Anal* 16:371-78.

Klesges, Robert C., James M. Malott, Pamela F. Boschee, and Jill M. Weber. 1986. The effects of parental influences on children's food intake, physical activity, and relative weight. *International Journal of Eating Disorders* 5:335-46.

Klesges, Robert C., Risa J. Stein, Linda H. Eck, Terry R. Isbell, and Lisa M. Klesges. 1991. Parental influence on food selection in young children and its relationships to childhood obesity. *Am J Clin Nutr* 53:859-64.

Koivisto, Ulla-Kaisa, Jan Fellenius, and Per-Olow Sjöden. 1994. Relations between parental mealtime practices and children's food intake. *Appetite* 22:245-57.

Kremers, Stef P., Johannes Brug, Hein de Vries, and Rutger C. M. E. Engels. 2003. Parenting style and adolescent fruit consumption. *Appetite* 41:43-50.

Kuczmarski, Robert L., Cynthia L. Ogden, S. Guo, L. Grummer-Strawn, Katherine M. Flegal, Z. Mei, Rong Wei, L. R. Curtin, A. F. Roche, and Clifford L. Johnson. 2002. *2000 CDC growth charts for the United States: Methods and development*, pp. 1-190. Hyattsville, MD: National Center for Health Statistics.

la Fleur, Susanne E., Susan F. Akana, Sotara L. Manalo, and Mary F. Dallman. 2004. Interaction between corticosterone and insulin in obesity: Regulation of lard intake and fat stores. *Endocrinology* 145:2174-85.

Lamborn, Susie D., Nina S. Mounts, Laurence Steinberg, and Sanford M. Dornbusch. 1991. Patterns of competence and adjustment among adolescents from authoritative, authoritarian, indulgent, and neglectful families. *Child Development* 62:1049-65.

Leung, Alexander K. C., and William L. M. Robson 1994. The toddler who does not eat. *Am Fam Physician* 49:1789-92, 799-800.

Lewin, Adam R., Amanda D. Heidgerken, Gary R. Geffken, Laura B. Williams, Eric A. Storch, Kenneth M. Gelfand, and Janet H. Silverstein. 2006. The relation between family factors and metabolic control: The role of diabetes adherence. *J Pediatr Psychol* 31:174-83.

Lumeng, Julie C., and Lori M. Burke. 2006. Maternal prompts to eat, child compliance, and mother and child weight status. *J Pediatr* 149:330-35.

Maccoby, Eleanor, and J. Martin. 1983. Socialization in the context of the family: Parent-child interaction. In *Handbook of child psychology: Socialization, personality and social development*, ed. E. Hetherington, 1-101. New York: Wiley.

McKenzie, Thomas L., James F. Sallis, Philip R. Nader, Thomas L. Patterson, John C. Elder, Charles C. Berry, Joan W. Rupp, Catherine J. Atkins, Michael J. Buono, and Julie A. Nelson. 1991. BEACHES: An observational system for assessing children's eating and physical activity behaviors and associated events. *J Appl Behav Anal* 24:141-51.

Mendelson, Beverly K., Donna R. White, and Evelyn Schliecker. 1995. Adolescents' weight, sex, and family functioning. *Int J Eat Disord* 17:73-79.

Moens, Ellen, Caroline Braet, and Barbara Soetens. 2007. Observation of family functioning at mealtime: A comparison between families of children with and without overweight. *J Pediatr Psychol* 32:52-63.

Nanni, Giulio, Simona Scheggi, Benedetta Leggio, Silvia Grappi, Flavio Masi, Riccardo Rauggi, and Maria Graziella De Montis. 2003. Acquisition of an appetitive behavior prevents development of stress-induced neurochemical modifications in rat nucleus accumbens. *J Neurosci Res* 73:573-80.

Neumark-Sztainer, Dianne, Peter J. Hannan, Mary Story, Jillian Croll, and Cheryl Perry. 2003. Family meal patterns: Associations with sociodemographic characteristics and improved dietary intake among adolescents. *J Am Diet Assoc* 103:317-22.

Newman, Joan, and Alan Taylor. 1992. Effect of a means-end contingency on young children's food preferences. *J Exp Child Psychol* 53:200-216.

Nicklas, Theresa A., Tom Baranowski, Janice C. Baranowski, Karen W. Cullen, LaTroy Rittenberry, and Norma Olvera. 2001. Family and child-care provider influences on preschool children's fruit, juice, and vegetable consumption. *Nutrition Reviews* 59:224-35.

Ogden, Cynthia L., Margaret D. Carroll, Lester R. Curtin, Margaret A. McDowell, Carolyn J. Tabak, and Katherine M. Flegal. 2006. Prevalence of overweight and obesity in the United States, 1999-2004. *Jama* 295:1549-55.

Ogden, Cynthia L., Katherine M. Flegal, Margaret D. Carroll, and Clifford L. Johnson. 2002. Prevalence and trends in overweight among US children and adolescents, 1999-2000. *Jama* 288:1728-32.

Orlet Fisher, Jennifer, Barbara J. Rolls, and Leann L. Birch. 2003. Children's bite size and intake of an entree are greater with large portions than with age-appropriate or self-selected portions. *Am J Clin Nutr* 77:1164-70.

Pecoraro, Norman, Faith Reyes, Francisca Gomez, Aditi Bhargava, and Mary F. Dallman. 2004. Chronic stress promotes palatable feeding, which reduces signs of stress: Feedforward and feedback effects of chronic stress. *Endocrinology* 145:3754-62.

Powers, Scott W., Kelly C. Byars, Monica J. Mitchell, Susana R. Patton, Debbie A. Standiford, and Lawrence M. Dolan. 2002. Parent report of mealtime behavior and parenting stress in young children with type 1 diabetes and in healthy control subjects. *Diabetes Care* 25:313-18.

Radziszewska, Barbara, Jean L. Richardson, Clyde W. Dent, and Brian R. Flay. 1996. Parenting style and adolescent depressive symptoms, smoking, and academic achievement: Ethnic, gender, and SES differences. *J Behav Med* 19:289-305.

Reinaerts, Evelien, Jascha de Nooijer, Math Candel, and Nanne de Vries. 2007. Explaining school children's fruit and vegetable consumption: The contributions of availability, accessibility, exposure, parental consumption and habit in addition to psychosocial factors. *Appetite* 48:248-58.

Rhee, Kyung E., Julie C. Lumeng, Danielle P. Appugliese, Niko Kaciroti, and Robert H. Bradley. 2006. Parenting styles and overweight status in first grade. *Pediatrics* 117:2047-54.

Rippe, James M., Suellyn Crossley, and Rhonda Ringer. 1998. Obesity as a chronic disease: Modern medical and lifestyle management. *Journal of the American Dietetic Association* 98:S9-S15.

Robinson, Thomas N., Michaela Kiernan, Donna M. Matheson, and K. Farish Haydel. 2001. Is parental control over children's eating associated with childhood obesity? Results from a population-based sample of third graders. *Obes Res* 9:306-12.

Rolls, Barbara J., Dianne Engell, and Leann L. Birch. 2000. Serving portion size influences 5-year-old but not 3-year-old children's food intakes. *J Am Diet Assoc* 100:232-34.

Rolls, Barbara J., Erin L. Morris, and Liane S. Row. 2002. Portion size of food affects energy intake in normal-weight and overweight men and women. *Am J Clin Nutr* 76:1207-13.

Rolls, Barbara J., Liane S. Row, Tanja V. E. Kral, Jennifer S. Meengs, and Denise E. Wall. 2004. Increasing the portion size of a packaged snack increases energy intake in men and women. *Appetite* 42:63-69.

Rolls, Barbara J., Liane S. Row, and Jennifer S. Meengs. 2006. Larger portion sizes lead to a sustained increase in energy intake over 2 days. *J Am Diet Assoc* 106:543-49.

Rolls, Barbara J., Liane S. Row, Jennifer S. Meengs, and Denise E. Wall. 2004. Increasing the portion size of a sandwich increases energy intake. *J Am Diet Assoc* 104:367-72.

Saelens, Brian E., Michelle M. Ernst, and Leonard H. Epstein. 2000. Maternal child feeding practices and obesity: A discordant sibling analysis. *Int J Eat Disord* 27:459-63.

Sanders, Matther R. 1999. Triple P—Positive Parenting Program: Towards an empirically validated multilevel parenting and family support strategy for the prevention of behavior and emotional problems in children. *Clin Child Fam Psychol Rev* 2:71-90.

Schmitz, Kathryn H, Leslie A. Lytle, Glenn A. Phillips, David M. Murray, Amanda S. Birnbaum, and Martha Y. Kubik. 2002. Psychosocial correlates of physical activity and sedentary leisure habits in young adolescents: The Teens Eating for Energy and Nutrition at School study. *Prev Med* 34:266-78.

Scott, Stephen, Quentin Spender, Moira Doolan, Brian Jacobs, Helen Aspland. 2001. Multicentre controlled trial of parenting groups for childhood antisocial behaviour in clinical practice. *BMJ* 323:194-98.

Sen, Bisakha. 2006. Frequency of family dinner and adolescent body weight status: Evidence from the National Longitudinal Survey of Youth, 1997. *Obesity (Silver Spring)* 14:2266-76.

Stein, Richard I., Leonard H. Epstein, Hollie A. Raynor, Colleen K. Kilanowski, and Rocco A. Paluch. 2005. The influence of parenting change on pediatric weight control. *Obes Res* 13:1749-55.

Steinberg, Laurence, Susie Lamborn, Nancy Darling, Nina S. Mounts, and Sanford M. Dornbusch. 1994. Over-time changes in adjustment and competence among adolescents from authoritative, authoritarian, indulgent, and neglectful families. *Child Development* 65:754-70.

Steinberg, Laurence, Susie Lamborn, Sanford M. Dornbusch, and Nancy Darling. 1992. Impact of parenting practices on adolescent achievement: Authoritative parenting, school involvement, and encouragement to succeed. *Child Development* 63:1266-81.

Taveras, Elsie M., Sheryl L. Rifas-Shiman, Catherine S. Berkey, Helaine R. H. Rockett, Alison E. Field, A. Lindsay Frazier, Graham A. Colditz, and Matthew W. Gillman. 2005. Family dinner and adolescent overweight. *Obes Res* 13:900-906.

Tibbs, Tiffany, Debra Haire-Joshu, Kenneth B. Schechtman, Ross C. Brownson, Marilyn S. Nanney, Cheryl Houston, and Wendy Auslander. 2001. The relationship between parental modeling, eating patterns, and dietary intake among African-American parents. *J Am Diet Assoc* 101:535-41.

Valtolina, Giovanni G., and Elena Marta. 1998. Family relations and psychosocial risk in families with an obese adolescent. *Psychol Rep* 83:251-60.

van der Horst, Klazine, Stef Kremers, Isabel Ferreira, Amika Singh, Anke Oenema, and Johannes Brug. 2007. Perceived parenting style and practices and the consumption of sugar-sweetened beverages by adolescents. *Health Educ Res* 22 (2): 295-304.

Videon, Tami M., and Carolyn K. Manning. 2003. Influences on adolescent eating patterns: the importance of family meals. *J Adolesc Health* 32:365-73.

Wardle, Jane, Lucy Cooke, E. Leigh Gibson, Manuela Sapochnik, Aubrey Sheiham, and Margaret Lawson. 2003. Increasing children's acceptance of vegetables; a randomized trial of parent-led exposure. *Appetite* 40:155-62.

Wardle, Jane, M. L. Herrera, Lucy Cooke, and E. Leigh Gibson. 2003. Modifying children's food preferences: The effects of exposure and reward on acceptance of an unfamiliar vegetable. *Eur J Clin Nutr* 57:341-48.

Webster-Stratton, Carolyn, and Mary Hammond. 1997. Treating children with early-onset conduct problems: A comparison of child and parent training interventions. *J Consult Clin Psychol* 65:93-109.

———. 1998. Conduct problems and level of social competence in Head Start children: Prevalence, pervasiveness, and associated risk factors. *Clin Child Fam Psychol Rev* 1:101-24.

Webster-Stratton, Carolyn, M. Jamila Reid, and Mary Hammond. 2001. Preventing conduct problems, promoting social competence: A parent and teacher training partnership in head start. *J Clin Child Psychol* 30:283-302.

———. 2004. Treating children with early-onset conduct problems: Intervention outcomes for parent, child, and teacher training. *J Clin Child Adolesc Psychol* 33:105-24.

Wilkins, Stephanie C., Olivia W. Kendrick, Kathleen R. Stitt, Nick Stinett, and Virginia A. Hammarlund. 1998. Family functioning is related to overweight in children. *J Am Diet Assoc* 98:572-74.

Wysocki, Tim, Huxtable Karen, T. R. Linscheid, and Wendy Wayne. 1989. Adjustment to diabetes mellitus in preschoolers and their mothers. *Diabetes Care* 12:524-29.

Zeller, Meg H., Jennifer Reiter-Purtill, Avani C. Modi, Joeanne Gutzwiller, Kathryn Vannatta, and W. Hobart Davies. 2007. Controlled study of critical parent and family factors in the obesigenic environment. *Obesity (Silver Spring)* 15:126-36.

As people became aware of the epidemic of childhood obesity, policy makers and public health practitioners called for the schools to change their environments to encourage healthy eating and increased physical activity. This article describes recent policy developments and clarifies what can and cannot be expected of schools based on existing and emerging evidence for prevention of childhood obesity.

Keywords: childhood obesity; prevention; energy balance; school environment; wellness policies

Children's Healthy Weight and the School Environment

By
LAURA C. LEVITON

Concern about the recent increase in the percentage of overweight children has led many policy makers and the public to call for changes in schools to address the problem. This chapter outlines the promise and limitations of schools in preventing childhood obesity. While schools are unlikely to reverse the epidemic of childhood obesity by themselves, they are an important venue for prevention, in concert with a comprehensive community-wide effort.

The schools seem like an obvious choice for prevention, since more than 97 percent of

Laura C. Leviton has been a senior program officer of the Robert Wood Johnson Foundation since 1999. She has been a professor at two schools of public health, where she collaborated on the first randomized experiment on HIV prevention, and later on two large place-based randomized experiments on improving medical practices. She received the 1993 award from the American Psychological Association for Distinguished Contributions to Psychology in the Public Interest. She was appointed by the Secretary of the U.S. Department of Health and Human Services to the National Advisory Committee on HIV and STD Prevention of the Centers for Disease Control and Prevention (CDC). She was president of the American Evaluation Association in the year 2000 and has coauthored two books: Foundations of Program Evaluation *and* Confronting Public Health Risks. *She is interested in all aspects of evaluation methodology and practice.*

DOI: 10.1177/0002716207308953

children five years and older spend six to eight hours a day there for nine to ten months a year (Institute of Medicine 2006; Trust for America's Health 2006). The policies that affect factors within schools can be monitored more readily than the wide variety of policies affecting community environments (Institute of Medicine 2006). Advocates have noted disturbing trends in school environments and are calling for reversal of those trends (e.g., Action for Healthy Kids 2007). They have called for reforms to restore time spent on recess and physical education, to limit "competitive foods" (foods of little nutritional value that compete with the school breakfast and lunch), and to improve healthy offerings in the school cafeteria.

There is also a public perception that schools should initiate efforts to prevent childhood obesity. A recent national poll revealed that 87 percent of respondents believed schools should address the problem (Research!America 2006). Other polls consistently mirror this trend (Napier 2006; Stein 2004). Public health professionals agree: a survey of state health department chronic disease directors (who have responsibility for preventing obesity) rated school-based approaches as the highest priority to prevent childhood obesity (Trust for America's Health 2006; Segal and Gadola 2008 [this volume]). In line with these perceptions, federal and state policy makers are requiring changes to make the school environment conducive to preventing obesity. The environmental factors in school seem readily apparent and somewhat easier to change than the many forces in communities that are contributing to the problem.

At the same time, there are limits to what schools can do about the problem. Historically, health promotion has never been a priority of the schools. School health services are often criticized for poor planning, a lack of clear goals, and failure to keep up with the changing needs of students. Schools are often hard-pressed financially, forcing them to make difficult choices about programs to save or cut, including physical education. Schools have been forced into an almost exclusive focus on improving achievement scores (the "No Child Left Behind" legislation is merely the most recent pressure). The focus on achievement has consumed limited time in the school day, forcing out many activities that are not seen as directly supporting student achievement (Pedulla et al. 2003; Stecher and Barron 2001, Trust for America's Health 2006). Finally, school personnel often suffer from "innovation fatigue": they have seen many changes come and go (Troman and Woods 2001). Control over school program implementation depends on cooperation at several levels: the district level, the school facilities, and the individual teacher or staff person (Berends, Bodilly, and Kirby 2002). Without staff buy-in, who will implement any reforms to prevent childhood obesity?

Fortunately, these obstacles can be overcome. Recent innovations for school programming and experiences in policy reform suggest that the obstacles to changing the environment are not as great as we feared, and some perceived obstacles are not well founded in actual experience.

Population-Wide Improvements Require
Environmental Changes

Prevention, not treatment of obesity, is the goal of school interventions. In framing the childhood obesity problem, prevention needs to be clearly differentiated from medical treatment for children who are already obese. People do not usually differentiate prevention and treatment, and this poses a challenge for school settings. Focus groups conducted by the Robert Wood Johnson Foundation indicate that the public—and many policy makers—automatically think that weight loss is the answer to the problem. With that focus come associated concerns about encouraging eating disorders and other problems.

In framing the childhood obesity problem, prevention needs to be clearly differentiated from medical treatment for children who are already obese. People do not usually differentiate prevention and treatment, and this poses a challenge for school settings.

The Institute of Medicine (2005) noted that prevention helps children who are not obese to maintain a healthy weight and is therefore appropriate for school interventions. Treatment (weight loss) is best accomplished under a doctor's supervision. A healthy school environment can help support weight loss and, provided that adequate follow-up and treatment are available, may be helpful in screening for overweight (Institute of Medicine 2005). The school nurse can play a role by following through with medical recommendations and supporting behavior change (Costante 2001). Finally, there is some reason to be concerned that obesity prevention in the schools may increase stigma, teasing, and victimization of overweight children—but effective staff training programs can minimize these problems (Puhl and Latner 2007). Well-conducted programs in Arkansas have seen no increase in teasing (Raczynski et al. 2007).

Prevention requires small but consistent changes in schools. Recent statistical modeling suggests that normal-weight children need only small daily changes to achieve a balance between calories consumed and calories expended through physical activity (Hill et al. 2003; Wang et al. 2006). Normal weight children consume (or fail to expend) between 110 and 165 excess calories every day, leading to an excess weight gain of ten pounds over ten years. In contrast, overweight children consume between 700 and 1,000 calories in excess of what is required for normal growth, leading to a gain of fifty-eight excess pounds over ten years (Wang et al. 2006). It is plausible that school environments can assist prevention, because the required changes in the energy balance are relatively small. Treatment of obesity that includes weight loss requires a scale of behavior modification that is beyond the power of most school environments, however.

Prevention requires environmental changes to achieve consistent effects. Environmental interventions engineer behavior change to make it automatic or to minimize opportunities for individual choices or habits. Environmental interventions may also enable individual choices and habits that are otherwise more difficult (Green and Kreuter 2005). When environmental interventions are available, public health professionals usually prefer them to interventions that depend on human error and individual choices. For example, clean drinking water is greatly preferred to individual purification systems or purchase of bottled water, and engineered safety protections at the workplace are greatly preferred to safety rules that are subject to human error. Environmental interventions can apply to entire populations, not just to targeted individuals (Leviton, Rhodes, and Chang 2007). They also have more consistent effects, and in the case of childhood obesity it is the daily, consistent balance in energy that is required. Recently health promotion has turned away from a strict focus on direct intervention or health education with individuals, to what is termed the ecological approach. This approach recognizes many levels of influence on individual health and behavior, including individual factors, community, organizations, society, industry and agriculture, policy, environment, and interpersonal factors. These all have reciprocal influences; interventions are generally more powerful when tailored to several levels at the same time (Green and Kreuter 2005).

Focus groups conducted for Robert Wood Johnson Foundation indicate that many health professionals do not understand the ecological approach to obesity prevention, relying instead on didactic approaches or, at most, experiential learning. Yet as seen below, most school-based programs that focus solely on individual change have relatively small effects or no effect on obesity-related behaviors, while programs that include environmental changes generally have larger effects.

A variety of environmental changes are needed in schools. No quick fixes or single policy solutions exist for the school environment. For example, many policy makers have focused on limiting sweetened beverages at school (Institute of Medicine 2005). Indeed, good evidence suggests that reducing their consumption will help to restore energy balance (James et al. 2004; Vartanian, Schwartz,

TABLE 1
NATIONAL SURVEYS OF SCHOOL POLICIES AND ENVIRONMENTS

Every year the Youth, Education, and Society (YES) component of the Robert Wood
   Johnson–supported program "Bridging the Gap" reports on policies and environment for
   physical activity and nutrition in middle and high schools.
Every six years the Centers for Disease Control and Prevention (CDC) supports SHPPS: the
   School Health Policies and Programs Study, which examines the school environment for
   physical activity, health education, and nutrition (results for 2006 were not available at the
   time of this writing).
In 1996, 2002, and 2004, the CDC also supported surveys using the School Health Profile,
   which covers physical education and health education in middle and high schools.
Every seven years the U.S. Department of Agriculture (USDA) supports the School
   Nutrition Dietary Assessment Study (SNDA), which monitors the quality of reimbursable
   school breakfast and lunch (results for 2005 are only now being reported).
In 2005, the U.S. Department of Education also conducted a survey of elementary school
   administrators concerning physical activity and nutrition (Parsad and Lewis 2006).

and Brownell 2007). After all, one can of sweetened soda has about 155 calories, which is about enough to restore a day's energy balance all by itself. However, while limiting soda is a good idea, it is probably not sufficient by itself to prevent obesity throughout the schools. Not all children want a can of soda; some consume too many calories outside of school hours, and some children consume fewer calories but are overly sedentary. The statistical simulations deal in averages, meaning the energy balance needs vary among a population of children. Prevention will be best served when children's environment gives them a variety of opportunities to consume healthy food and to be physically active.

Negative Environmental Forces Stimulate a Call for Action

Surveillance of policies and school environments. If a variety of small changes in the schools are required, then the schools are generally going in the wrong direction. Survey data (see Table 1) have revealed some disturbing features of the school environment. Note, however, that because these surveys all used somewhat different methods, we should use caution in inferring any direct comparison or conclusion about trends.

Physical activity. The School Health Policies and Programs Study (SHPPS) revealed that, in 2000, slightly fewer than one-half of elementary schools required physical education in grades one through five, while only 25 percent required it in eighth grade and 5 percent required it in twelfth grade. In 2005, the U.S. Department of Education reported that 99 percent of elementary schools provided physical education, and the annual survey conducted by Youth, Education, and Society (YES) indicated that physical education was provided in 86 percent of eighth grades, 53 percent of tenth grades, and 21 percent of twelfth grades (Johnston et al. 2006). This appears to be a striking improvement and consistent across surveys, but merely having physical education is not sufficient. The Institute of Medicine (2005) recommended daily physical education, yet according to SHPPS 2000, only 8 percent of elementary schools and 6 percent of middle and high schools meet this requirement (Burgeson et al. 2001). According to the U.S. Department of Education in 2005, however, daily physical education was offered by a somewhat larger percentage of elementary schools: between 17 and 22 percent depending on grade level. The 2005 YES survey indicated that the average number of days of physical education in middle and high school was four days per week and the average number of minutes was fifty-four (Johnston et al. 2006).

Healthy food offerings. The food environments of schools are correlated with weight status—where school policies support frequent snacking and the availability of foods high in calories and fat, children's body mass index (BMI) is greater (Kubik, Lytle, and Story 2005). Two general forces affect the food environment: whether the school food service follows the U.S. Department of Agriculture (USDA) dietary guidelines, and whether competitive foods, those that "compete" with the school breakfast and lunch, are present.

The USDA has a powerful effect on school environments through reimbursement of school breakfast and lunch: 99 percent of all public schools and 83 percent of all private and public schools participate in the program (Story, Kaphingst, and French 2006). Since 1995, school breakfasts and lunches have been required to meet the USDA dietary guidelines—yet according to the 1998 School Nutrition Dietary Assessment Study (SNDA), more than 75 percent of schools had not yet met the guidelines for fat content.[1] The USDA provides training on nutritious food service, but in 2005 fewer than half of the schools responding to the YES survey were participating in such training (Johnston et al. 2006); even where they did so, their ability to follow the guidelines may still be in question. The general conclusion is that the USDA-funded School Lunch and Breakfast are better than they were in 1995, but there is still room for improvement in terms of fat and calorie content, use of fresh fruits and vegetables, skim milk, and whole grains (Story, Kaphingst, and French 2006).

Of most concern, however, are competitive foods. Because the cafeteria foods are often unappetizing, competitive foods displace consumption of healthy foods, and unfortunately they are often high in calories and fat (Story, Kaphingst, and French 2006). The 2000 SHPPS revealed that 43 percent of elementary schools, 74 percent of middle schools, and 98 percent of high schools sell competitive foods in snack bars, school stores, and vending machines and for fund-raising (Wechsler et al. 2001). By 2005, according to the U.S. Department of Education, 94 percent of public elementary schools reported offering food for sale outside the school breakfast and lunch (Parsad and Lewis 2006). For middle and high schools in 2005, 81 percent of schools offered soft drinks for sale at some point during the school day (Johnston et al. 2006). The preliminary findings of the 2005 SNDA are that 38 percent of all schools have vending machines near the cafeteria, and 68 percent have no restrictions on the types of food sold (Frost and McKinney 2006). The 2004 School Health Profile survey indicated that in the twenty-seven states studied, 94.5 percent of middle and high schools sold sweetened drinks through vending machines (Institute of Medicine 2005), a pattern entirely consistent with the 2005 YES survey (Johnston et al. 2006). Advocates call for making the school breakfast and lunch more appetizing, making competitive foods healthier, or eliminating competitive foods altogether.

Because schools are held accountable for student test scores, any subject that is not tested gets a lower priority, and as a result health education, physical education, and recess have been pushed out of the curriculum.

What maintains these unhealthy school environments? Story, Kaphingst, and French (2006) have analyzed the reasons for the rise in competitive foods and the decline in physical activity in schools.

1. School food service often needs to be self-supporting, and in 2000 the USDA only reimbursed 51 percent of the cost of a meal. The easiest way for schools to make up the difference is to offer the popular competitive foods, and competitive foods do not have to meet USDA nutritional requirements.
2. School districts come to rely on the revenues from competitive foods not only to support food service, but also academic and extracurricular activities. Also, school districts negotiate "pouring rights," exclusive contracts for the sale of soft drinks. Companies offer incentives to school districts in the form of lump-sum payments and a percentage of the profits (see Graff 2008 [this volume]).
3. The vending machines and school stores are more attractive to students when their lunch period is scheduled as early as 10 a.m., when they have insufficient time to eat, and face long lines in cramped and unpleasant cafeterias. However, scheduling and space are usually not under the food service's control.
4. Because schools are held accountable for student test scores, any subject that is not tested gets a lower priority, and as a result health education, physical education, and recess have been pushed out of the curriculum.
5. Students often do not have transportation to take advantage of sports or other physical activity before and after schools.

Story, Kaphingst, and French (2006) outlined several approaches to deal with these obstacles. Indeed, as states and school districts introduce reforms to address obesity, it is becoming clear that some of the feared consequences are simply without foundation. Properly conducted physical education does not detract from academic test scores (at least in the case of one curriculum; see Sallis et al. 1999), and Story, Kaphingst, and French cited some evidence that physical activity is associated with achievement: several studies examining the relationship between achievement scores and physical activity or physical education policies, and one study indicating that fourth-graders had trouble concentrating on days without recess. In addition, Wharton, Long, and Schwartz (forthcoming) challenged the fear that school districts will lose revenue from food service reforms. They conducted a systematic review of the effect on school revenues when school districts limited competitive foods and put nutritional standards into place. Contrary to expectations, most schools do not lose revenue, and some schools saw an increase in USDA School Lunch participation. Technical assistance and ideas for overcoming the problems of school food service are abundant (Story, Kaphingst, and French 2006; Wharton, Long, and Schwartz forthcoming).

The Evidence Base: What Might the Schools Achieve for Prevention?

The role of controlled studies. Controlled studies of school-based prevention are important because they indicate whether reversing the trend in prevalence of childhood obesity is feasible and suggest the directions that policy and environmental change should take. Ideally, a local school district or state department of education would mandate that schools implement evidence-based programs and environmental interventions to combat childhood obesity. The Centers for Disease Control and Prevention (CDC) Task Force on Community Preventive Services has conducted several systematic reviews to determine which kinds of school intervention are effective and for what purpose (CDC 2005a, 2005b). However, the evidence to definitively guide school changes is simply not available in many cases.

Obesity prevention. The Task Force on Community Preventive Services recently concluded that there was insufficient evidence to support school-based programs for obesity prevention (Story, Kaphingst, and French 2006). In contrast, the direct relationship between physical activity and obesity prevention is much more clear. A systematic review by Strong et al. (2005) examined both experimental and quasi-experimental studies of health effects of physical activity on children's body mass index. Moderately intense physical activity for thirty to sixty minutes a day led to a reduction in percent body fat for overweight children and youth. No reduction in body fat percentage occurred in normal-weight children in these studies. However, it is important to bear in mind that prevention means maintaining the weight of normal-weight children, so one might not expect to see a change in those with normal weight.

Changing children's diet. The Community Preventive Services Task Force has concluded that evidence is mixed and more research is needed to determine whether school-based intervention will change children's diet (CDC 2005b). Nutrition education by itself is not generally effective in getting children to make healthier choices. One controlled study of British school children did find that a five-session curriculum aimed at reducing sweetened soda consumption did reduce children's drinking of these sodas and the prevalence of overweight in the treatment schools (James et al. 2004). However, the methods of this study are flawed (French 2004). Multicomponent intervention studies have been some-what more successful. For example, the High 5 Project was a randomized exper-iment including classroom, cafeteria, and family involvement—it produced relatively large changes in children's consumption of fruits and vegetables (Reynolds et al. 2000). Consuming more fruits and vegetables is not by itself suf-ficient to prevent overweight; however, they can give a sense of fullness and may therefore displace the more calorie-dense "junk foods."

Changing the school food environment, that is, the price, promotion, and availability of foods, has been found effective in changing children's choices of food during the school day. However, very little research has focused on the effects of the school food environment on children's overall eating behavior or on prevalence of overweight (Story, Kaphingst, and French 2006). Healthy food environments are associated with lower body mass index (Kubik, Lytle, and Story 2005), but this finding concerns an association, not a causal connection, between healthy school environments and lower body mass index. It is correlational, not causal, because families may self-select into schools with these environments or a third, unknown variable may be responsible for both the food environment and lower body mass index. To the best of my knowledge, no randomized experiment to date has tested the causal relationship.

Increasing physical activity. Enhanced physical education, which uses creden-tialed teachers, is effective in increasing children's physical activity (CDC 2005a). An important policy reform is the choice of an evidence-based physical education curriculum. SPARK (Sports, Play and Active Recreation for Kids) is one such cur-riculum. It provides for physical education specialists and teacher training in phys-ical education. In a quasi-experiment, children receiving instruction from specialists or trained teachers were more physically active at the end of two years than were comparison students (Sallis et al. 1997). Physical activity outside of school hours was unaffected. There were no significant effects on body mass index (Sallis et al. 1993). SPARK had no adverse effect on academic achievement (Sallis et al. 1999). At the end of one and a half years, specialists were withdrawn, and at four years the teachers were still implementing SPARK at 88 percent of its previ-ous quality (McKenzie et al. 1997). Although this finding argues for using creden-tialed physical education teachers, the fact that SPARK continued to be implemented at this level is notable. SPARK has been adopted and its use sustained in school districts all over the country (Dowda et al. 2005).

While advocates are urging schools to restore recess time in elementary and middle schools, the characteristics of recess are critically important. Children are more active generally at school when there is equipment such as basketball hoops, improvements in playgrounds, and supervision to organize active games (Sallis et al. 2001; Stratton and Mullan 2005; Verstraete et al. 2006).

Reducing screen time. Television and video games may be implicated in the rise in prevalence of childhood obesity, because too much time in these sedentary activities replaces physical activity and because many children snack while viewing television. In one study, elementary school children were given a six-month curriculum to reduce television, videotape, and video game use. They significantly reduced these activities, as well as eating while watching television, and significantly reduced their BMI (Robinson 1999). The "We Can!" initiative of the National Institutes of Health (www.nichd.nih.gov/news/resources/spotlight/042407_wecan.cfm) includes limiting screen time as an important evidence-based practice for the schools. The Community Preventive Services Task Force is currently undertaking a systematic review of this topic.

Multicomponent interventions. Programs that cover both nutrition and physical activity should, in theory, be more effective than single component interventions. The Planet Health intervention was a randomized experiment testing health outcomes of a two-year school-based health education intervention for sixth to eighth graders. It integrated health education into four major subjects as well as physical education, and focused on reduced television viewing, eating fewer high-fat foods, eating more fruits and vegetables, and increased physical activity. Body mass index declined for girls but not boys; girls ate more fruits and vegetables and consumed fewer calories. For both boys and girls, television viewing declined (Gortmaker et al. 1999). However, Planet Health primarily involves individual health education to change knowledge and attitudes; it does not have a strong environmental component.

Other well-conducted multicomponent interventions were not successful in changing the prevalence of overweight. Two well-conducted studies intervened with third- to fifth-grade children: Child and Adolescent Trial for Cardiovascular Health (CATCH) and the Pathways study for American Indian schoolchildren. These programs changed food offerings in schools, enhanced the physical education curriculum, and offered health education. Although they were school based, they also provided family education to promote lifestyle change beyond the school walls. CATCH was successful in changing children's eating and physical activity but had no effect on body mass index (Luepker et al. 1996). Pathways changed some aspects of diet as well as knowledge and attitudes but had no effect on physical activity or body mass index (Caballero et al. 2003).

Making sense of the evidence. What, then, is one to do with the mixed findings from these studies? First, it is worth keeping in mind that society overall was changing toward the increasing prevalence of children's overweight at the same time that these studies aimed to affect children's behavior through the schools (Ogden et al. 2002). The schools, like society as a whole, were engineering physical activity out of the environment, luring children with sedentary video games, expanding portion sizes, and increasing the availability of junk foods during the day. In the face of such changes, even a comprehensive program might not be effective—little changes making for an energy imbalance were mounting up.

Second, the school environment itself may have defeated prevention efforts. A key principle of health promotion is to focus on the ecology in which health behavior takes place (Green and Kreuter 2005). It is likely that the presence of junk food, limited time for physical activity, and other features of the school environment undercut the health message in some of these programs and contributed to energy imbalance.

The Community Preventive Services Task Force must use the most stringent criteria of effectiveness. Yet the epidemic will not wait. At the moment, the Task Force must deal with a paucity of well-controlled studies, variation in outcome measures, variation in student ages, variation in the models being implemented, and variation in the implementation of the models being tested. Even the most casual reader of the available studies can see reason for optimism in school-based approaches, suggestions about where to put effort, and reasons to discount some findings.

Furthermore, the correlational evidence concerning the environment is more consistent and positive than the evidence from controlled studies of effectiveness. School environments are associated with weight status and related behavior. A logic model or theory of change is required, and it provides a much greater sense of optimism. While the logic model itself needs a test, it still provides a guide to action. An abbreviated logic model might be as follows:

- The physical activity connection:
  o *If* time is made for physical education and supervised recess, *then* kids are more physically active;
  o *if* they are more physically active, *then* they expend more calories and are closer to achieving an energy balance.
- The food environment connection:
  o *If* schools limit competitive foods *and* provide appetizing school meals that meet dietary guidelines, in appealing circumstances with sufficient time to eat,
  o *then* they will consume appropriate calories and come closer to achieving an energy balance.
- The school environment:
  o *If* schools have a healthy environment for eating and physical activity,
  o *and* community and family environments are also healthy,
  o *then* children will achieve an energy balance and maintain healthy weight.

What Is Being Done?

As policy and environmental approaches are proposed and endorsed, we are seeing a familiar pattern: local initiatives take the lead, followed by state and federal actions. The reasons are understandable: as in the case of tobacco, local decision makers are in a better position to take some risks and try new things

(Lawrence W. Green, personal communication on the evolution of policy advocacy in prevention policies, January 20, 2006). Advocates would say that for the competitive foods issue in particular, the food industry has hampered progress (Story, Kaphingst, and French 2006).

Federal action. Resources have been provided for some time for training and technical assistance (Institute of Medicine 2005). The CDC has long provided funding and technical assistance to states to implement the coordinated school health program model, emphasizing physical education and nutrition and a healthy school environment (www.cdc.gov/HealthyYouth/CSHP/). The USDA offers a variety of resources to states to assist school food service to meet the mandated dietary guidelines (http://teamnutrition.usda.gov/grants.html).

The Child Nutrition and WIC Reauthorization Act of 2004 mandated that by fall of 2006, all schools participating in the USDA School Lunch and School Breakfast programs were required to establish and implement wellness policies. The wellness policies would set forth requirements for physical education, health education, and nutrition and ensure that school meals meet the federal dietary guidelines. However, with only $4 million appropriated to implement the policies, this is essentially an unfunded mandate for the schools.

The 2007 Farm Bill is under consideration at the time of this writing. It is a wide-ranging set of laws that touch every aspect of the food systems of this country. Public health advocates, nutrition experts, and the USDA have recommended several changes in the law to improve the food environment of schools. These include enforcing the requirements that school food service meet the federal dietary guidelines, authorizing new resources to train food service employees, and authorizing $500 million over the next ten years to provide fruit and vegetable snacks to students (e.g., American Public Health Association 2007; Institute of Medicine 2007). These changes are sorely needed because so many schools have failed to meet the federal dietary guidelines for so long.

National voluntary efforts. Action for Healthy Kids (AFHK) is a public–private partnership of more than fifty national organizations and government agencies organized in 2002 to combat childhood obesity through changes in school. Through 51 Teams in every state and the District of Columbia, AFHK works through thousands of volunteer parents, school and health care personnel, and citizens. It provides model projects and policies and shares suggestions about how to engage schools, and develop parent and youth advocates. Local volunteers make sure that school districts have oversight and person power to implement obesity prevention strategies (AFHK 2007).

The Alliance for a Healthier Generation is a national partnership between the American Heart Association and the William J. Clinton Foundation on childhood obesity prevention. In 2006, the Alliance launched the Healthy Schools program, which focuses on helping schools to create healthier environments. The Alliance provides relationship managers, who work regionally with individual school districts to assist them, and it provides virtual technical assistance online. The Alliance developed standards for policy, program, and practice based on the best evidence for physical activity and healthy eating. These standards serve as the basis for a recognition program.[2] The relationship managers assist the schools with planning and assessment, but also in identifying resources. For example, by buying equipment and supplies together, schools can reduce expenses they may incur when changing practices and programs. In May 2007, 230 schools received technical assistance from a relationship manager, and another 900 schools enrolled in the virtual support program. The Alliance plans to include another 6,400 schools that serve primarily low-income and minority children who suffer disproportionately from the obesity epidemic.

State-level changes. State legislatures and departments of education have been active in the past few years in passing new laws and regulations on the school environment. Since the 2004 federal requirement for school wellness policies, the level of activity has increased. Many states have their own wellness policies, which the school districts have emulated. The Robert Wood Johnson Foundation Web site (www.rwjf.org) publishes Balance, a series of tracking reports on state legislation and regulations relevant to childhood obesity. A 2006 annual report is now available (Health Policy Tracking Service 2006). These reports indicate that the states are generally increasing the required time for physical education and recess; raising standards for physical education and nutrition education; increasing compliance with the USDA dietary guidelines in school service; and most notably, limiting access to foods of limited nutritional value in vending machines, school stores, and cafeterias. However, the quality of the state laws is also a matter of concern: public health advocates worry that the requirements can be considerably watered down.

The quality of the state laws is also a matter of concern: public health advocates worry that the requirements can be considerably watered down.

The National Cancer Institute has developed assessment measures for state policies on school physical activity and nutrition that takes into account a variety of features of the school environment and assigns points for the quality of each (Mâsse, Frosh, et al. forthcoming; Mâsse, Chriqui, et al. forthcoming). While other organizations have also ranked the quality of state policies, these assessment measures have the advantage that that they were developed through an expert consensus process.

Local district changes. According to the USDA, 56 percent of schools were not subject to a wellness policy in 2005 (Frost and McKinney 2006). Districts were to have written and implemented wellness policies by the beginning of the 2006-2007 school year. Federal surveys have not been conducted, yet from the available evidence progress has been slow. AFHK (2007) reviewed a sample of policies from 256 school districts in forty-nine states between summer 2006 and February 2007. Although the sample was not representative, it did include urban, rural, and suburban schools and small, medium, and large school districts. AFHK assessed the policies to determine whether they met the minimum requirements of the law, and also compared the policies to the AFHK model policy. The policies generally addressed the elements required by the law (the range was 78 percent requiring meals that adhere to the dietary guidelines, to 88 percent establishing school health councils or wellness teams). However, only 15 percent required physical education that meets national standards and 35 percent required qualified staff for physical education; 58 percent included requirements for recess and activities outside school hours. Nutrition education was required to be incorporated into health education and the general curriculum in more than 60 percent of policies, while 40 percent required teacher training for nutrition education. Almost 85 percent of the policies address nutrition standards for competitive foods in vending machines and student stores, and 56 percent state that competitive foods must meet or exceed the dietary guidelines.[3] Most serious, however, was the lack of attention in most school policies to planning for implementation and evaluation.

Implementation is clearly the largest challenge to wellness policies in the schools. For example, Samuels and associates (2006) examined six California school districts that had passed policies limiting sweetened beverages and snacks high in sugar and fat on school campuses. The policies had only been partially implemented at the time of the case studies. In the same way, schools in the state of Arkansas, which passed ambitious legislation in 2004, were making some progress by 2007 but were far from satisfying the law (Raczynski et al. 2007). And schools' general failure to implement the USDA dietary guidelines for school meals led to strong advocacy for reform in the pending Farm Bill. Implementation is incremental in schools, so that continued supports will be needed. The voluntary efforts of AFHK, the Alliance for a Healthier Generation, government agencies, and youth-serving organizations can all work to provide this support.

Conclusions

The school environment can contribute to an overall energy balance in children's lives. The evidence is far from definitive, but the correlational evidence is striking, and there is just enough in the way of causal tests of effectiveness for some optimism. At a minimum, schools can reverse decades of policies and environmental changes that have helped to produce the epidemic of overweight. Monitoring data indicates they may well have done so. Of course, the schools cannot reverse the epidemic by themselves. Moving beyond the school walls, coordinated efforts include farm-to-school programs, safe routes that permit children to walk to school, use of the school facility by community organizations for active after-school time, and a host of other efforts that have not been touched on here (Story, Kaphingst, and French 2006). To change the school environment, however, will take time and effort. The available evidence is that implementation is the key, and implementation is a long, hard road for any school program.

Notes

1. Findings from School Nutrition Dietary Assessment Study (SNDA) III on this point are not available at the time of this writing.

2. The recognition criteria can be found at www.healthiergeneration.org/schools.aspx?id=76&ekmensel =1ef02451_10_12_76_2.

3. Other important features of the school policies can be found at the Action for Healthy Kids Web site: http://www.actionforhealthykids.org.

References

Action for Healthy Kids. 2007. *Local wellness policies one year later: Showing improvements in school nutrition and physical activity*. Skokie, IL: Action for Healthy Kids. http://actionforhealthykids.org/ pdf/WP%20Analysis%20May%202007.pdf (accessed July 11, 2007).

American Public Health Association. 2007. Farm Bill reauthorization: Making the case for public health priorities in the Farm Bill. http://www.apha.org/NR/rdonlyres/C21C2A6E-3071-470E-B001-1F2E05953145/0/2007FarmBillReauthorizationFactSheet.pdf (accessed July 10, 2007).

Berends, M., Susan J. Bodilly, and Sheila Nataraj Kirby. 2002. *Facing the challenges of whole-school reform: New American Schools after a decade*. Rand Corporation Monograph Reports. Santa Monica, CA: Rand Corporation. www.rand.org/pubs/monograph_reports/MR1498/ (accessed July 6, 2007).

Burgeson, C. R., H. Wechsler, N. D. Brener, J. C. Young, and C. G. Spain. 2001. Physical education and activity: Results from the School Health Policies and Programs Study 2000. *Journal of School Health* 71 (7): 279-93.

Caballero, B., T. Clay, S. M. Davis, B. Ethelbah, B. Holy Rock, T. Lohman, J. Norman, M. Story, E. J. Stone, L. Stephenson L., and J. Stevens for the Pathways Study Research Group. 2003. Pathways: A school-based, randomized controlled trial for the prevention of obesity in American Indian school-children. *American Journal of Clinical Nutrition* 78:1030-38.

Centers for Disease Control and Prevention (CDC). 2005a. *Enhanced physical education classes in schools are recommended to increase physical activity among young people*. The Community Guide to Preventive Services. Atlanta, GA: CDC. http://www.thecommunityguide.org/pa/pa-int-school-pe.pdf (accessed July 9, 2007).

———. 2005b. *More evidence is needed to determine the effectiveness of school-based programs to improve the nutritional status of children and adolescents*. The Community Guide to Preventive Services. Atlanta, GA: CDC. http://www.thecommunityguide.org/nutrition/nutr-int-schools.pdf (accessed July 9, 2007).

Costante, C. C. 2001. School health nursing: Framework for the future, Part I. *Journal of School Nursing* 17 (1): 3-11.

Dowda, M., F. James, J. F. Sallis, T. L. McKenzie, P. Rosengard, and H. W. Kohl III. 2005. Evaluating the sustainability of SPARK physical education: A case study of translating research into practice. *Research Quarterly for Exercise and Sport* 76 (1): 11-19.

French, S. 2004. School soft drink intervention study: Too good to be true? *British Medical Journal* 329 (7462): E315-16.

Frost, A., and P. McKinney. 2006. FNS school meals . . . do they measure up? Presentation posted to the USDA Web site. http://www.fns.usda.gov/oane/menu/Presentations/SNA-ANC2006.pdf (accessed July 9, 2007).

Gortmaker, S. L., K. Peterson, J. Wiecha, A. M. Sobol, S. Dixit, M. K. Fox, and N. Laird. 1999. Reducing obesity via a school-based interdisciplinary intervention among youth: Planet Health. *Archives of Pediatric and Adolescent Medicine* 153 (4): 409-18.

Graff, S. K. 2008. First Amendment implications of restricting food and beverage marketing in schools. *Annals of the American Academy of Political and Social Science* 615: 158-77.

Green, L. W., and M. Kreuter. 2005. *Health promotion planning: An educational and ecological approach.* New York: McGraw-Hill.

Health Policy Tracking Service. 2006. *Balance: A report on state action to promote nutrition, increase physical activity and prevent obesity.* Issue 3. Princeton, NJ: Robert Wood Johnson Foundation. http://www.rwjf.org/programareas/resources/product.jsp?id=15950&pid=1138&gsa=1.

Hill, J. O., H. R. Wyatt, G. W. Reed, and J. C. Peters. 2003. Obesity and the environment: Where do we go from here? *Science* 299 (5608): 853-55.

Institute of Medicine. 2005. *Preventing childhood obesity: Health in the balance.* Washington DC: National Academy Press.

———. 2006. *Progress in preventing childhood obesity: How do we measure up?* Washington, DC: National Academy Press.

———. 2007. Nutrition standards for foods in schools: Opening statement by Virginia Stallings. April 25. http://www8.nationalacademies.org/onpinews/bydate.aspx (accessed July 10, 2007).

James, J., P. Thomas, D. Cavan, and D. Kerr. 2004. Preventing childhood obesity by reducing consumption of carbonated drinks: Cluster randomised controlled trial. *British Medical Journal* 328 (7450): 1237-41.

Johnston, L. D., P. M. O'Malley, J. Delva, J. G. Bachman, and J. E. Schulenberg. 2006. *Youth Education and Society: Results on school policies and programs, overview of key findings, 2005.* Ann Arbor: University of Michigan. http://www.yesresearch.org/publications/reports/schoolreport2005.pdf (accessed July 19, 2007).

Kubik, M. Y., L. A. Lytle, and M. Story. 2005. Schoolwide food practices are associated with body mass index in middle school students. *Archives of Pediatric and Adolescent Medicine* 159 (12): 1111-14.

Leviton, L. C., S. D. Rhodes, and C. Chang. 2007. Public health: Policy, practice, and perceptions. In *Health care delivery in the United States*, 9th ed., ed. A. R. Kovner, J. R. Knickman, and S. Jonas, chap. 4. New York: Springer.

Luepker, R. V., C. L. Perry, S. M. McKinlay, P. R. Nader, G. S. Parcel, E. J. Stone, L. S. Webber, J. P. Elder, H. A. Feldman, C. C. Johnson, S. H. Kelder, and M. Wu. 1996. Outcomes of a field trial to improve children's dietary patterns and physical activity. The Child and Adolescent Trial for Cardiovascular Health. CATCH collaborative group. *Journal of the American Medical Association* 275:768-76.

Mâsse, L. C., J. F. Chriqui, J. F. Igoe, A. A. Atienza, J. Kruger, H. W. Kohl, M. Frosh, and A. L. Yaroch. Forthcoming. Development of a system for measuring state physical education-related policies. *American Journal of Preventive Medicine*, Special Supplement

Mâsse, L. C., M. Frosh, J. F. Chriqui, A. L. Yaroch, T. Agurs-Collins, H. M. Blanck, A. A. Atienza, M. L. McKenna, and J. F. Igoe. Forthcoming. Development of a measurement system to assess the extensiveness of state school nutrition-environment policies. *American Journal of Preventive Medicine*, Special Supplement.

McKenzie, T. L., J. F. Sallis, B. Kolody, and F. N. Faucette. 1997. Long-term effects of a physical education curriculum and staff development program: SPARK. *Research Quarterly for Exercise and Sport* 68 (4): 280-91.

Napier, M. 2006. *What does America think about childhood obesity?* Robert Wood Johnson Foundation Research Highlight Number 3. www.rwjf.org/files/research/Obesity_ResearchHighlight_3_0604.pdf (accessed July 6, 2007).

Ogden, C. L., K. M. Flegal, M. D. Carroll, and C. L. Johnson. 2002. Prevalence and trends in overweight among US children and adolescents, 1999-2000. *Journal of the American Medical Association* 288 (14): 1772-73.

Parsad, B., and L. Lewis. 2006. *Calories in, calories out: Food and exercise in public elementary schools, 2005* (NCES 2006–057). U.S. Department of Education. Washington, DC: National Center for Education Statistics.

Pedulla, J. J., L. M. Abrams, G. F. Madaus, M. K. Russell, M. A. Ramos, and J. Miao. 2003. *Perceived effects of state-mandated testing programs on teaching and learning: Findings from a national survey of teachers*. Boston: Boston College, National Board on Educational Testing and Public Policy, Lynch School of Education.

Puhl, R. M., and J. D. Latner. 2007. Stigma, obesity and the health of the nation's children. *Psychological Bulletin* 133 (4): 557-80.

Raczynski, J. M., M. Phillips, Z. Bursac, R. A. Kahn, L. Pulley, D. West, R. L. Craig, S. F. Elliott V. L. Evans, H. Gauss, B. E. E. Montgomery, and A. G. Philyaw. 2007. *Year three evaluation: Arkansas Act 1220 of 2003 to combat childhood obesity*. Little Rock, AR: University of Arkansas for Medical Sciences. http://www.uams.edu/coph/reports/2006Act1220_Year3.pdf (accessed July 11, 2007).

Research!America. 2006. *Obesity cited number-one kids' health issue*. www.researchamerica.org/polldata/2006/endocrinepoll.pdf (accessed July 6, 2007).

Reynolds, K. D., F. A. Franklin, D. Binkley, J. M. Raczynski, K. F. Harrington, K. A. Kirk, and S. Person. 2000. Increasing the fruit and vegetable consumption of fourth-graders: Results from the High 5 Project. *Preventive Medicine* 30 (4): 309-19.

Robinson, T. N. 1999. Reducing children's television viewing to prevent obesity: A randomized controlled trial. *Journal of the American Medical Association* 282 (16): 1561-67.

Sallis, J. F., T. L. Conway, J. J. Prochaska, T. L. McKenzie, S. J. Marshall, and M. Brown. 2001. The association of school environments with youth physical activity. *American Journal of Public Health* 91 (4): 618-20.

Sallis, J. F., T. L. McKenzie, J. E. Alcaraz, B. Kolody, N. Faucette, and M. F. Hovell. 1997. The effects of a 2-year physical education program (SPARK) on physical activity and fitness in elementary school students. Sports, Play and Active Recreation for Kids. *American Journal of Public Health* 87 (8): 1328-34.

Sallis J. F., T. L. McKenzie, J. E. Alcaraz, B. Kolody, M. F. Hovell, and P. R. Nader. 1993. Project SPARK. Effects of physical education on adiposity in children. *Annals of the New York Academy of Science* 29 (699): 127-36.

Sallis, J. F., T. L. McKenzie, B. Kolody, M. Lewis, S. Marshall, and P. Rosengard. 1999. Effects of health-related physical education on academic achievement: Project SPARK. *Research Quarterly for Exercise and Sport* 70 (2): 127-34.

Samuels, S. E., L. Craypo, M. Boyle, S. Stone-Francisco, and L. Schwarte. 2006. *Improving school food environments through district-level policies: Findings from six California case studies*. Oakland, CA: Samuels and Associates. www.rwjf.org/files/research/60285_CAEImprovFoodExSum.pdf (accessed July 11, 2007).

Segal, L. M., and E. A. Gadola. 2008. Generation O: Addressing childhood overweight before it's too late. *Annals of the American Academy of Political and Social Science* 615: 195-213.

Stecher, B. M., and S. Barron. 2001. Unintended consequences of test-based accountability when testing in "milepost" grades. *Educational Assessment* 7 (4): 259–82.

Stein, A. 2004. *Measuring public support for childhood obesity prevention interventions*. www.rwjf.org/pr/product.jsp?id=18149&topicid=1024&gsa=8 (accessed July 6, 2007).

Story, M., K. M. Kaphingst, and S. French. 2006. The role of schools in obesity prevention. *The Future of Children* 16 (1): 109-42.

Stratton, G., and E. Mullan. 2005. The effect of multicolor playground markings on children's physical activity level during recess. *Preventive Medicine* 41:828-33.

Strong, W., R. Malina, C. Blimkie, S. Daniels, R. Dishman, B. Gutin, A. Hergenroeder, A. Must, P. Nixon, and J. Pivarnik. 2005. Evidence based physical activity for school-age youth. *Journal of Pediatrics* 146 (6): 732-37.

Troman, G., and P. Woods. 2001. *Primary teachers' stress*. London: Routledge.

Trust for America's Health. 2006. *F as in fat: How obesity policies are failing in America*. Washington, DC: Trust for America's Health. http://healthyamericans.org/reports/obesity2006/ (accessed June 29, 2007).

Vartanian, L. R., M. B. Schwartz, and K. D. Brownell. 2007. Effects of soft drink consumption on nutrition and health: A systematic review and meta-analysis. *American Journal of Public Health* 97 (4): 667-75.

Verstraete, S. J., G. M. Cardon, D. L. R. De Clercq, and I. M. M. De Bourdeaudhuij. 2006. Increasing children's physical activity levels during recess periods in elementary schools: The effects of providing game equipment. *European Journal of Public Health* 16:415-19.

Wang, Y. C., G. L. Gortmaker, A. M. Sobol, and K. M. Kuntz. 2006. Estimating the energy gap among US children: A counterfactual approach. *Pediatrics* 118 (6): 1721-33.

Wechsler, H., N. D. Brener, S. Kuester, and C. Miller. 2001. Food service and foods and beverages available at school: Results from the School Health Policies and Programs Study 2000. *Journal of School Health* 71 (7): 313-24.

Wharton, C. M., M. Long, and M. Schwartz. Forthcoming. Changing nutrition standards in schools: The emerging impact on school revenue. *Journal of School Health*.

Childhood Overweight and the Built Environment: Making Technology Part of the Solution rather than Part of the Problem

By
AMY HILLIER

The changing nature of how children engage with their physical environment is one factor in the dramatic increase in childhood overweight. Children today are engaging much less with the world outside their homes in terms of physical activity and much more in terms of eating. Technological innovations in media have contributed to these changes, keeping children inside and sedentary during more of their playtime and exposing them to highly coordinated advertising campaigns. But researchers are increasingly looking to technology for solutions to understand how children interact with their built environments and to make changes that promote healthy living. This article reviews many of these innovations, including the use of geospatial technologies, accelerometers, electronic food and travel diaries, and video games to promote physical activity and healthy eating. It also explores some of the other possibilities for harnessing the potential of technology to combat the childhood overweight epidemic.

Keywords: childhood overweight; childhood obesity; built environment; geographic information systems; GIS; global positioning systems; GPS; technology

The idea that children used to eat a made-from-scratch dinner at home with their families before running outside to play may have taken on mythic power in the context of the current childhood overweight epidemic. But fifty years ago, who would have imagined the obesegenic environments we would create for them, in part with the help of technology? Who would have imagined that, at the extreme, our children would be sitting in the backseat of climate-controlled minivans watching movies on personal DVD players while eating take-out

Amy Hillier is an assistant professor of city and regional planning at the University of Pennsylvania School of Design. In addition to city planning courses, she teaches for Penn's Urban Studies Program, the School of Social Policy & Practice, and the Master of Urban Spatial Analytics program. She is also a senior fellow at the Leonard Davis Institute of Health Economics. Her research uses GIS and spatial statistics to analyze geographic disparities in housing and health.

DOI: 10.1177/0002716207308399

fast-food meals featuring the same animated characters they are watching on their screens?

The changing nature of how children engage with their environment is one factor in the dramatic increase in childhood overweight. Children today are engaging much less with the world outside their homes in terms of physical activity and much more in terms of eating. Technological innovations, including the Internet, sophisticated video games, and the many at-home television and movie options, have contributed to these changes. As a result, children spend on average nearly four hours a day watching television, DVDs, and prerecorded shows and playing video games. Over the course of a week, their exposure to media (including music) is equivalent to a full-time job (Rideout, Roberts, and Foehr 2005). The American Medical Association suggested that for some children—perhaps more than 5 million—extensive use of video games may constitute an addiction (Associated Press 2007).

In addition to keeping children inside and sedentary during more of their play-time, these media expose them to highly coordinated advertising campaigns, many of which target children (Gantz et al. 2007; Kelly 2005). Gantz et al. (2007) estimated that children ages eight to twelve see approximately seventy-six hundred television food ads a year, and two out of three parents say their children have asked them to buy foods that they have seen advertised on television (Rideout 2004). Children and adults, alike, have responded to aggressive food marketing and the convenience of eating out. The proportion of calories Americans of all ages consume from foods obtained away from home increased from 18 percent in 1974 to 32 percent in 1996 to about half of all calories in 2004 (Stewart, Blisard, and Jolliffe 2006; Lin, Frazão, and Guthrie 1999).

At the same time researchers document these trends, they are increasingly looking to technology to better understand how children interact with their built environments and to make changes that promote healthy living. This article reviews many of these innovations, including the use of geospatial technologies such as geographic information systems (GIS) and global positioning systems (GPS), accelerometers, electronic food and travel diaries, digital audio players, Web sites, and cell phones. First, it explores the idea of the built environment, reviews the research on the influence of the built environment on physical activity and eating, and considers the technological changes that have made children more sedentary. After describing many of the innovative uses of technology to address the problem of childhood overweight, it offers an agenda for making technology—and children—a bigger part of the solution.

What Is the "Built Environment"?

"Built environment" is used here to describe everything that children encounter when they step outside their door in their immediate neighborhood area. It is based on a spatial conception of environment that imagines that children

spend much of their time near their homes. Previous research has defined the
built environment to include physical structures, parks, recreation facilities,
transportation infrastructure, and, more generally, land use patterns and urban
design (Sallis and Glanz 2006; Transportation Research Board 2005; Handy et al.
2002; Frank, Engelke, and Schmid 2003). The availability of food, from fast-food
restaurants and convenience stores to supermarkets, and the prevalence of outdoor advertising have also been considered part of the built environment (Sallis
and Glanz 2006; Roux 2003).

Increased attention to the impact of the built environment signals a common
theoretical orientation toward ecological thinking more than a standardized operational definition. Researchers increasingly conceptualize obesity as a multilevel
problem, referring to factors beyond the individual that affect health as "neighborhood influences" (Booth, Pinkston, and Poston 2005), "residential environment" (Roux 2003), "macroenvironment" (King et al. 2002), and "structural
mechanisms" (Cohen, Scribner, and Farley 2000). "Built environment" and
"environment" are not always synonymous, as some researchers have broken this
larger concept of environment into components. For example, Cohen, Scribner,
and Farley (2000) have identified four different factors that potentially affect
health: availability of healthful (e.g., fruits and vegetables) and harmful (e.g., gun
and alcohol) products, physical structures, social structures, and cultural and
media messages. The modifier "built" may imply something more specific than
the broad concept used here, which incorporates physical, social, media, and
access factors, but referring to the "built environment" is a helpful reminder that
we humans are complicit in all of its ill health effects.

What Do We Know about the Impact of the Built Environment?

Physical Activity

A growing body of research, much of it sponsored by Robert Wood Johnson
Foundation's Active Living by Design Program and published in a series of special journal issues, provides evidence of a link between the built environment and
physical activity (Robert Wood Johnson Foundation 2007). This includes dozens
of studies about land use, urban design, zoning, sprawl, smart growth, transit-
oriented development, new urbanism, walkability, and access to and use of parks
and trails. Several experts in the fields of planning, transportation, physical activity, and health have systematically reviewed this literature (Sallis and Glanz 2006;
Transportation Research Board 2005; Heath, Hebert, and Lancaster 2006;
Handy et al. 2002). Recognizing that there are some inconsistent findings, they
conclude that (1) areas with mixed land use, greater residential and commercial
densities, grid street networks, and sidewalks are associated with more walking,
biking, and public transportation usage; and (2) children with access to parks,

recreation facilities, and programs are more physically active than children without access.

Food Access

A smaller and less coordinated, but still substantial, collection of research has shown that food access, in the form of supermarkets, fast-food restaurants, and convenience stores, varies considerably by neighborhood. Low-income and ethnic minority neighborhoods have fewer supermarkets and less access to fresh fruit, produce, and other healthy foods (Zenk et al. 2005; Rose and Richards 2004; Horowitz et al. 2004; Morland et al. 2002) and greater access to fast-food restaurants (Lewis et al. 2005; Block, Scribner, and DeSalvo 2004) and alcohol outlets (Morland et al. 2002). Fewer studies have linked food access to eating behavior, but several studies have shown that the availability of healthful products predicts healthier eating (Laraia et al. 2004; Rose and Richards 2004; Morland, Wing, and Roux 2002; Cheadle et al. 1993).

Outdoor Ads, Crime, and Safety

Outdoor advertising has received even less attention from researchers, but the results are similar: areas with racial minorities and low-income populations have more ads for alcohol and tobacco (Kwate and Lee 2007; Hackbarth et al. 2001).[1] One study documented a link between exposure to outdoor alcohol ads and alcohol intentions among youth (Pasch et al. 2007). Studies on the impact of neighborhood safety on physical activity and weight status have produced less consistent results, but some have shown that parent perceptions of crime and traffic safety influence physical activity levels and weight status of their children, most likely indirectly as their concerns about children keep them inside and thus more sedentary (Lumeng et al. 2006; Timperio et al. 2005).

Racial and Income Disparities

Racial and income disparities characterize all of these issues—physical activity, eating, food access, outdoor advertising, and crime—as well as overweight among children and adults (Day 2006; Kumanyika and Grier 2006; Taylor et al. 2006). Researchers hypothesize that differences in environment caused by residential segregation account for much of the disparity (Kawachi and Berkman 2003). In addition to being exposed to more fast-food restaurants and convenience stores (Lewis et al. 2005; Block, Scribner, and DeSalvo 2004), fewer supermarkets and healthy food options (Zenk et al. 2005; Rose and Richards 2004; Horowitz et al. 2004; Morland et al. 2002), and having less access to physical activity settings (Powell, Slater, and Chaloupka 2004), ethnic minorities and low-income children watch more television and movies than their white peers (Rideout et al. 2000; Kumanyika and Grier 2006). Research has also shown that television shows targeting black audiences have more food commercials (Tirodkar and Jain 2003) and are more likely to promote candy, soda, and fast food than general audience programs (Henderson and Kelly 2005).

Racial and income disparities characterize all of these issues—physical activity, eating, food access, outdoor advertising, and crime—as well as overweight among children and adults. Researchers hypothesize that differences in environment caused by residential segregation account for much of the disparity.

Limitations of Previous Research

Researchers are quick to point out the many limitations of this body of research on physical activity and eating, including the fact that none of it documents a definitive causal link between the built environment and weight status (Sallis and Glanz 2006; Transportation Research Board 2005). Most of the research on the built environment has not focused on children (Krizek, Birnbaum, and Levinson 2004) or racial minorities (Kumanyika and Grier 2006). Most studies have not used random assignment or natural experiments, making it impossible to determine the impact of neighborhood self-selection (Sallis and Glanz 2006; Roux 2003). Most studies have been cross-sectional, while exposure and access are hypothesized to matter over time (Transportation Research Board 2005; Roux 2003). Little research has been conducted to determine how individual characteristics, other than gender, mediate the impact of the environment (Lewis et al. 2002; Miller, Stewart, and Brown 2002) and how children actually spend their time (Krizek, Birnbaum, and Levinson 2004). Despite increasing use of GIS and attention to physical environment, researchers give little attention to the influence of geographic scale (Roux 2003; Heath, Hebert, and Lancaster 2006). "Scale" refers to the size of the geographic area that influences behavior. For example, does violent crime within a census tract, zip code, or neighborhood affect residents, or does it need to occur on the block where people live in order to matter? The list of limitations goes on and on, but to summarize, more research on children, including racial minorities, is needed to determine (1) how they interact with their environments over time; (2) the choices they are making about food, travel, and physical activity; and (3) how those choices affect their weight status.

How Is Technology Part of the Problem?

Access to Media Technologies

New technologies offer children an increasing array of entertainment options that involve staying indoors and being sedentary. Children today have unprecedented access to technology. For half of all children, the TV is on in their household "most of the time," and for children in two-thirds of all households, it is usually on during meals. Two-thirds of children ages eight to eighteen have a TV in their bedroom (Rideout, Roberts, and Foehr 2005). What experts are calling "screen time"—time spent in front of video games, computers, and TV—fills much of the time between school and sleep.

New Media Content and Formats

The content of that screen time is transforming rapidly, with video games evolving from the crude Atari Pac-Man of the 1980s to EA Sports's lifelike Madden NFL Football. The average cost of producing a video game jumped from $40,000 in the early 1990s to $10 million in 2004 because of three-dimensional graphics, artificial intelligence, and sound effects that make games more sophisticated and entertaining (Crandall and Sidak 2006). Today, children can play video games anywhere—in the car, during worship services, while shopping with parents—thanks to a plethora of mobile options including Nintendo's GameBoy Advance line, which offers five hundred different game options (Liz 2004).

What children watch on television and how they watch has also changed, as the number of channels and movie options has mushroomed. Over the past fifteen years, the percentage of U.S. households with cable television has increased from 60 to 85 percent (Dietz and Strasburger 1991; Cabletelevision Advertising Bureau 2006), and 55 percent of children have access to premium cable channels (Rideout, Roberts, and Foehr 2005). Digital video recorders (DVRs) such as TiVo allow users to record programs based on their preferences and watch at their convenience, while high-definition and plasma TV sets continue to improve the experience—and cost—of watching TV.

What children play on video game consoles and watch on TV and how they play and watch has changed considerably, but the greatest revolution has taken place with the Internet. In particular, online communities that allow visitors to customize sites and interact with other people have drawn in adults and children in unprecedented numbers. Social networking sites such as MySpace and Facebook attract children as early as middle school by allowing them to customize their own site with photographs, videos, and information about their friends. YouTube allows visitors to post their homemade videos in an accessible format, creating new opportunities for everything from *Saturday Night Live* skits (Steinberg 2007) to presidential debates (Seelye 2007). MySpace, MySpace email, Facebook, and YouTube all ranked among the top eleven Web sites in 2006, representing nearly 12 percent of all Internet usage (Hitwise 2007).

Beyond video games, TV, and computers, children and adults increasingly walk around with high-tech digital audio players and cell phones. Between 2001 and 2007, Apple sold 100 million iPods, by far the most popular of the MP3 players (Apple 2007b). Cell phones feature flash cameras, camcorders, GPS, text-messaging, e-mail, Internet access, video games, and music downloads. "Family plans" and cell phones designed for children encourage adults and children, alike, to consider personal phones indispensable. Most of these technologies can be integrated. For example, Apple depends upon its iTunes Store Web site to generate revenue when iPod users download individual songs, and Apple TV will allow users to view anything on their computer through their TV sets, including the full catalog of YouTube videos (Apple 2007a). This new environment is leading companies to merge their boardrooms as well as their technology. Fox Interactive Media Corporation, which oversees all Internet operations for Fox News Corporation, paid $580 million in 2005 for MySpace (*Sidney Morning Herald* 2005). Apple and Google have also hinted at a merger (Markoff 2006). Rather than competing head to head to increase their market share, these corporations are finding it more effective to join forces.

Advertising

Children have their greatest exposure to advertising through broadcast and cable television, and much of what they see advertised is food. U.S. food manufacturers spend 75 percent of their advertising budgets and U.S. fast-food restaurants spend 95 percent of their advertising budgets on television (Gallo 1999). Fast-food restaurants regularly partner with movies aimed at children and advertise special promotions on TV. In the summer of 2007, McDonald's Happy Meals featured toys from Sony Animation's "Surfs Up" along with collector glasses, Swamp Sludge McFlurry, and Minty Mudbath Shake for DreamWorks' "Shrek's Treketh to Adventure." The movie industry does not stop with promotions for fast-food restaurants. In addition to McDonalds, DreamWorks listed Frito-Lay Cheetos (cheese curls that turn your mouth green), Sierra Mist diet soda, Yoplait Yogurt (yogurt tubes with swamp riddles), Sargento cheese, Nestle ice cream (sludge fudge and swamp pops), M&M candies (ogre-sized peanut butter and chocolate candies), Kellogg's, and Kraft macaroni & cheese as *Shrek III* partners (DreamWorks 2007). Many food manufacturers also partner with toy companies, feature video games and kids' clubs on their Web sites, and sell advertising directly in movies through product placement (Story and French 2004).

While television is the most ubiquitous form of advertising for children, outdoor advertising has become increasingly creative in how it uses technology. Outdoor advertising is a $6.8 billion industry (Outdoor Advertising Association of

America 2007a) and includes everything from billboards to street furniture, bus shelters, and bus and building wraps. Digital billboards represent a small proportion of all billboards (approximately 500 out of 450,000 billboard in the United States), but technological innovations are making new forms of advertising possible, including real-time updates of anything from lottery jackpots to mortgage interest rates (Outdoor Advertising Association of America, Inc. 2007a) and billboards featuring digital ink that requires less energy and cost than conventional digital billboards (Outdoor Advertising Association of America 2007b).

Cities across the United States have buses wrapped in vinyl advertisements, and the outdoor advertising industry is threatening to wrap buildings and other large outdoor features with ads on the model of Times Square. Nomad Worldwide, a leader in ad wraps, boasted that it sees a "world of blank canvasses" and has "proven that any surface can be conquered—billboards, scaffolding, wallscapes, barricades, building wraps, and construction sites" (Nomad 2007). While these building wraps do not all feature unhealthy foods, an unlicensed building wrap in downtown Philadelphia that generated significant attention from advocates and the media featured a Dunkin' Donuts ad (Slobodzian 2007).

Summary of the Problem

The time children spend indoors is increasingly consumed by media technology, from television to computer games and the Internet. Increasingly sophisticated computer, television, and audio options keep them sedentary during much of their free time while exposing them to coordinated advertising campaigns disproportionately promoting unhealthy foods. Many of these technologies are now portable, meaning that media technologies can also occupy time spent away from home. High-tech outdoor advertising is relatively new, but the possibilities for "wrapping" all aspects of our built environment, including things that move, like busses, seem endless and promise even more exposure to unhealthy foods. When children and families do spend time out of the home, it is increasingly to purchase fast-food meals and snacks. While not the sole cause of the childhood overweight epidemic, the increasing role of media technology in the lives of children explains, in part, how the equation between physical activity and food consumption has become so out of balance.

How Can Technology Be Part of the Solution?

While children spend much of their time with these various technologies, most research on children's physical activity and eating still relies on paper-and-pencil measures for observing children and surveying communities. This low-tech approach may provide a more appropriate choice in many situations, saving researchers money and time and potentially providing as good if not better data than high-tech options. But all of the technological improvements in the past ten years provide limitless opportunities for researchers to advance our understanding of how children interact with the built environment and how to intervene to reduce childhood overweight. The Robert Wood Johnson Foundation's Active Living by Design and Healthy Eating Programs and the National Institutes of Health's Improving Diet and Physical Activity Assessment initiative have provided significant funding for researchers to create new or adapt existing instruments for handheld personal digital assistants (PDAs) and tablet PCs and to incorporate GIS and GPS.

Technology for Measuring the Built Environment

Geospatial technologies including GIS and GPS are increasingly used by researchers to model the built environment. Because exposure is generally conceptualized to relate to physical proximity (Austin et al. 2005; Pasch et al. 2007), knowing what resources and conditions exist near where children spend time is critical to understanding their exposure. GPS is the favored tool for field data collection because location information can be acquired anywhere (in theory) using satellites, while GIS depends upon pregenerated map layers of features like buildings, streets, and administrative areas.

GIS has been used extensively in research on the impact of the built environment on childhood overweight. Most research has used vector GIS to represent basic physical infrastructure such as roads, sidewalks, and transit lines, or administrative units such as census tracts and zip codes to display demographic information, but GIS is capable of providing much higher levels of spatial analyses than simple visual overlays. The Twin Cities Walking Study, which integrates paper-and-pencil survey data with extensive and well-documented GIS data, provides one example of the more sophisticated modeling GIS makes possible (Forsyth 2007; Forsyth et al. 2006). The study uses GIS measures of road networking that incorporate direction and speed rather than just simple street centerline files provided by the U.S. Census Bureau that only show street locations, names, and classifications. The study also uses GIS to calculate area and dissimilarity indexes to determine land use mix rather than simply showing color-coded land use maps.

In addition to vector GIS, the Twin Cities Walking Study uses raster GIS, which represent map layers using regularly shaped cells to denote a continuous surface and provide more flexibility in analyzing data. Using raster GIS, it is also possible to calculate slope and viewsheds, two factors that may be related to the walkability of a neighborhood (Forsyth 2007; Forsyth et al. 2006). Raster GIS has also been used to create continuous measures of environmental conditions that are not dependent upon aggregations of administrative units like census tracts. Hillier et al. (2003) computed kernel densities of housing code violations, housing demolitions, and tax delinquent properties using raster GIS.

Examples of using GPS to measure the built environment are rarer. In developing the Path Environment Audit Tool (PEAT), Troped et al. (2006) used GPS to map paths and trails in eastern Massachusetts. Students at California State Polytechnic University used GPS with handheld computers and digital cameras to map assets in San Jose's poorest neighborhoods (Ulrich 2005). Digital and disposable cameras provide tools for documenting neighborhood conditions. In the Health of Philadelphia Photo-Documentation Project (Cannuscio and Asch 2006), researchers gave students and community members disposable cameras to document elements of their neighborhood that facilitate or create barriers to health. Cell phones are increasingly equipped with digital cameras that allow for convenient—if not high-quality—photographs in the field. Digital cameras provide another option. A study of outdoor advertising in Austin, Los Angeles, and Philadelphia (Hillier et al. n.d.) used digital cameras and GPS devices to record the location and content of outdoor advertisements. Data showing the location of outdoor ads and photographs of the ads can then be displayed along with other map layers, as shown in Figure 1. New digital GPS cameras integrate the functionality of handheld GPS with digital cameras, making it possible to stamp photographs with location information (Ellison 2006).

Handheld computers, referred to as "pocket PCs," and PDAs are also being used in neighborhood assessments. The Physical Activity Resource Assessment (PARA) instrument for inventorying physical activity resources in an urban setting was originally designed for paper and pencil, but a handheld computer version is in development (Lee et al. 2005). In addition to survey instruments, PDAs can be used with GIS to facilitate field data collection. A study of the location of corner stores and other places where children purchase food on the way to and from school used PDAs equipped with GIS software (Fitzgerald 2005).

Technology for Measuring Physical Activity

Numerous researchers have also developed tools that use new technologies to measure physical activity with funding from the Robert Wood Johnson Foundation's Active Living Program (Robert Wood Johnson Foundation 2007). The System for Observing Play and Recreation in Communities (SOPARC), created to determine the number of people in parks and the types of activities in which they are engaged, was also developed originally as a paper-and-pencil instrument, but the newest version will use PDAs to record information (McKenzie et al. 2006).

While GPS can be used to identify resources and conditions within the built environment, it also holds promise for measuring physical activity. A 1997 study (Schultz and Chambaz 1997) concluded that GPS could be used to record information about physical activity in a nonintrusive and continuous manner anywhere outside because satellite readings are available worldwide. More recently, Rodriguez, Brown, and Troped (2005) used GPS in conjunction with accelerometers to track the locations where study participants were physically active. SOPARC will also use GPS to validate self-reported and observed physical activity (McKenzie et al. 2006).

Other technology has been used to measure physical activity and movement. In the Trial of Activity for Adolescent Girls (TAAG), study participants attached

FIGURE 1
MAPPING OUTDOOR ADS WITH DIGITAL PHOTOGRAPHS
AND DEMOGRAPHIC DATA

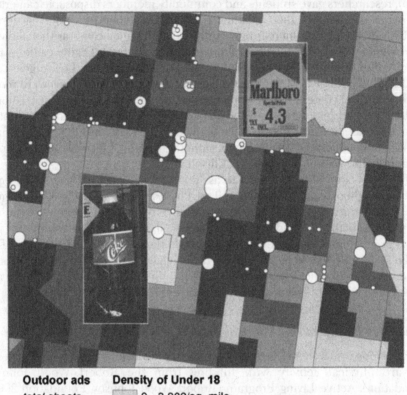

Outdoor ads   **Density of Under 18**

total sheets

○ 1   0 - 3,000/sq. mile

○ 5   3,001 - 6,000/sq. mile

○ 10   6,001 - 10,000/sq. mile

         10,001 - 15,000/sq. mile

         15,001 - 30,000/sq. mile

accelerometers to belts around their waist to measure moderate to vigorous physical activity at thirty-second intervals. Results showed that girls who lived closer to their schools engaged in more physical activity (Cohen et al. 2006). Another study used accelerometers, self-reported television watching, and GIS data to determine that neighborhood characteristics influence boys' physical activity more than girls' physical activity (Roemmich et al. 2007). In a very different type of study, Lindsey et al. (2006) used infrared monitors to measure traffic along multiple trail locations to determine aggregate, rather than individual, activity levels.

Technology for Measuring Eating and Travel Behavior

Even more than physical activity measures, measures of eating have relied on paper-and-pencil surveys. New tools that utilize technology are emerging, however. The National Cancer Institute is developing a Web-based instrument for self-administered twenty-four-hour food recalls called Automated Self-Administered 24-Hour Recall (ASA24) (National Cancer Institute 2007). Together with researchers at the University of Pennsylvania, the author hopes to develop Food and Environment Diaries for Urban Places (FED-UP), a video-game-like food and travel diary that students would complete online using a map interface (Hillier and Volpe n.d.). Children would be asked to collect information during their trip to and from school, using cell phone text-messaging and digital photography to record what they purchase and eat. This information would be transmitted wirelessly to their online account. GPS devices would be used to record the paths children take to and from school or to verify self-reported travel behavior. Children would then review and complete the records of their daily trips online.

Instruments like ASA24 and FED-UP hold the potential of capturing much more detailed self-reported data than traditional food frequencies and food recalls, with images to help identify specific products and portion sizes. By making these instruments available online, study participants can input data regularly without need for an interviewer. FED-UP would have the additional benefit of recording spatial information about where children purchase and consume food and understanding how children interact with their environment. In a pilot study, we used a customized GIS created using ArcPad software for handheld computers to record the route that students reported taking (Hillier and Volpe n.d.). As Figure 2 demonstrates, this data on routes can be mapped with information about crime, housing, land use, and demographics using GIS.

Several applications for mapping routes on the Internet have been developed using Google Maps, including Gmaps Pedometer and walkrunjog.net, and could be adapted for travel diary research. The Space-Time Adolescent Risk Study (STAR) (Wiebe 2006) of young adult gunshot victims is using a combination of Internet mapping, GIS, and tablet PCs (laptop computers with screens that lie flat and can be "drawn" on with a stylus) to allow gunshot victims to show where they were leading up to their shooting.

Smart card technology provides another tool. Data acquired by supermarkets when purchases are scanned and linked to customer accounts can be analyzed at the individual or aggregate level to understand food behavior (Bucklin and Gupta 1999). The same technology has been used to determine (Lambert et al. 2005) and limit (Snyder 2006) what children eat in school cafeterias.

Technology for Improving the Built Environment

Policy makers, software companies, and government officials have found ways to use technology to reshape the built environment. For example, GIS and spatial modeling are being used to design healthier and more livable communities

FIGURE 2
HYPOTHETICAL ROUTES TO SCHOOL WITH
CONCENTRATION OF CRIME

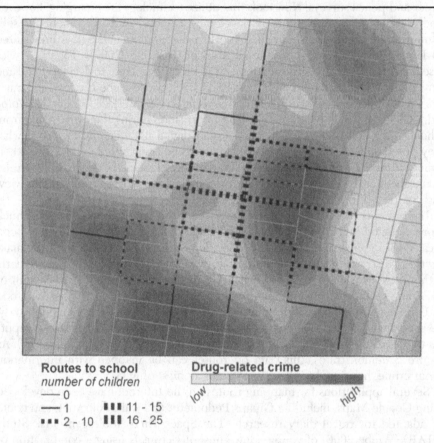

consistent with the research findings about walkability and mixed land use. CommunityViz integrates GIS technology with 3D modeling to analyze the impact of development choices (Placeways 2007). The integration of GIS with agent-based modeling, a technique for modeling complex behaviors with multiple interactions (Bonabeau 2002), also holds promise for predicting the impact of certain built environment changes on children's behavior.

Public safety efforts rely heavily on GIS and other high-tech approaches to fighting crime and reducing vehicular accidents. The New York City Police Department popularized CompStat, a GIS-intensive accountability management system for geographically targeting delivery of police services (Walsh 2001). Red-light cameras that automatically photograph the license plate of vehicles that enter an intersection after a traffic light turns red are significantly reducing the number of vehicles running red lights, which is a major cause of motor vehicle and pedestrian accidents (Retting, Ferguson, and Farmer 2007; Federal Highway Administration and National Highway Traffic Safety Administration 2005). Research has shown that parent perceptions of crime and traffic safety influence their children's levels of physical activity (Lumeng et al. 2006; Timperio et al. 2005), so reducing crime and traffic accidents may reduce parent concerns and increase physical activity among children.

Policy makers, software companies, and government officials have found ways to use technology to reshape the built environment. For example, GIS and spatial modeling are also being used to design healthier and more livable communities consistent with the research findings about walkability and mixed land use.

Technology for Improving Eating

New technologies have also been adapted to educate children and adults to change their eating habits. At least two computer games have been developed to encourage healthy eating—Squire's Quest (Baranowski et al. 2003) and the United States Department of Agriculture's MyPyramid Blast-Off Game (U.S. Department of Agriculture 2007). The development budgets for these projects pale in comparison with the millions of dollars that for-profit companies invest in new games, but they represent early efforts to engage children through familiar technology. Digital audio players, online videos, wikis, blogs, "mosh-pits," and other Web2.0 applications are being used by health professionals for clinical education and sharing of health resources (*Journal of the American Medical Association* 2007; Maag 2006; Trier 2007; Skiba 2007; Boulos, Maramba, and Wheeler 2006; Cebeci and Tekdal 2006). All of these hold promise for educating children and parents about healthy living as well as teaching researchers about best practices.

Cellular telephones provide an additional technology with potential for changing behavior. Phones designed for children like Verizon's Migo and the Disney phone allow parents to use the built-in GPS to monitor where their children are, restrict phone numbers dialed and received, and pre-program emergency numbers or "family alert" test messages for young children. In addition to reducing parent concerns about children being outside the home, this technology could be used to send children reminders about healthy eating and physical activity or track their travel and food consumption.

Technology for Improving Physical Activity

In addition to these educational applications, a number of new technologically based games have emerged that hold promise for reengaging children in physical activity and the outdoors. Geocaching, played primarily by adults, involves a series of clues such as GPS coordinates for finding "caches," usually watertight boxes with a logbook and small objects for trading. Players post information about new hunts on an official game Web site that by June 2007 included information about more than four hundred thousand "caches" (Groundspeak 2007). This treasure hunt game could be adapted for children in urban communities, having them move through parks, travel to child-friendly institutions, and learn about GPS technology.

Cell phones can also be used to promote physical activity. Recently, they have been used to provide information during self-guided walking tours. The Cross/Walks project in Philadelphia provides prerecorded messages about the history of the Fabric Row section of South Philadelphia that can be accessed by cell phone (Iverson 2007). Tours like these could be designed by children for children, incorporating historical content as well as commentary on personal landmarks, creating an outdoor version of MySpace.

New "activity-promoting" video games also hold promise for converting sedentary screen time to active screen time (Lanningham-Foster et al. 2006). These include Nintendo's Wii, a game console featuring a wireless controller that can detect motion (Nintendo 2007) and Sony Eye Toy, which uses a USB camera to incorporate images and movements of the player into the game (Sony Computer Entertainment 2007). Dance Dance Revolution (DDR), a Japanese invention with the motto "Where exercise gets fun," uses arrows to instruct players to step on one of four places on a dance pad in rhythm with a song (DDRgame.com 2007). DDR began as an arcade game, but dance pads that plug into the television are now available, as well as a "practice pad" that does not use technology but can be used outside (DDRgame.com 2007). A future outdoor version for parks, school playgrounds, or even sidewalks that uses digital audio players, cell phone displays, or PDAs to instruct the dancer might revolutionize recess, outdoor play, and trips to and from school (Lanningham-Foster et al. 2006). Table 1 compares these different technologies used to measure and improve eating behavior and physical activity.

The challenges involved in capitalizing on these new technologies for research, education, reshaping the built environment, and engaging children in physical activity and healthy eating are considerable. Developing new technologies or even adapting existing ones pose significant costs relating to hardware acquisitions and training. Obtaining consistent readings from GPS in different weather and built

(text continues on page 76)

TABLE 1

COMPARISON OF TECHNOLOGIES

Technology	Examples	Use	Availability	Strengths	Limitations	Cost
Geospatial						
Geographic information systems (GIS)	Twin Cities Walking Study (Forsyth et al. 2006); Food and Exercise Diaries for Urban Places (FED-UP) (Hillier and Volpe n.d.)	Measure built environment and travel behavior	Widely available at academic institutions and government agencies; more limited use in nonprofits	Can be applied to many different data types; highlights spatial relationships	Difficult to model movement or change over time; requires training to use	Some open source (free) software, but $500 or more for most popular software; PC needed
Global positioning systems (GPS)	Path Environment Audit Tool (PEAT) (Troped et al. 2006); Trial of Activity for Adolescent Girls (TAAG) (Cohen et al. 2006)	Measure built environment, travel behavior; encourage physical activity (GPS treasure-hunting games)	Widely available in wrist or hand-held versions, in cell phones, and car navigation systems	Identifies location without street address	May not work in all conditions (weather, tall buildings); requires training	$100 or more
GPS cameras	No published studies	Measure built environment and eating behavior	New technology not widely available	Stamps photographs with location information (for mapping)	May not work in all conditions (weather, tall buildings); requires training	$800 or more
Online interactive mapping	Space-Time Adolescent Risk Study (STAR) (Wiebe 2006); FED-UP (Hillier and Volpe n.d.)	Measure travel and eating behavior	Wherever Internet is available	Widespread access; ease of use; can be adapted for different applications	Not designed for research; may require customization	Free unless customization required

(continued)

71

TABLE 1 (CONTINUED)

Technology	Examples	Use	Availability	Strengths	Limitations	Cost
Photography						
Disposable cameras	Health of Philadelphia Photo-Documentation Project (Cannuscio and Asch 2006)	Measure built environment, food behavior, and physical activity	Widespread; available at drug stores, convenience stores, etc.	Inexpensive; easy to use; good for fieldwork if loss of or damage to camera is concern	Image quality may not be comparable to more expensive cameras	Less than $10 plus film-processing fees
Digital cameras	Five-City Billboard Study (Hillier et al. n.d.)	Measure built environment, food behavior, and physical activity	Widely available	Easy to use; generate high-quality images in digital format	Require charged batteries; ease of use may encourage taking too many photos	$200 or more (varies widely)
Red-light cameras	Roosevelt Blvd., Philadelphia (Gambardello 2007)	Promote traffic safety	Limited to dangerous intersections in certain cities	Reduce red-light running and increase pedestrian and vehicular safety	Expensive to install	$50,000 or more
Digital audio recordings						
MP3 downloads	Journal of the American Medical Association (2007); nursing education (Maag 2006)	Education and training for professionals or children	More common for commercial music than educational material	Convenient to listen to; MP3 players are very common	Limited control over setting in which recording is heard	None if software for recording and digital audio player for listening are available
Podcasts	(Boulos, Maramba, and Wheeler 2006)	Education and training for professionals or children	More common for nonresearch uses	Convenient to listen to or watch; can incorporate audio and video	Limited control over setting in which recording is heard	None if software for recording and digital audio player for listening are available

Cellular phones						
Telephone calls	Cross/Walks: Weaving Fabric Row (Iverson 2007)	Promote physical activity through narrated walking tours	Limited examples of tours but near universal access to cell phone service in urban areas	Widespread access to cell phones and cell phone service; ease of use	Cell phone service not reliable	$35/month or more plus cost of phone
Text messages	FED-UP (Hillier and Volpe n.d.)	Measure travel and food behavior	Nonresearch usage is widespread	Widespread access to cell phones and cell phone service; ease of use	Depends upon self-report; can only capture a limited amount of information	Available with most cell phone services; requires cell phone and cell phone service
Digital photographs	FED-UP (Hillier and Volpe n.d.)	Measure travel and food behavior	Nonresearch usage is widespread	Convenience; ease of use; widespread access	Poor-quality images	Available with most cell phone services; requires cell phone and cell phone service
Monitors of movement and consumption						
Accelerometers	TAAG (Cohen et al. 2006; Roemmich et al. 2007)	Measure physical activity	Used widely in research	Provide reliable and valid measures of movement; do not depend on self-report	Data recorded is difficult to interpret	$100 or more

(continued)

TABLE 1 (CONTINUED)

Technology	Examples	Use	Availability	Strengths	Limitations	Cost
Infrared monitors	Trail monitoring (Lindsey et al. 2006)	Measure physical activity	Used widely for nonresearch applications	Measure movement without needing people or cameras; nonintrusive	Provides no data about who is moving	$200 or more
Smart cards	Supermarket scanner data (Bucklin and Gupta 1999); school cafeterias (Lambert et al. 2005; Snyder 2006)	Measure eating behavior; promote healthy eating	Widely used in supermarkets	Widely available; convenient; easy to use	Privacy issues	Cards are inexpensive but scanning system required
Computers						
Educational computer games	Squires Quest (Baranowski et al. 2003); MyPyramid Blastoff (U.S. Department of Agriculture 2007)	Promote healthy eating	Limited use in research setting	Fun for children	Expensive to develop; rarely as sophisticated and engaging as commercial products	Free to play; tens of thousands of dollars to develop
Physically active computer games	Dance Dance Revolution (DDRgame.com 2007); Wii (Nintendo 2007)	Promote physical activity	Used widely by children in arcades and at home	Fun for children	Commercial products developed to be entertaining rather than healthy	$30 or more; $250 or more for game console

Personal digital assistants (PDAs)	System for Observing Play and Recreation in Communities (SOPARC) (McKenzie et al. 2006)	Measure the built environment	Used widely for personal and business use but not for research	Widely available; convenient size	Small screen and small processor limit functionality	$200 or more
Tablet PCs	STAR (Wiebe 2006)	Measure built environment and travel behavior	Limited usage outside of research	Ease of use; feels more like computer game than conventional PC	Much larger and more expensive than PDA	$2,000 or more
Internet						
Internet Web sites	Automated Self-Administered 24-Hour Recall (ASA24) (National Cancer Institute 2007)	Measure eating behavior	Wherever Internet connection is available	Accessibility; easy to use; can be customized	Expensive to develop interactive site	
Wikis	(Boulos, Maramba, and Wheeler 2006)	Education and training for professionals or children	Wherever Internet connection is available	Interactive	Limited control over content	Free or low cost
Blogs	(Boulos, Maramba, and Wheeler 2006)	Education and training for professionals or children	Wherever Internet connection is available	Easy to use	Limited control over content	Free or low cost

environment conditions, having reliable wireless Internet access, and interpreting data generated from accelerometers are among the known challenges. Establishing the reliability and validity of these new instruments requires attention beyond getting them to work. The current generation of researchers did not grow up with multipurpose cell phones or Web2.0 applications like blogs and wikis, so using them for research is often not instinctive. The ability of these new technologies to track and influence individual behavior also poses serious questions about human subjects, research ethics, and privacy. Clearly, applying technology more consistently and more effectively to combat childhood overweight requires much more than technical expertise.

An Agenda for Moving Forward

What researchers know about the role of the built environment on childhood overweight is fairly limited. Mixed-use and high-density areas with less crime and greater traffic safety where children have access to recreation facilities promote physical activity (Sallis and Glanz 2006; Transportation Research Bureau 2005; Heath, Hebert, and Lancaster 2006; Handy et al. 2002). Depending upon where they live, children have very different access to healthy foods (Zenk et al. 2005; Rose and Richards 2004; Horowitz et al. 2004; Morland et al. 2002). Media from TV to the Internet to computer games pervade their time, limiting their active and outdoor play and exposing them to messages promoting unhealthy foods (Rideout, Roberts, and Foehr 2005; Gantz et al. 2007; Kelly 2005). To date, technology has contributed more to this problem than to its solution, but many technological innovations and applications hold promise for reversing this pattern. So how do researchers and public health advocates ensure that this happens?

To date, technology has contributed more to this problem than to its solution, but many technological innovations and applications hold promise for reversing this pattern.

Making Children Part of the Solution

Part of the answer involves a conceptualization of childhood overweight that makes children active participants in developing solutions. We must meet children where they are, and that means understanding why they are so interested in Wii, DDR, MySpace, YouTube, cell phones, text-messaging, and other technologies that distinguish their childhoods dramatically from previous generations. These technologies use sophisticated graphics and multimedia and allow children to participate and shape their own fun. What else do children like? What makes these things fun? How can the features of these new technologies that engage children be adapted for research, teaching, and promoting physical activity? Who better to ask than children?

Participatory research that includes children as agents of change and not passive research participants is one approach (Sloane et al. 2003; Hackbarth et al. 2001). Partnerships with schools must respect the pressure on teachers to meet curricular standards and improve test scores, but privately funded technological enrichment activities may be welcome through after-school programs, computer classes, health classes, or physical education programming. Such partnerships should also leave technological devices and software like GIS, GPS, and accelerometers with teachers for use with other projects, such as mapping school grounds and conducting science experiments. Social marketing provides another opportunity. Nintendo and EA Sports know what children like because they ask them and spend time learning about their preferences. The Food Trust, a Philadelphia-based nonprofit food research and advocacy group, used this approach to develop healthy snack foods as part of its Corner Store Campaign. The Food Trust hired a firm specializing in social marketing to work with children to design a new line of baked corn chips under the name "Slam Dunk" (Food Trust 2007).

Making Media Corporations Part of the Solution

The companies that create the most successful video games, cell phones, and Web sites must be viewed as potential allies in the fight against childhood overweight. The limited amount of funding available from private foundations and government institutes make it unlikely that most technological applications that researchers develop on their own will compete with $10 million video games (although YouTube and MySpace offer two examples of creative media that are relatively inexpensive). With some form of subsidy or public recognition, might a shoe company develop affordable shoes for children that have built-in pedometers and light up when personal activity goals are met? Which phone service might develop a cell phone scanner that allows children and adults to scan bar codes to determine how food items fit within individual dietary plans and federal nutrition guidelines? Which food company might develop a system for producing Web-based personal food reports that track smart card food purchases and suggest alternative foods? For example, the report might suggest 100 percent juice as a substitute for artificially sweetened beverages and provide coupons from manufacturers to try new products. It is unlikely that researchers and health advocates can develop and distribute new technologies like these on a large scale without the help of the entertainment industries.

Advocates must continue to file lawsuits and shame food companies like Kellogg's into changing the way they market to children (Martin 2007) or the beverage industry into changing how it serves children at school (Warner 2005). City planners and local governments must continue to use technology to design healthier communities. Legislators must continue to support laws that make it easier for supermarkets to locate in underserved areas (Clark 2004). But there are limits to our ability to eliminate health risks and reshape the environment in which children live. Ultimately, we need to help children make better choices over their life course, creating what King et al. (2002) described as "choice-enabling" environments. This means that all children need to have access to healthy foods and recreation; then we can focus on helping them to make good choices. They must see evidence that their choices can make a difference for themselves and for society, that childhood overweight is a problem, and that the problem is not intractable. Children will inherit this overweight epidemic, with all of its health and financial implications. We should enlist their help, including their interest and skills in technology, now.

Note

1. The tobacco industry voluntarily stopped advertising on billboards in 1999, but this only eliminated large-format outdoor ads.

References

Apple, Inc. 2007a. Apple TV. http://www.apple.com/appletv/ (accessed July 15, 2007).
———. 2007b. 100 million iPods sold. http://www.apple.com/pr/library/2007/04/09ipod.html (accessed July 15, 2007).
Associated Press. 2007. Video game addiction: A new diagnosis? *New York Times*, June 21. http://www.nytimes.com/aponline/us/AP-Video-Game-Addiction.html?_r=1&oref=slogin (accessed July 15, 2007).
Austin, S. B., S. J. Melly, B. N. Sanchez, A. Patel, S. Buka, and S. L. Gortmaker. 2005. Clustering of fast-food restaurants around schools: A novel application of spatial statistics to the study of food environments. *American Journal of Public Health* 95 (9): 1575-81.
Baranowski, T., J. Baranowski, K. W. Cullen, T. Marsh, N. Islam, I. Zakeri, L. Honess-Morreale, and C. deMoor. 2003. Squire's Quest! Dietary outcome evaluation of a multimedia game. *American Journal of Preventive Medicine* 3 (24): 52-61.
Block, J. P., R. A. Scribner, and K. B. DeSalvo. 2004. Fast food, race/ethnicity, and income: A geographic analysis. *American Journal of Preventive Medicine* 27 (3): 211-17.
Bonabeau, E. 2002. Agent-based modeling: Methods and techniques for simulating human systems. *Proceedings of the National Academy of Sciences* 99 (3): 7280-87.
Booth, K., M. M. Pinkston, and C. Poston. 2005. Obesity and the built environment. *Journal of the American Dietetic Association* 105 (5): S110-17.
Boulos, N. K., I. Maramba, and S. Wheeler. 2006. Wikis, blogs and podcasts: A new generation of Web-based tools for virtual collaborative clinical practice and education. *BMC Medical Education* 6 (41). http://www.biomedcentral.com/content/pdf/1472-6920-6-41.pdf (accessed July 15, 2007).
Bucklin, R. E., and S. Gupta. 1999. Commercial use of UPC scanner data: Industry and academic perspectives. *Marketing Science* 18 (3): 247-73.
Cabletelevision Advertising Bureau. 2006. http://www.onetvworld.org/main/cab/research/2007TVFacts/index.shtml (accessed September 17, 2007).

Cannuscio, C. C., and D. Asch. 2006. *Health of Philadelphia Photo-documentation Project*. Funded proposal to the Robert Wood Johnson Foundation Health and Society Scholars Research and Education Fund, University of Pennsylvania, Philadelphia.

Cebeci, Z., and M. Tekdal. 2006. Using podcasts as audio learning objects. *Interdisciplinary Journal of Knowledge and Learning Objects* 2:47-57.

Cheadle, A., B. M. Psaty, S. Curry, E. Wagner, P. Diehr, T. Koepsell, and A. Kristal. 1993. Can measures of the grocery store environment be used to track community-level dietary changes? *Preventive Medicine* 22 (3): 361-72.

Clark, V. 2004. Plan would add supermarkets in city. *Philadelphia Inquirer*, May 5, p. B04.

Cohen, D. A., S. Ashwood, M. Scott, A. Overton, K. R. Evenson, C. C. Voorhees, A. Bedimo-Rung, and T. L. McKenzie. 2006. Proximity to school and physical activity among middle school girls: The Trial of Activity for Adolescent Girls Study. *Journal of Physical Activity and Health* 3(Suppl. 1): S129-38.

Cohen, D. A., R. A. Scribner, and T. A. Farley. 2000. A structural model of health behavior: A pragmatic approach to explain and influence health behaviors at the population level. *Preventive Medicine* 30 (2): 146-54.

Crandall, R. W., and J. G. Sidak. 2006. *Video games: Serious business for America's economy*. Washington, DC: Entertainment Software Association.

Day, K. 2006. Active living and social justice: Planning for physical activity in low-income, black, and Latino communities. *Journal of the American Planning Association* 72 (1): 88-99.

DDRgame.com. 2007. http://www.ddrgame.com/ (accessed July 15, 2007).

Dietz, W. H., and V. C. Strasburger. 1991. Children, adolescents, and television. *Current Problems in Pediatric and Adolescent Health Care* 21 (1): 8-31.

DreamWorks. 2007. *Shrek the Third*, partners and promotions. http://www.shrek.com/main.html (accessed July 15, 2007).

Ellison, C. 2006. Navman unveils GPS/camera combo. *PC Magazine*, April 3. http://www.pcmag.com/article2/0,1895,1945433,00.asp (accessed July 15, 2007).

Federal Highway Administration and National Highway Traffic Safety Administration. 2005. Red light camera systems operational guidelines. Publication No. FHWA-SA-05-002. Washington, DC: Federal Highway Administration and National Highway Traffic Safety Administration.

Fitzgerald, S. 2005. Junk-food geography. *Philadelphia Inquirer*, May 23, p. B1.

Food Trust. 2007. Corner Store Campaign. http://www.thefoodtrust.org/php/programs/corner.store.campaign.php (accessed July 15, 2007).

Forsyth, A., ed. 2007. Environment and physical activity: GIS Protocols Version 4.1. June. n.p.

Forsyth, A., K. H. Schmitz, M. Oakes, J. Zimmerman, and J. Koepp. 2006. Standards for environmental measures using GIS: Toward a protocol for protocols. *Journal of Physical Activity and Health* 3 (Suppl. 1): S241-57.

Frank, L. D., P. O. Engelke, and T. L. Schmid. 2003. *Health and community design: The impact of the built environment on physical activity*. Washington, DC: Island.

Gallo, A. E. 1999. Food advertising in the United States. In *America's eating habits: Changes and consequences*, ed. USDA/Economic Research Service, 173-80. Washington, DC: U.S. Department of Agriculture.

Gambardello, J. A. 2007. On the boulevard, cameras result in dramatic change. *Philadelphia Inquirer*, January 30, p. B01.

Gantz, W., N. Schwartz, J. R. Angelini, V. Rideout, and Kaiser Family Foundation. 2007. *Food for thought: Television food advertising to children in the U.S.* Menlo Park, CA: Kaiser Family Foundation.

Groundspeak. 2007. Geocaching—The official website of the global GPS cache hunt site. http://www.geocaching.com/ (accessed July 15, 2007).

Hackbarth, D. P., D. Snopp-Wyatt, D. Katz, J. Williams, B. Silvestri, and M. Pfleger. 2001. Collaborative research and action to control the geographic placement of outdoor advertising of alcohol and tobacco products in Chicago. *Public Health Reports* 116:558-67.

Handy, S. L., M. G. Boarnet, R. Ewing, and R. E. Killingsworth. 2002. How the built environment affects physical activity: Views from urban planning. *American Journal of Preventive Medicine* 23 (2S): 64-73.

Heath, G. W., K. A. Hebert, and K. Lancaster. 2006. The effectiveness of urban design and land use and transport policies and practices to increase physical activity: A systematic review. *Journal of Physical Activity and Health* 3 (Suppl. 1): S55-S76.

Henderson, V. R., and B. Kelly. 2005. Food advertising in the age of obesity: Content analysis of food advertising on general market and African American television. *Journal of Nutrition Education and Behavior* 37 (4): 191–96.

Hillier, A., D. P. Culhane, T. E. Smith, and C. D. Tomlin. 2003. Predicting housing abandonment with the Philadelphia Neighborhood Information System. *Journal of Urban Affairs* 25 (1): 91-105.

Hillier, A., and S. Volpe. n.d. FED-UP with childhood obesity: Using maps to create food and exercise diaries. In *PhillyDotMap*, ed. C. D. Tomlin, D. P. Culhane, and S. Kinnevy. Manuscript in preparation.

Hillier, A., A. K. Yancey, B. Cole, J. D. Williams, and W. McCarthy. n.d. Three-city study of the concentration of outdoor advertisements around schools, parks, and child care organizations. Manuscript.

Hitwise. 2007. Hitwise US—Top 20 websites—May 2007. http://www.hitwise.com/datacenter/rankings .php (accessed July 15, 2007).

Horowitz, C. R., K. A. Colson, P. L. Hebert, and K. Lancaster. 2004. Barriers to buying healthy foods for people with diabetes: Evidence of environmental disparities. *American Journal of Public Health* 94 (9): 1549-54.

Iverson, H. 2007. Cross/Walks: Weaving fabric row. http://www.cross-walks.org (accessed July 15, 2007).

Journal of the American Medical Association. 2007. http://jama.ama-assn.org/ (accessed September 17, 2007).

Kawachi I., and L. F. Berkman. 2003. Introduction. In *Neighborhoods and health*, ed. I. Kawachi and L. F. Berkman, 1-17. New York: Oxford University Press.

Kelly, B. 2005. To quell obesity, who should regulate food marketing to children? *Globalization and Health* 1 (9): 1-3.

King, A. C., D. Stokols, E. Talen, G. S. Brassington, and R. Killingsworth. 2002. Theoretical approaches to the promotion of physical activity: Forging a transdisciplinary paradigm. *American Journal of Preventive Medicine* 23 (Suppl. 2): 15-25.

Krizek, K. J., A. S. Birnbaum, and D. M. Levinson. 2004. A schematic for focusing on youth in investigations of community design and physical activity. *American Journal of Health Promotion* 19 (1): 33-38.

Kumanyika, S., and S. Grier. 2006. Targeting interventions for ethnic minority and low-income populations. *The Future of Children* 16 (1): 187-207.

Kwate, N. O. A., and T. H. Lee. 2007. Ghettoizing outdoor advertising: Disadvantage and panel density in black neighborhoods. *Journal of Urban Health* 84 (1): 21-31.

Lambert, N., J. Plumb, B. Looise, T. Johnson, J. Harvey, C. Wheeler, M. Robinson, and P. Rolfe. 2005. Using smart card technology to monitor the eating habits of children in a school cafeteria: 1. Developing and validating the methodology. *Journal of Human Nutrition and Dietetics* 18 (4): 243-54.

Lanningham-Foster, L., T. B. Jensen, R. C. Roster, A. B. Redmond, B. A. Walker, D. Heinz, and J. A. Levine. 2006. Energy expenditure of sedentary screen time compared with active screen time for children. *Pediatrics* 118 (6): e1831-e1835.

Laraia, B. A., A. M. Siega-Riz, J. S. Kaufman, and S. J. Jones. 2004. Proximity of supermarkets is positively associated with diet quality index for pregnancy. *Preventive Medicine* 39 (5): 869-75.

Lee, R. E., K. M. Booth, J. Y. Reese-Smith, G. Regan, and H. H. Howard. 2005. The Physical Activity Resource Assessment (PARA) instrument: Evaluating features, amenities and incivilities of physical activity resources in urban neighborhoods. *International Journal of Behavioral Nutrition and Physical Activity* 2 (13). http://www.ijbnpa.org/content/pdf/1479-5868-2-13.pdf (accessed July 15, 2007).

Lewis, B. A., B. H. Marcus, R. R. Pate, and A. L. Dunn. 2002. Psychosocial mediators of physical activity behavior among adults and children. *American Journal of Preventive Medicine* 23 (2S): 26-35.

Lewis, L. B., D. C. Sloane, L. M. Nascimento, A. L. Diamant, J. J. Guinyard, A. K. Yancey, and G. Flynn, for the REACH Coalition of the African Americans Building a Legacy of Health Project. 2005. African Americans' access to healthy food options in South Los Angeles restaurants. *American Journal of Public Health* 95 (4): 668-73.

Lin, B.-H., E. Frazão, and J. Guthrie. 1999. *Away-from-home foods increasingly important to quality of American diet.* Agriculture Information Bulletin no. 749. Washington, DC: U.S. Department of Agriculture, Food and Drug Administration, U.S. Department of Health and Human Services.

Lindsey, G., Y. Han, J. Wilson, and J. Yang. 2006. Neighborhood correlates of urban trail use. *Journal of Physical Activity and Health* 3 (Suppl. 1): S139-57.

Liz, J. 2004. Nintendo releases GBA sales milestones. http://www.pgnx.net/news.php?page=full&id=4968 (accessed July 15, 2007).

Lumeng, J. C., D. Appugliese, H. J. Cabral, R. H. Bradley, and B. Zuckerman. 2006. Neighborhood safety and overweight status in children. *Archives of Pediatric & Adolescent Medicine* 160 (1): 25-31.

Maag, M. 2006. Podcasting and MP3 players: Emerging education technologies. *CIN: Computers, Informatics, Nursing*, January/February. http://www.cinjournal.com/pt/re/cin/issuelist.htm;jsessionid=GndQbhtkTKTnpWrKR0GG4vQld308r5c58t5y4Vlnbk8HF0S4LT1p!-1754492629!181195629!8091!-1.

Markoff, J. 2006. An Apple-Google friendship, and a common enemy. *New York Times*, August 31. http://www.nytimes.com/2006/08/31/technology/31valley.html?ex=1182657600&en=f949f273bed56887&ei=507.

Martin, A. 2007. Kellogg to phase out some food ads to children. *New York Times*, June 14. http://www.nytimes.com/2007/06/14/business/14kellogg.html?ex=1182916800&en=d06674b72800ffeb&ei=5070 (accessed July 15, 2007).

McKenzie, T. L., D. A. Cohen, A. Sehgal, S. Williamson, and D. Golinelli. 2006. System for Observing Play and Recreation in Communities (SOPARC): Reliability and feasibility measures. *Journal of Physical Activity and Health* 3 (Suppl. 1): S208-22.

Miller, Y. D., G. T. Stewart, and W. J. Brown. 2002. Mediators of physical activity behavior change among women with young children. *American Journal of Preventive Medicine* 23 (2S): 98-103.

Morland, K., S. Wing, and A. D. Roux. 2002. The contextual effects of the local food environment on residents' diets: The Atherosclerosis Risk in Communities Study. *American Journal of Public Health* 92 (11): 1761-67.

Morland, K., S. Wing, A. D. Roux, and C. Poole. 2002. Neighborhood characteristics associated with the location of food stores and food service places. *American Journal of Preventive Medicine* 22 (1): 23-29.

National Cancer Institute. 2007. Development of a Web-based Automated Self-Administered 24-Hour Recall (ASA24). http://riskfactor.cancer.gov/tools/instruments/asa24.html (accessed July 15, 2007).

Nintendo. 2007. Wii. http://wii.nintendo.com/ (accessed July 15, 2007).

Nomad Worldwide, LLC. 2007. http://www.nonadww.com (accessed July 15, 2007).

Outdoor Advertising Association of America. 2007a. Digital billboards. http://www.oaaa.org/government/billboards.asp (accessed July 15, 2007).

————. 2007b. Your message here, in a flash. http://www.oaaa.org/presscenter/release.asp?RELEASE_ID=1363 (accessed July 15, 2007).

Pasch, K. E., K. A. Komro, C. L. Perry, M. O. Hearst, and K. Farbakhsh. 2007. Outdoor alcohol advertising near schools: What does it advertise and how is it related to intentions and use of alcohol among young adolescents? *Journal of Studies on Alcohol and Drugs* 68 (4): 587-96.

Placeways. 2007. CommunityViz. http://www.placeways.com/ (accessed July 15, 2007).

Powell, L. M., S. Slater, and F. J. Chaloupka. 2004. The relationship between community physical activity settings and race, ethnicity, and socioeconomic status. *Evidence-Based Preventive Medicine* 1 (2): 135-44.

Retting, R. A., S. A. Ferguson, and C. A. Farmer. 2007. *Reducing red light running through longer yellow signal timing and red light camera enforcement: Results of a field investigation*. Washington, DC: Insurance Institute for Highway Safety, Federal Highway Administration.

Rideout, V. 2004. *Parents, media and public policy: A Kaiser Family Foundation survey*. Menlo Park, CA: Kaiser Family Foundation.

Rideout, V., U. G. Foehr, D. F. Roberts, and M. Brodie. 1999. *Kids & media @ the new millennium*. Menlo Park, CA: Kaiser Family Foundation.

Rideout, V., D. F. Roberts, and Ulla Foehr. 2005. *Generation M: Media in the lives of 8–18 year-olds*. Menlo Park, CA: Henry J. Kaiser Family Foundation.

Robert Wood Johnson Foundation. 2007. *Active living by design. Special issues*. http://www.activelivingbydesign.org/inded.php?id=225 (accessed July 15, 2007).

Rodriguez, D. A., A. L. Brown, and P. J. Troped. 2005. Portable global positioning units to complement accelerometry-based physical activity monitors. *Medicine & Science in Sports & Exercise* 37 (Suppl. 11): S572-81.

Roemmich, J. N., L. H. Epstein, S. Raja, and L. Yin. 2007. The neighborhood and home environments: Disparate relationships with physical activity and sedentary behaviors in youth. *Annals of Behavioral Medicine* 33 (1): 29-38.

Rose, D., and R. Richards. 2004. Food store access and household fruit and vegetable use among participants in the US Food Stamp Program. *Public Health Nutrition* 7 (8): 1081-88.

Roux, A. V. 2003. Residential environments and cardiovascular risk. *Journal of Urban Health* 80 (40): 569-89.

Sallis, J. F., and K. Glanz. 2006. The role of built environments in physical activity, eating, and obesity in childhood. *The Future of Children* 16 (1): 89-108.

Schultz, Y., and A. Chambaz. 1997. Could a satellite-based navigation system (GPS) be used to assess the physical activity of individuals on earth? *European Journal of Clinical Nutrition* 51 (5): 338-39.

Seelye, K. Q. 2007. YouTube passes debates to a new generation. *New York Times*, June 14. http://www.nytimes.com/2007/06/14/us/politics/14youtube.html (accessed July 15, 2007).

Sidney Morning Herald. 2007. MySpace users uneasy about Fox. August 3. http://www.smh.com.au/news/breaking/myspace-users-uneasy-about-fox/2005/08/02/1122748641767.html (accessed July 15, 2007).

Skiba, D. J. 2007. Nursing education 2.0: YouTube. *Nursing Education Perspectives* 28 (2): 101-2.

Sloane, D. C., A. L. Diamant, L. B. Lewis, A. K. Yancy, G. Flynn, L. M. Nascimento, W. J. McCarthy, J. J. Guinyard, and M. R. Cousineau. 2003. Improving the nutritional resource environment for healthy living through community-based participatory research. *Journal of General Internal Medicine* 18 (7): 568-75.

Slobodzian, J. A. 2007. SEPTA's giant ad plans: The agency wants to wrap two stories of its buildings. *Philadelphia Inquirer*, May 21. http://www.philly.com/inquirer/local/20070521_SEPTAs_giant_ad_plans.html (accessed July 15, 2007).

Snyder, S. 2006. In the lunch line, parents can have a say. *Philadelphia Inquirer*, February 21, p. A1.

Sony Computer Entertainment, Inc. 2007. Sony eye toy. http://www.eyetoy.com (accessed July 15, 2007).

Steinberg, J. 2007. Censored "SNL" sketch jumps bleepless onto the Internet. *New York Times*, December 21. http://www.nytimes.com/2006/12/21/arts/television/21sket.html?ex=1324357200&en=dc7ed33c84bcb2fd&ei=5088&parner=rssnyt&emc=rss (accessed July 15, 2007).

Stewart, H., N. Blisard, and D. Jolliffe. 2006. *Let's eat out: Americans weigh taste, convenience, and nutrition.* United States Department of Agriculture Economic Information Bulletin no. 19. Washington, DC: U.S. Department of Agriculture.

Story, M., and S. French. 2004. Food advertising and marketing directed at children and adolescents in the US. *International Journal of Behavioral Nutrition and Physical Activity* 1 (3). http://www.ijbnpa.org/content/pdf/1479-5868-1-3.pdf (accessed July 15, 2007).

Taylor, W. C., W. S. C. Poston, J. Jones, and K. Kraft. 2006. Environmental justice: Obesity, physical activity, and healthy eating. *Journal of Physical Activity and Health* 3 (Suppl. 1): S30-S54.

Timperio, A., J. Salmon, A. Telford, and D. Crawford. 2005. Perceptions of local neighbourhood environments and their relationship to childhood overweight and obesity. *International Journal of Obesity* 29 (2): 170-75.

Tirodkar, M. A., and A. Jain. 2003. Food messages on African American television shows. *American Journal of Public Health* 93 (3): 439-41.

Transportation Research Board. 2005. Does the built environment influence physical activity? TRB Special Report 282. Washington, DC: Transportation Research Board.

Trier, J. 2007. "Cool" engagements with YouTube: Part 1. *Journal of Adolescent & Adult Literacy* 50 (5): 408-12.

Troped, P. J., E. K. Cromley, M. S. Fragala, S. J. Melly, H. H. Hasbrouck, S. L. Gortmaker, and R. C. Brownson. 2006. Development and reliability and validity testing of an audit tool for trail/path characteristics: The Path Environment Audit Tool (PEAT). *Journal of Physical Activity and Health* 3 (Suppl. 1): S158-75.

Ulrich, T. 2005. How computer maps will help the poor. *Christian Science Monitor*, October 12. http://www.csmonitor.com/2005/1012/p13s02-legn.html (accessed July 15, 2007).

U.S. Department of Agriculture. 2007. MyPyramid Blast Off Game. http://www.mypyramid.gov (accessed July 15, 2007).

Walsh, W. 2001. Compstat: An analysis of an emerging police managerial paradigm. *Policing: An International Journal of Police Strategies & Management* 24 (3): 347-62.

Warner, M. 2005. Critics say soda policy for schools lacks teeth. *New York Times*, August 22. http://www.nytimes.com/2005/08/22/business/22soda.html?ex=1282363200&en=a685e9de086c15d0&ei=5088&partner=rssnyt&emc=rss (accessed July 15, 2007).

Wiebe D. 2006. Space-Time Adolescent Risk Study (STAR). National Institutes of Health R01 AA014944, 2006-2008. Washington, DC: National Institutes of Health.

Zenk, S. N., A. J. Schulz, B. A. Israel, S. A. James, S. Boa, and M. L. Wilson. 2005. Neighborhood racial composition, neighborhood poverty, and the spatial accessibility of supermarkets in metropolitan Detroit. *American Journal of Public Health* 95 (4): 660-67.

Childhood Obesity Prevention: Successful Community-Based Efforts

By
LAURE DeMATTIA
and
SHANNON LEE DENNEY

One out of every three children is overweight. Obesity is linked to increased risks of diseases such as type 2 diabetes, liver disease, hypertension, and heart disease. As the numbers of children with chronic disease goes up, so will the strain on the U.S. health care system, including the cost of health care. The Ecological Model of Childhood Overweight allows one to consider how an individual child's weight is influenced by characteristics ranging from the individual to the society. This article focuses on community characteristics that interact with children's weight status. It reviews community-based programs and whether they are successfully slowing the rate of childhood obesity, including demonstrations of recipe preparation, community gardens, and school-based curricula. It concludes with suggestions for intervention efforts and funding priorities focusing on high-risk populations of low-income overweight women of childbearing years. Interventions that occur during preconception may be true primary prevention of childhood obesity.

Keywords: community; childhood obesity; interventions

C hildhood obesity continues to be a major and increasing public health problem. The rates of childhood obesity have tripled since the 1960s, with more than 33.3 percent of children now at risk for obesity, defined as having a body mass index (BMI) between the 85th and 95th percentiles.[1] According to Ogden et al. (2006)

Laure DeMattia is a community family physician. She recently completed a Primary Care Research Fellowship at the Medical College of Wisconsin, where she serves as assistant clinical professor for Family and Community Medicine. She has authored several peer-reviewed articles on prevention and treatment of childhood obesity. She also has been a clinician for Children's Hospital of Wisconsin's NEW Kids program and serves on the Milwaukee County Nutrition and Physical Activity Coalition.

Shannon Lee Denney is an adjunct instructor at the University of Wisconsin–Milwaukee. She received her Juris doctorate from the University of Oklahoma and her master's in communication from the University of Wisconsin–Milwaukee. She has focused the majority of her research on ethics and communication.

DOI: 10.1177/0002716207309940

17 percent of today's children already have BMIs higher than the 95th percentile. The resulting excess weight puts children at risk for complicating diseases such as type 2 diabetes (Fagot-Campagna 2000), hyperinsulinemia (Klein et al. 2004), hypertension (Gidding et al. 1995), dyslipidemia (Gidding et al. 1995), joint abnormalities (Taylor et al. 2006), polycystic ovarian syndrome (Gulekli et al. 1993), nonalcoholic fatty liver disease (Clark, Brancati, and Diehl 2002), and sleep disturbances (Mallory, Fiser, and Jackson 1989). These complications or comorbidities are likely to persist into adulthood (American Academy of Pediatrics 2003).

If a child is obese at the age of four, he or she will have a 20 percent likelihood of being overweight as an adult. By adolescence, the likelihood of remaining overweight as an adult reaches 80 percent (Guo and Chumlea 1999). Annual hospital costs related to childhood obesity totaled $127 million from 1997 to 1999 (in 2001 constant U.S. dollars), up from $35 million from 1979 to 1981 (Wang and Dietz 2002). As these overweight and obese children age, their health will continue to deteriorate and will further burden our health care system. Their ability to care for themselves and live independently will decrease, their chronic medical conditions will increase, and they will incur greater health care costs compared to their normal weight peers (Sturm, Ringel, and Andreyeva 2004).

---

*These data should be disconcerting
enough to spur a national movement
to reverse the trend of the "obesity epidemic."
While it may seem inequitable for the nation
to incur the cost of prevention for what is
largely considered an individual's problem, the
taxpayers' current cost is astonishing.*

These data should be disconcerting enough to spur a national movement to reverse the trend of the "obesity epidemic." While it may seem inequitable for the nation to incur the cost of prevention for what is largely considered an individual's problem, the taxpayers' current cost is astonishing. According to the U.S. Department of Health and Human Services (2001), the total costs of obesity in 2000 were $117 billion. Using current 2007 U.S. population data, this is an additional $387 per person per year (U.S. Census Bureau 2007). Unless Americans can reverse this epidemic, this figure will continue to increase.

According to an Institute of Medicine report, *Preventing Childhood Obesity: Health in the Balance* (2004), it is a national duty to take steps to reverse the obesity trend. A committee that included representatives from various disciplines (nutrition, physical activity, obesity prevention, pediatrics, family medicine, public health, public policy, health education, community development, and behavioral epidemiology) convened in response to the report to develop ways to address the increasing numbers of children who are overweight. This committee analyzed data from a survey of programs focused on childhood obesity during the years 2004 to 2006 from a national registry called Shaping America's Youth.[2] They also gathered information through three regional symposia and completed a comprehensive literature review. The Institute of Medicine compiled this information into a follow-up to the 2004 report, *Progress in Preventing Childhood Obesity: How Do We Measure Up?* (Institute of Medicine 2006).

The conclusions of the report are as follows:

1. While the country has responded to the obesity epidemic, the current level of investment does not match the scale of the problem.
2. Various entities are implementing programs, policies, and interventions, but researchers need to produce evidence-based approaches that will guide national action.
3. Current evidence is not sufficient to complete a comprehensive assessment of the progress that the nation has made. Researchers should use best practices in the short term with the goal of developing a larger evidence base with which to develop initiatives that can be used in various settings.
4. Evaluation needs to occur at multiple levels and settings. This layered information will help guide improvements to childhood obesity efforts. Surveillance, monitoring, and research are all components of evaluation.
5. We need short term, intermediate, and long term evaluation in order to have a sustained improvement of the childhood obesity epidemic. (Institute of Medicine 2006, p. 8)

The overriding conclusion of the committee is that we have a greater chance of success in addressing the childhood obesity epidemic if public, private, and voluntary organizations would combine and share respective resources to create a coordinated and sustained effort. To this end, one recommendation is to have industry, communities, and schools build partnerships with government, academia, and foundations to strengthen the evaluation process and expedite creating a more comprehensive evidence base with which to develop better long-term practices.

Despite the government's efforts to influence individual behaviors that lead to expression of childhood obesity, success has been limited. In 2001, a survey from the Centers for Disease Control and Prevention (CDC) demonstrated that the majority of adults (54.6 percent) did not engage in physical activity most days of the week (CDC 2003). More recently, a national public opinion poll showed that 99 percent of Americans believe exercise is vital to preserving health (International Health, Racquet and Sportsclub Association 2007), but less than half of all Americans get the recommended amount of physical activity each day.

FIGURE 1
ECOLOGICAL MODEL OF CHILDHOOD OBESITY

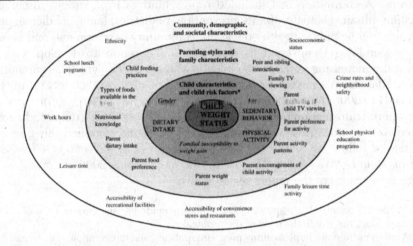

SOURCE: Davison and Birch (2001). Reprinted with permission from Blackwell Publishing. The original figure can be accessed at http://www.blackwell-synergy.com/loi/obr

Ecological Considerations in Childhood Obesity

The Ecological Systems Theory states that individual change cannot be completely explained without considering the ecological niche in which the individual exists (Bronfenbrenner 1986). The Ecological Model of Childhood Overweight, developed by University at Albany and Pennsylvania State University researchers Davison and Birch (2001), focuses specifically on characteristics that could affect an individual child's weight status in relation to the multiple environments in which that child is embedded (see Figure 1). This model is ideal for looking at the combined effects of society, family, and individual factors that would amplify or illuminate the causes of childhood obesity.

The first system is the individual child's genetic environment. Children have different rates of growth and energy requirements, which vary by sex and age. This variability reveals itself in many studies where results of weight change are difficult to interpret because the study groups contain children of large age ranges and/or do not account for gender (Epstein, Paluch, and Raynor 2001). Additionally, if a child has two overweight parents (hence genetic susceptibility), a slight increase in dietary intake of the genetically susceptible child may show a larger increase in weight gain compared to the child with no familial obesity (Francis et al. 2007).

The next system that influences a child's weight status is the family environment. The parents contribute both the genetic factors and behaviors that will influence the expression of obesity in their child. Parental overweight predicts higher BMI in girls and risk for disinhibited eating (Francis et al. 2007). A study by Wrotniak et al. (2005) showed that parental modeling of healthy behaviors improves weight loss in overweight youth participating in a family-based program where both parents and children are actively trying to lose weight. These behaviors included parental prioritization of family activity, limiting the family's amount of screen time (including television, computers, and video games), and limiting access to high-calorie, low-nutrient-value foods. Family systems require individuals to change their behaviors to affect the weight status of the child. So far, the home has been the focus for the majority of current programs and interventions.

The Ecological Model forces us to take into account the larger community in which the child lives. Studies often cite barriers to adopting healthy behaviors, such as lack of accessibility of recreational opportunities, decreased access to healthy food options, and lack of time to implement physical activity (International Health, Racquet and Sportsclub Association 2007). A coordinated community approach to obesity intervention is often the missing component necessary to supporting lifestyle changes that influence childhood obesity. This article will first focus on the modifiable community characteristics of neighborhood and school environments and the promising programs that can address these characteristics. Then, it will lay the groundwork for further studies and research within the community context.

Coordinated Community Efforts

National legislation has been slow to react to the escalation of childhood obesity. While the majority of legislation efforts are at the level of the individual states, there have been some actions at the federal level. Congress and President George W. Bush enacted The Child Nutrition and WIC Reauthorization Act of 2004. The law requires every school district that participates in the National School Lunch Program to bring parents, teachers, and administrators together to adopt and oversee a school wellness policy that addresses healthy nutrition and physical activity (U.S. Congress 2004). The main push in state legislation change has focused on school physical activity requirements and updating nutritional standards. In 2006, at least thirty-one states introduced or amended bills to improve schools' nutrition environment and physical activity. Eleven states adopted such legislation (Robert Wood Johnson Foundation 2006).

Community efforts outside of legislation are occurring at the grassroots and academic levels. The coordination of these endeavors can improve the benefits for all parties involved through sharing resources that otherwise may not be available to smaller groups, building relationships with groups already embedded in the community, and reducing redundancy of ineffective programs. One program that has been successful in taking an ecological approach to childhood obesity is the Consortium to Lower Obesity in Chicago Children (CLOCC). This consortium has been successful at bringing together hundreds of academic, government, and grassroots organizations to take on childhood obesity. The consortium has an ongoing public health campaign, provides technical assistance for communities, allocates seed money quarterly to help local organizations secure funds from outside funding entities, and has committed to six areas of Chicago by providing implementation grants.

The Ecological Model states that ethnicity, socioeconomic status, work demands, school lunch programs, school PE programs, neighborhood safety, accessibility to recreational facilities, and access to convenience foods and restaurants are factors that influence an individual child's weight. Factors that are not modifiable include ethnicity, socioeconomic status, and work demands. These unmodifiable factors interact with more controllable characteristics, however, including neighborhood safety, access to convenience foods, school physical education, and curriculum. Modifiable characteristics can be grouped into two categories, neighborhood and school, and will be the focus of the remainder of the article.

Neighborhood Environments

Safety

The neighborhood as we know it today is very different from the traditional European model. Communities once sought to keep industrial areas separate from residential spaces to protect the property and health of residents. Indeed, today's zoning requirements derive from a Supreme Court Case in 1926, *Ambler Realty v. Village of Euclid*, which nominally recognized the health basis of zoning business separate from residences (Schilling and Linton 2005). The current theory is that mixed use of land may help reduce obesity. Urban sprawl increases the probability of chronic disease, possibly by providing fewer opportunities for physical activity and appealing to less active people who are drawn to car-friendly areas (Sturm and Cohen 2004). However, the study of the built environment is a relatively new field and little research has focused on children (see Hillier 2008 [this volume]).

Neighborhood safety can influence the physical activity levels of children. Parents report concerns about neighborhood safety more frequently on behalf of girls (17.6 percent) than for boys (14.6 percent) and are reported more frequently by Hispanic parents (41.2 percent) than by non-Hispanic white (8.5 percent) and non-Hispanic black (13.3 percent) parents (Burdette and Whitaker 2005). Overall, parents with lower incomes and education levels report more barriers to allowing their children to play outside. Perceptions about neighborhood safety can also affect the amount of time children watch TV (Burdette and Whitaker 2005). Children whose mothers reported the least safe neighborhood conditions had the highest percentage of screen time (greater than two hours).

In 1969, about half of all students walked or bicycled to school (Federal Highway Administration 1972). In 2002, fewer than 15 percent of all school trips used active means of transportation (*Morbidity and Mortality Weekly Report* 2003). A 2004 survey of parents by the CDC explored the barriers to walking to school for children aged five to eighteen. The top reasons were distance and safety (CDC 2005). Safe Routes to School (SR2S) is a national program started in 2005 that is making progress in changing those numbers. SR2S provides funding to communities to develop programs and projects related to bicycle/pedestrian safety to bring back walking to school. The city of Milwaukee, for example, began with this project in 2005 and had six pilot schools. Through Milwaukee's Neighborhood School Initiative and SR2S, the city decided to build six new schools from the ground up, expand nineteen existing schools, and renovate fifteen other existing schools (Introduction to Safe Routes to School 2007). Returning to neighborhood schools increases the potential of children to walk to and from school and the possibility of parents walking their children to school. This small increase in physical activity has the potential to affect the increase in weight gain we have seen in our community.

Access to Healthy Food: Grocery and Convenience Stores

Neighborhoods without a grocery store are associated with reduced access to fresh fruits and vegetables (Baker et al. 2006; Zenk et al. 2005). Baker et al.'s (2006) cross-sectional study of an upper Midwest portion of the country showed that areas where there were neighborhoods with a varied racial distribution or high poverty among whites had fewer stores that offered fruits and vegetables, compared with higher income neighborhoods. This study also reported that, regardless of income, predominantly African American areas had less access to fruits and vegetables. The authors of this research acknowledge that it is difficult to argue in a correlational study that increasing access to fruits and vegetables translates into increased intake. Morland, Diez Roux, and Wing (2006) described a large-scale cross-sectional study of 10,763 adults that found that respondents from communities with access to supermarkets had lower prevalence of obesity, while those with greater access to convenience stores had increased prevalence of obesity.

While additional characteristics contribute to obesity in neighborhoods without grocery stores, the nutritional limitations of being dependent upon groceries from convenience stores deserve special attention. Efforts are under way at the government and grassroots level to make buying fruits and vegetables more convenient. Governor Ed Rendell of Pennsylvania launched a program to form public-private partnerships that improve access to healthy foods. The program encourages supermarket development in low-income areas by awarding grants and loans exceeding $2 billion to those willing to invest into these areas (Robert Wood Johnson Foundation 2006). In 2005, Nevada legislature passed Senate Bill 229 into law, which provided a temporary tax incentive for locating or expanding grocery stores in the southern part of the state (Robert Wood Johnson Foundation 2006).

Another dedicated effort trying to improve the availability of fruits and vegetables in urban settings is Growing Power, Inc. Growing Power is an urban farm located in Milwaukee, Wisconsin, that is developing community food systems throughout the nation. Their mission as a nonprofit organization and land trust is to support people from diverse backgrounds and the environment in which they live by helping to provide equal access to healthy, high-quality, safe, and affordable food. They implement this mission by providing hands-on training, on-the-ground demonstration, outreach, and technical assistance through the development of Community Food Systems, which help people grow, process, market, and distribute food in a sustainable manner. They have multiple outreach programs that have helped to develop more than twenty-five urban gardens, partnered with schools to bring children back to the connection between land and food, and recultivated land that otherwise stood vacant. They have completed training workshops in California, Illinois, Minnesota, Massachusetts, Mississippi, and Blackfeet Nation in Montana as well as Toronto, Canada (Growing Power 2007).

Restaurants and Fast Food

American families are eating more outside their homes now than at any other period in history. Families spend almost 50 percent of total food dollars at restaurants and on fast food (Institute of Medicine 2004). Bowman and colleagues (2004) reported that 30.3 percent of children aged four to nineteen consumed at least one meal per day that was fast food. This study also established that children who ate fast food, compared to those who did not, consumed more total calories (187 kcal/day) (Bowman et al. 2004).

While the restaurant industry has begun to increase its healthy alternatives, many restaurants are resisting change. New York City and Seattle have passed regulations that require chain restaurants to label menus with calorie information for use at point of sale. The Subway chain has led the way in compliance, while a restaurant association representing multiple companies in New York is suing the city in federal court (Center for Science in the Public Interest 2007).

Breastfeeding

The American Academy of Pediatrics encourages breastfeeding a child through the first year of life (Gartner et al. 2005). The World Health Organization (2003) sets a goal for every child to be breastfed for the first two years of life. In addition to numerous other breastfeeding benefits for both the mother and the child, one of the most important benefits is the reduction of obesity risks in children. According to the Growing Up Today Study (GUTS), which studied children of the women who participated in the Nurses' Health Study II, the length and exclusivity of breastfeeding is associated with reduced risk of childhood obesity (Mayer-Davis et al. 2006). The researchers found that breastfed children had a lower incidence of being overweight, even factoring in the mothers' characteristics of being overweight and/or diabetic. The researchers found that siblings in the same home with the same genetics had different outcomes depending on the degree to which they were breastfed (Mayer-Davis et al. 2006). In another study published in *Obesity*, Li and his fellow researchers (2007) found that breastfeeding for at least four months decreased both early-onset (age two years) and late-onset (age twelve years) overweight.

Even with this knowledge, the breastfeeding rates in the United States are dismal. According to Li et al. (2005), in 2002 only 71.4 percent of babies were breastfed initially. Only 13.3 percent of babies were exclusively breastfed until the age of six months, and only 16.1 percent of babies were nursed until their first birthday. Breastfeeding rates remain low, despite all the evidence that breast-feeding can reduce obesity as well as other diseases. Women face a variety of bar-riers to breastfeeding, however. These barriers fall into two broad categories: work and social pressure.

To protect breastfeeding in the workplace, it is necessary to change overt poli-cies and implicit attitudes working against it. Breastfeeding must be protected against discrimination on a federal level. Under *Derungs v. Wal-Mart Stores* (2004), breastfeeding is ruled as unprotected under the Pregnancy Discrimination Act (PDA). The PDA was enacted as an amendment to Title VII of the Civil Rights act of 1967 and was meant to broaden the meaning of sex dis-crimination in employment to protect pregnant women against discrimination. The Sixth Circuit specifically ruled in *Derungs* that breastfeeding was not con-templated in the PDA, and therefore denial of breastfeeding could not be con-sidered discrimination based on sex (*Derungs* 2004; Whelen 2005).

Under the Breastfeeding Promotion Act, introduced to the 110th Congress (HR 2236) in the spring of 2007, U.S. Representative Carolyn Maloney (D-NY) proposed three things. The first is an amendment to the PDA to insert just two words, "including lactation," and providing for its definition. This would make it illegal for an employer to discriminate against a breastfeeding woman. She also provides for a tax credit for employers who facilitate breastfeeding or expressing mothers. Finally, she provides that breast pumps can be classified as medical equipment and will have to meet government standards. The federal government can show that it is serious about encouraging breastfeeding by amending Title VII to protect the practice in employment and in public.

A much harder challenge is changing the implicit attitudes of discrimination against nursing mothers. As difficult as it is for a pumping and working mother to express milk at work in a cubicle (Mieszkowski 2007), it is that much harder for a mother to express milk while working at McDonald's or Wal-Mart (Gebel 2007). Not only is privacy a complication, but also employers and coworkers may be intolerant. If we change the law, workplace tolerance may improve (Baldwin and Friedman 1999).

Another conflict of attitudes is in society's support of breastfeeding. As Baldwin and Friedman pointed out in their 1999 article in *Mothering*, breast-feeding has skipped several generations and is now seen as a "lifestyle choice" rather than as the most appropriate way to feed a baby. This means that women are being asked to remove themselves from public spaces when they attempt to nurse their babies. This particular issue was the basis for the *Derung* case. Ms. Derung was one of three mother plaintiffs who were asked to leave Wal-Mart while feeding their babies. Ms. Derung was breastfeeding her son on a bench outside of the layaway department when a Wal-Mart employee told her that she could not feed her baby there, and that she would have to remove herself to the restroom or outside to breastfeed the baby. The other two mothers (Gore and Baird) in the *Derungs* case were in other Ohio Wal-Mart stores when employees told them that they could not nurse their babies inside the store. Other notable recent cases occurred in Victoria's Secret stores in Massachusetts and Wisconsin and aboard a Delta flight from Vermont (Mishra 2006). As long as society sees breastfeeding as an exception or a lifestyle choice, intolerance will continue. States need to pass laws that exempt breastfeeding from public indecency statutes and that affirmatively assert the right for mothers to breastfeed anywhere they need (Wagget and Waggot 1005).

School Environment

The school environment is an ideal location for education, intervention against inactivity and poor nutritional intake, and monitoring of BMI. The schools have a triple opportunity in the classroom, gymnasium, and cafeteria. Several random-ized control trials have been able to show benefits in reducing childhood obesity through different curriculum interventions. Robinson, Gortmaker, and Dennison have each developed curriculum-based programs that have been successful in reducing sedentary behavior, improving nutritional intake, and decreasing BMI across the age spectrum of preschoolers (Dennison et al. 2004) to middle-school-aged children (Robinson 1999; Robinson et al. 2003; Gortmaker et al. 1999).

The school environment is an ideal location for education, intervention against inactivity and poor nutritional intake, and monitoring of BMI. The schools have a triple opportunity in the classroom, gymnasium, and cafeteria.

Curriculum

Hip Hop to Health (Dennison et al. 2004) is a curriculum that aims to reduce television viewing time and increase fruit and vegetable intake in preschool-aged children. The intervention tried to involve parents in the practice of reduced television viewing by informing them of the potential risk screen time has on children and asking the parents to support a no-TV week at home. This program measured a decrease in BMI of the preschoolers in the intervention group and an increase in the BMI of the control group, though the differences were statistically insignificant (Dennison et al. 2004). Sedentary behaviors in the intervention group, however, were reduced significantly.

Planet Health (Gortmaker et al. 1999) is an integrated interdisciplinary curriculum designed as an overweight prevention program first used in the Boston Public Schools. It was designed for children in sixth and seventh grade. Researchers tested this intervention in five schools, with five additional schools serving as controls, for a total participation of 1,295 students. After adjusting for age, ethnicity, intervention status, and baseline BMI measurements, children in intervention schools were less likely to be overweight than in control schools (odds ratio = .47, p = .03). Teachers found this program easy to use; it benefited the teachers in unforeseen ways such as improved health behaviors and improved teaching due to exposure to new teaching methods. Challenges remained, however, such as the perception of a lack of curriculum reinforcement in school meals, vending machines, and the children's homes (Wiecha et al. 2004).

Robinson developed interventions for both curricula during school and after-school programming (Robinson 1999; Robinson et al. 2003). In 1999, he randomly assigned one of two schools in San Jose, California, to receive an eighteen-lesson, six-month classroom curriculum for eight- to ten-year-olds aimed to reduce TV, videotape, and video game use. This curriculum change was successful at lowering the BMI by 0.45 points after adjusting for baseline BMI, age, and sex. Girls Health Enrichment Multisite Studies (GEMS) comprise a group of interdependent studies focusing on reducing obesity in African American girls as they progress through puberty. Stanford GEMS is an ongoing study that concluded in the fall of 2007. A twelve-week pilot study focused on increasing physical activity through after-school dance classes and reducing sedentary behavior via lessons on selective viewing of television and TV time managers. While the intervention group's TV viewing significantly decreased compared to the control, no significant difference in BMI occurred between the two groups (Robinson et al. 2003).

Nutrition

The Milwaukee program, Youth Take Charge, is an after-school pilot program developed to increase fruit and vegetable intake among school-aged children. Evaluated via a descriptive process, it shows promise in changing knowledge and behavior regarding fruit and vegetable intake (Johansen and Greer 2006). Through collaboration of multiple partners including the Milwaukee Health Department and the Milwaukee County Nutrition Physical Activity Coalition, nutritionists have middle school children initially taste test several recipes with fruits and vegetables and rate them. In the pilot program of 2006, researchers trained twenty-one adolescent youths to present a mock demonstration to their peers. These twenty-one children rated six recipes with fruits or vegetables as the main ingredient. The six recipes were rated as the best-tasting 47 to 71 percent of the time and worst-tasting 5 to 25 percent of the time. Several youths then completed a demonstration for preschool children at the Northside YMCA after-school program, farmers markets, the Wisconsin State Fair, and YMCA sports camps.

Children serving as peer role models addresses several factors that have been associated with decreased fruit and vegetable intake, self-efficacy, social normative behavior, and peer modeling surrounding fruit and vegetable intake. Granner and colleagues (2004) reported that as adolescents increased in age their self-efficacy for eating fruits and vegetables decreased and peers modeling of eating fruits and vegetables decreased. While this program was carried out as a pilot program, it has the potential to be replicated on a larger scale through the school system and to transform the normative beliefs of fruit and vegetable intake in the younger classes while increasing the self-efficacy of the older children who participate as the peer models (Johansen and Greer 2006).

Increasing fruits and vegetables in children's diets is one way to displace energy-dense, low-nutrient foods that contribute to excess calorie intake and childhood obesity. The responsibility for this task can no longer be perceived as solely an individual choice. Parents, schools, and after-school settings need to work together to ensure that the environments in which each child operates are undergoing changes to reduce barriers to making healthy choices.

Parents, schools, and after-school settings need to work together to ensure that the environments in which each child operates are undergoing changes to reduce barriers to making healthy choices.

Conclusion

National momentum to reverse childhood obesity is evident. Small victories are being realized across the country. Arkansas reduced the rate of increase in childhood obesity over a three-year period (Arkansas Center for Health Improvement 2006). The Coordinated Approach to Child Health (Coleman et al. 2005), a Texas-based program, is preventing an increase of overweight in low-income schools with predominantly Hispanic children. In addition, Shape Up Somerville (Economos et al. 2007) was the first community-based obesity prevention program to show a decrease in weight over one year for first-through third-graders.

Small victories aside, we still are living in a country that faces a future where this generation of children may not outlive their parents. Research has led us to conclude that early intervention and prevention are more effective and less costly than treatment of adolescent or adult obesity. The treatment of obesity for many people is not a covered benefit through their insurance companies. Increasing our national investment in research dollars, policy change, program funding, and health care benefits aimed at the prevention and early intervention of childhood obesity will change the environment to support individual behaviors that reduce the risk of obesity and improve the health of our country.

Specific policies that will help support individual behavior changes include the following:

1. Develop tax incentives for schools that implement Safe Routes to School Programs.
2. Improve accessibility to grocery stores and farmers markets by supporting incentives for vendors.
3. Introduce regulation by the Food and Drug Administration requiring that all chain restaurants place clear calorie information at point of sale.
4. Promote breastfeeding and adopt laws to protect a mother's ability to pump or breast-feed at work, including an amendment to Title VII of the Civil Rights Act of 1964 to include workplace protection of breastfeeding. In addition, state legislatures need to change existing law to specifically exclude breastfeeding from indecency statutes.
5. Mandate incorporating physical activity into school curriculum for all students.

Future Research and Funding Focus

The federal government has stated that it is a national priority to reduce child-hood obesity. While we need to see moneys directed at prevention efforts for all age ranges, high-priority populations are women of childbearing age who are of a lower socioeconomic status. Over the past decade, evolving research has shown that fetal malnutrition and maternal prepregnancy obesity are placing children at a lifelong risk of obesity (Oken and Gillman 2003). Excessive pregnancy weight gain also puts children at risk of obesity (Li et al. 2007). Therefore, we need to begin the prevention of childhood obesity at prenatal counseling. Following up in the postnatal time period will potentially help parents learn about appropriate portion size and food choice. Targeting lower-income and overweight mothers for weight-loss classes can improve the fat intake, portion size, and food choice of their young children, as was shown by Klohe-Lehman and colleagues (2007). While this study only showed a modest effect of weight loss for the mothers, it did show significant improvement in their children's dietary intake while main-taining normal growth in height and weight. The subjects were recruited from Women Infants and Children (WIC) and public health clinics. These locations are potential areas for further intervention.

Historically, WIC has been a site for community health change. WIC was founded in 1974 to help prevent malnutrition and iron deficiency anemia. It has recently added produce vouchers for clients to improve nutritional intake and has multiple, funded grant projects aimed at reducing childhood obesity within high-risk populations. Loving Your Family Feeding Their Future, a Nutrition

Assistance Program, is a community level program that is trying to improve access to healthy food through individual education and subsidizing with food stamps (U.S. Department of Agriculture 2007).

Parent food choice, eating style, activity level, and screen time are all influences on how children will behave in relation to food intake and physical activity. Having children participate in healthy cooking classes at the school kitchen or neighborhood center would be an interesting community wide intervention. Ideally, parents would prepare the meal with their children, taste test the recipe, and then take away the additional portions to be eaten later in the week. This approach accomplishes multiple goals. Placing the activity in the school or community center offers the social support of peers for both parent and child. It is time saving because it allows the parents to come directly from work and prepare a healthy meal. Preparing the food together allows for modeling of preparation, and children are more likely to eat food that they have helped to prepare. Finally, taste testing in front of other peers influences children to try potentially novel foods.

Collaborating with community, government, and academia has changed public health outcomes in the past. Nationally, concerned individuals have influenced seat belt use, drunk driving, and the fight against smoking. Community members, as taxpayers and concerned stakeholders, have more immediate power to affect school lunch programs; school PE programs; neighborhood safety; and accessibility to recreational facilities, convenience foods, and restaurants. Many laypersons are already involved in activities that affect these environments, including the PTA and Neighborhood Watch. These organizations are already in place and can influence the community leaders and social networks to produce measurable outcomes and make sustainable changes that will reverse the current childhood obesity trend.

Notes

1. Body mass index (BMI) is a measure of weight in relation to height. The calculation of BMI is weight (kg) divided by height (m^2).

2. Shaping America's Youth (SAY) is a collaborative initiative that has established a clearinghouse of information on national programs that address the childhood obesity epidemic and is a platform that can unite the resources of all who may contribute to the fight on childhood obesity. SAY partners include the American Diabetes Association, the American Academy of Pediatrics, the American Obesity Association, and the Nutrition Department of the University of California–Davis, with sponsorship from Campbell Soup Company; Gerber Products Company; McNeil Nutritionals, LLC, a Johnson & Johnson company; and Nike, Inc.

References

American Academy of Pediatrics. 2003. Prevention of pediatric overweight and obesity. *Pediatrics* 112:424-30.

Arkansas Center for Health Improvement. 2006. Arkansas releases landmark data on childhood obesity. http://www.achi.net/BMI_Info/Docs/2006/Results06/National_Rept_BMI2006_press_kit+background_material.pdf (accessed August 30, 2007).

Baker, Elizabeth A., Mario Schootman, Ellen Barnidge, and Cheryl Kelly. 2006. The role of race and poverty in access to foods that enable individuals to adhere to dietary guidelines. *Preventing Chronic Disease* 3 (3): A76.

Baldwin, Elizabeth N., and Kenneth A. Friedman. 1999. Working it out: Breastfeeding at work. *Mothering*, March 1.

Bowman, Shanthy A., Steven L. Gortmaker, Cara B. Ebbeling, Mark A. Pereira, and David S. Ludwig, 2004. Effects of fast-food consumption on energy intake and diet quality among children in a national household survey. *Pediatrics* 113 (1): 112-18.

Bronfenbrenner, Urie. 1986. Ecology of the family as a context for human development: Research perspectives. *Developmental Psychology* 22:723-42.

Burdette, Hillary L., and Robert C. Whitaker. 2005. A national study of neighborhood safety, outdoor play, television viewing, and obesity in preschool children. *Pediatrics* 116:657-62.

Center for Science in the Public Interest. 2007. In Seattle, menu labeling is "in," trans fat is "out." http://www.cspinet.org/new/200707201.html (accessed September 20, 2007).

Centers for Disease Control and Prevention. 2003. Prevalence of physical activity, including lifestyle activities among adults—United States, 2000–2001. *Morbidity and Mortality Weekly Report* 52 (32): 764-69.

———. 2005. Barriers to children walking to or from school United States 2004. *Morbidity and Mortality Weekly Report.* www.cdc.gov/mmwr/preview/_mmwrhtml/mm5438a2.htm (accessed August 11, 2007).

Child Nutrition and WIC Reauthorization Act of 2004, PL 108-265, 2004 S 2507 (June 30, 2004).

Clark, Jeanne M., Fredrick L. Brancati, and Anna M. Diehl. 2002. Nonalcoholic fatty liver disease. *Gastroenterology* 122:1649-57.

Coleman, Karen J., Claire L. Tiller, Jesus Sanchez, Edward M. Heath, Oumar Sy, George Milliken, and David A. Dzewaltowski. 2005. Prevention of the epidemic increase in child risk of overweight in low-income schools: The El Paso coordinated approach to child health. *Archive of Pediatric Adolescent Medicine* 159:217-24.

Davison, Kirsten K., and Leann L. Birch. 2001. Childhood overweight: A contextual model and recommendations for future research. *Obesity Reviews* 2 (3): 159-71.

Dennison, Barbara A., Theresa J. Russo, Patrick A. Burdick, and Paul L. Jenkins. 2004. An intervention to reduce television viewing by preschool children. *Archives of Pediatric Adolescent Medicine* 158: 170-76.

Derungs v. Wal-Mart Stores, 374 F.3d 428, 430 (6th Cir. 2004).

Economos, Christina D., Raymond R. Hyatt, Jeanne P. Goldberg, Aviva Must, Elena N. Naumova, Jessica J. Collins, and Miriam E. Nelson. 2007. A community intervention reduces BMI *z*-score in children: Shape Up Somerville first year results. *Obesity* 15 (5): 1325-36.

Epstein, Leonard H., Rocco A. Paluch, and Hollie A. Raynor. 2001. Sex differences in obese children and siblings in family-based obesity treatment. *Obesity Research* 9:746-53.

Fagot-Campagna, Anne F. 2000. Emergence of type 2 diabetes mellitus in children: Epidemiological evidence. *Journal of Pediatric Endocrinology and Metabolism* 13:1395-1402.

Federal Highway Administration. 1972. Transportation characteristics of school children. Report no. 4, Nationwide Personal Transportation Study, Federal Highway Administration, Washington, DC.

Francis, Lori A., Alison K. Ventura, Michele Marini, and Leann Birch. 2007. Parent overweight predicts daughters' increase in BMI and disinhibited overeating from 5 to 13 years. *Obesity* 15:1544-53.

Gartner, Lawrence M., Jane Morton, Ruth A. Lawrence, Audrey J. Naylor, Donna O'Hare, Richard J. Schanler, and Arthur I. Eidelman. 2005. Breastfeeding and the use of human milk. *Pediatrics* 115:496-506. http://aappolicy.aappublications.org/cgi/reprint/pediatrics;115/2/496.pdf (accessed August 25, 2007).

Gebel, Erika. 2007. Got mother's milk? Advocates of breast-feeding try to boost the city's low rate of nursing. *Philadephia Inquirer*, August 20, State and Regional News section.

Gidding, Samuel S., Weihang Bao, Sathanur R. Srinivasan, and Gerald S. Berenson. 1995. Effects of secular trends in obesity on coronary risk factors in children: The Bogalusa Heart Study. *Journal of Pediatrics* 127 (6): 868-74.

Gortmaker, Samuel L., Karen E. Peterson, Jean Wiecha, Arthur M. Sobol, Sanjay Dixit, Mary K. Fox, and Nan Laird. 1999. Reducing obesity via a school-based interdisciplinary intervention among youth: Planet Health. *Archives of Pediatric Adolescent Medicine* 153:409-18.

Granner, Michelle L., Roger G. Sargent, Kristine S. Calderon, James R. Hussey, Alexandra Evans, and Ken W. Watkins. 2004. Factors of fruit and vegetable intake by race, gender, and age among young adolescents. *Journal of Nutrition Education and Behavior* 36 (4): 173-80.

Growing Power, Inc. 2007. Mission statement. http://www.growingpower.org/ (accessed August 11, 2007).

Gulekli, Bülent, Nilgün O. Turhan, Semih Senoz, Selahattin Kukner, Hawa Oral, and Oya Gokmen. 1993. Endocrinological, ultrasonographic and clinical findings in adolescent and adult polycystic ovary patients: A comparative study. *Gynelogical Endocrinology Journal* 7:273-77.

Guo, Shumei S., and William C. Chumlea. 1999. Tracking of body mass index in children in relation to overweight in adulthood. *American Journal of Clinical Nutrition* 70:145S-48S.

Hillier, Amy. 2008. Childhood overweight and the built environment· Making technology part of the solution rather than part of the problem. *Annals of the American Academy of Political and Social Science* 615: 56-82.

Institute of Medicine. 2004. *Preventing childhood obesity: Health in the balance.* Washington, DC: Institute of Medicine.

———. 2006. *Progress in preventing childhood obesity: How do we measure up?* Washington, DC: Institute of Medicine.

International Health, Racquet and Sportsclub Association. 2007. Current culture makes it hard for people to exercise, four out of five Americans say. http://cms.ihrsa.org/IHRSA/viewPage.cfm?pageId=3395 (accessed August 29, 2007).

Introduction to Safe Routes to School: The Health, Safety and Transportation Nexus. 2007. nmshtd.state .nm.us/upload/images/Safe_Routes_to_School/National%20SRTS%20pres%20print%20version.pdf (accessed August 11, 2007).

Johansen, Larry, and Yvonne Greer. 2006. Youth Take Charge! Final report. Presented at Wisconsin SE Regional Nutrition and Physical Activity Plan Forum, Milwaukee.

Klein, David J., Lisa Aronson Friedman, William R. Harlan, Bruce A. Barton, George B. Schreiber, Robert M. Cohen, Linda C. Harlan, and John A. Morrison. 2004. Obesity and the development of insulin resistance and impaired fasting glucose in black and white adolescent girls: A longitudinal study. *Diabetes Care* 27:378-83.

Klohe-Lehman, Deborah M., Jeanne Freeland-Graves, Kristine K. Clarke, Guowen Cai, V. Saroja Voruganti, Tracey J. Milani, Henry J. Nuss, Michael Proffitt, and Thomas M. Bohman. 2007. Low-income, overweight and obese mothers as agents of change to improve food choices, fat habits, and physical activity in their 1-to-3-year-old children. *Journal of the American College of Nutrition* 26 (3): 196-208.

Li, Chaoyang, Michael L. Goran, Harsohena Kaur, Nicole Nollen, and Jasjit Ahluwalia. 2007. Developmental trajectories of overweight during childhood: Role of early life factors. *Obesity* 15:760-71.

Li, Ruowei, Natalie Darling, Emmanuel Maurice, Lawrence Baker, and Laurence M. Grummer-Strawn. 2005. Breastfeeding rates in the United States by characteristics of the child, mother, or family: The 2002 National Immunization Study. *Pediatrics* 115 (1): e31-e37.

Mallory, George B., Jr., Debra H. Fiser, and Rodney Jackson. 1989. Sleep-associated breathing disorders in obese children and adolescents. *Journal of Pediatrics* 115:552-58.

Mayer-Davis, Elizabeth, Sheryl L. Rifas-Shiman, Li Zhan, Frank Hu, Graham A. Colditz, and Matthew W. Gillman. 2006. Breast-feeding and risk for childhood obesity: Does maternal diabetes or obesity status matter? *Diabetes Care* 29:2231-37.

Mieszkowski, Katharine. 2007. Breasts at work. *Salon.com*, August 22.

Mishra, Raja. 2006. Nursing mother's protest grows, nursing mother's complaint spurs plans to target Delta today, organizers target Delta today. *Boston Globe*, November 21, p. A1.

Morbidity and Mortality Weekly Report. 2003. Physical activity levels among children aged 9–13 years—United States, 2002. 52 (33): 785-88.

Morland, Kimberly, Ana V. Diez Roux, and Steve Wing. 2006. Supermarkets, other food stores, and obesity: The Atherosclerosis Risk in Communities Study. *American Journal of Preventive Medicine* 30 (4): 333-39.

Ogden, Cynthia L., Margaret D. Carroll, Lester R. Curtin, Margaret A. McDowell, Carolyn J. Tabak, and Katherine M. Flegal. 2006. Prevalence of overweight and obesity in the United States, 1999-2004. *Journal of the American Medical Association* 295:1549-55.

Oken, Emily, and Mathew W. Gillman. 2003. Fetal origins of obesity. *Obesity Research* 11:496-506.

Robert Wood Johnson Foundation. 2006. State action to promote nutrition, increase physical activity and prevent obesity. *Balance* 2:1-135. www.rwjf.org/pdf/Balance072006 (accessed August 29, 2007).

Robinson, Thomas N. 1999. Reducing children's television viewing to prevent obesity: A randomized controlled trial. *Journal of the American Medical Association* 282:1561-67.

Robinson, Thomas N., Joel D. Killen, Helena C. Kraemer, Darrell M. Wilson, Donna M. Matheson, William L. Haskell, Leslie A. Pruitt, Tiffany M. Powell, Ayisha S. Owens, Nikki S. Thompson, Natasha M. Flint-Moore, GeAndra J. Davis, Kara A. Emig, Rebecca T. Brown, James Rochon, Sarah Green, and Ann Varady. 2003. Dance and reducing television viewing to prevent weight gain in African-American girls: The Stanford GEMS pilot study. *Ethnicity and Disease* 13:S65-S77.

Schilling, Joseph, and Leslie S. Linton. 2005. The public health roots of zoning: In search of active living's legal genealogy. *American Journal of Preventative Medicine* 28 (2, Suppl. 2): 96-104.

Sturm, Roland, and Deborah A. Cohen. 2004. Suburban sprawl and physical and mental health. *Public Health* 118 (7): 488-96.

Sturm, Roland, Jeanne S. Ringel, and Tatiana Andreyeva. 2004. Increasing obesity rates and disability trends. *Health Affairs* 23:199-205.

Taylor, Erica D., Kelly R. Theim, Margaret C. Mirch, Samareh Ghorbani, Marian Tanofsky-Kraff, Diane C. Adler-Wailes, Sheila Brady, James C. Reynolds, Karim A. Calis, and Jack A. Yanovski. 2006. Orthopedic complications of overweight in children and adolescents. *Pediatrics* 117:2167-74.

U.S. Census Bureau. 2007. U.S. POPClock Projection. http://www.census.gov/population/www/popclockus .html (accessed August 11, 2007).

U.S. Congress. House. 2004. Committee on Education and the Workforce. The Child Nutrition and WIC Reauthorization Act Update. July. http://edworkforce.house.gov/democrats/hr3873cnupdate.html.

U.S. Department of Agriculture. 2007. Loving your family, feeding their future. http://foodstamp.nal.usda .gov/naldiplay (accessed August 28, 2007).

U.S. Department of Health and Human Services, Public Health Service, Office of the Surgeon General. 2001. *The Surgeon General's call to action to prevent and decrease overweight and obesity.* Washington, DC: Government Printing Office. http://www.surgeongeneral.gov/topics/obesity/calltoaction/fact_ glance.htm (accessed August 11, 2007).

Wagget, Gordon G., and Rega Richardson Waggett. 1995. Breast is best: Legislation supporting breast-feeding is an absolute bare necessity—A model approach. *Maryland Journal of Contemporary Issues* 6:71.

Wang, Guijing, and William H. Dietz. 2002. Economic burden of obesity in youths aged 6 to 17 years: 1979-1999. *Pediatrics* 109 (5): E81-E86.

Whelan, Brianne. 2005. Comment: For crying out loud: Ohio's legal battle with public breastfeeding and hope for the future. *American University Journal of Gender, Social Policy & the Law* 13:669.

Wiecha, Jean L., Alison M. El Ayadi, Bernard F. Fuemmeler, Jill E. Carter, Shirley Handler, Stacy Johnson, Nancy Strunk, Debra Korzec-Ramirez, and Steven L. Gortmaker. 2004. Diffusion of an integrated health education program in an urban school system: Planet Health. *Journal of Pediatric Psychology* 29 (6): 467-74.

World Health Organization. 2003. *Global strategy for infant and young child feeding.* Geneva, Switzerland: World Health Organization.

http://www.who.int/child-adolescent-health/New_Publications/NUTRITION/gs_iycf.pdf (accessed August 25, 2007).

Wrotniak, Brian H., Leonard H. Epstein, Rocco A. Paluch, and James A. Roemmich. 2005. The relationship between parent and child self-reported adherence and weight loss. *Obesity Research* 13 (6): 1089-95.

Zenk, Shannon N., Amy J. Schulz, Barbara A. Israel, Sherman A. James, Shuming Bao, and Mark L. Wilson. 2005. Neighborhood racial composition, neighborhood poverty, and the spatial accessibility of supermarkets in metropolitan Detroit. *American Journal of Public Health* 95 (4): 660-67.

SECTION TWO

Media and Culture

The Effects of Food Marketing on Children's Preferences: Testing the Moderating Roles of Age and Gender

By
ARIEL CHERNIN

A large body of research suggests that food marketing affects children's food preferences, short- and long-term dietary consumption, and purchase requests directed to parents. It is frequently argued that younger children are more susceptible to marketers' messages than older children because they do not understand the persuasive nature of advertising; however, little direct evidence supports this claim. Employing an experimental design, this study examined the influence of food marketing on children's preferences and tested whether age (and gender) moderated the effects of ad exposure. The sample consisted of 133 children between the ages of five and eleven. Results indicated that exposure to food commercials increased children's preferences for the advertised products. Age did not moderate this effect; younger and older children were equally persuaded by the commercials. Boys were more influenced by the commercials than girls. Implications for the study of food marketing to children are discussed.

Keywords: food marketing; advertising; children; persuasion

The authors of several large-scale literature reviews have concluded that exposure to food marketing affects children's food preferences and eating behavior (Hastings et al. 2003; Institute of Medicine 2006; Livingstone and Helsper 2004; Office of Communication [Ofcom] 2004; World Health Organization 2003; see Paliwoda and Crawford [2003] and Young [2003] for a more critical interpretation of the research literature). For example, the Institute of Medicine (2006) argued that there is "strong evidence" that commercials shape children's food preferences and short-term eating habits and increase the number of purchase requests children direct to parents. Similarly, Hastings et al. (2003) stated that food marketing "*can*

NOTE: This publication was made possible by grant number 5P50CA095856-04 from the National Cancer Institute. Its contents are solely the responsibility of the author and do not necessarily represent the official views of the National Cancer Institute.

DOI: 10.1177/0002716207308952

have and *is* having an effect on children, particularly in the areas of food preferences, purchase behavior, and consumption. It is also clear that these effects are significant, independent of other influences and operate at both brand and category level" (p. 182). It is also frequently suggested that children younger than eight years old are more susceptible to advertising than older children because they lack knowledge of persuasive intent; that is, they do not understand that commercials try to convince people to buy things (American Academy of Pediatrics 1995; Federal Trade Commission 1978; Institute of Medicine 2005; Kunkel et al. 2004). While knowledge of persuasive intent tends to increase with age (e.g., Blosser and Roberts 1985; Robertson and Rossiter 1974; Ward, Wackman, and Wartella 1977), little direct evidence supports the claim that younger children are inherently more persuasible than older children (Christenson 1985; Livingstone and Helsper 2004, 2006). This study examines the influence of food marketing on product preference and tests whether age and gender moderate any observed effects.

Background

A large body of research suggests that food marketing affects children's preferences, short- and long-term dietary consumption, and purchase requests. Both preference and short-term dietary consumption studies frequently employ experimental designs and examine the effect of exposure to advertising on product choice. These two types of studies differ, however, with respect to their operationalization of the dependent variable. In preference studies, children are typically asked to choose their favorite food(s) from a series of pictures, while in short-term dietary consumption studies, children's actual eating behavior is used as an indicator of choice (e.g., children select and eat a snack). In long-term dietary consumption research, children's exposure to food marketing is often linked to parent reports of children's regular eating habits. Purchase request studies examine the relationship between food marketing and children's requests for advertised products directed to parents. Research in each of these areas is reviewed below, beginning with the effects of food marketing on children's product preferences.

In Borzekowski and Robinson's (2001) widely cited study, children between the ages of two and six years old watched a television show with a series of food commercials or the same show without commercials. Children were then

Ariel Chernin is a postdoctoral fellow at the Center on Media and Child Health, Children's Hospital Boston, Division of Adolescent Medicine. She received her Ph.D. in communication from the Annenberg School for Communication at the University of Pennsylvania. This article presents research conducted as part of her dissertation, which was supervised by Dr. Robert Hornik. Her research interests include the effects of food marketing on children's eating habits, the link between media exposure and adolescents' sexual behavior, and the development and evaluation of media literacy curricula.

presented with pairs of similar products in picture form and asked to identify which of the two products they preferred in each pair (one product in each pair had been featured in the commercials). Borzekowski and Robinson found that the children who were exposed to the commercials selected the advertised products significantly more often than the children who did not see the commercials.

Goldberg, Gorn, and Gibson (1978) randomly assigned first-graders to watch a cartoon with either a series of commercials for highly sweetened snack and breakfast foods or several public service announcements (PSAs) promoting nutritious eating (a control group that did not watch television was also included in the study). All children were subsequently asked to choose several snacks and breakfast food items from a series of images of sugared and healthier options. Goldberg, Gorn, and Gibson reported that children who saw the commercials selected significantly more sugared foods than children who saw the PSAs or did not watch television.

Several studies have assessed food choice by directly observing children's eating behavior (e.g., Auty and Lewis 2004; Galst 1980; Gorn and Goldberg 1982; Jeffrey, McLellarn, and Fox 1982). In Gorn and Goldberg's (1982) two-week field experiment, children between the ages of five and eight years old watched a series of cartoons embedded with one of three types of ads: candy commercials, fruit commercials, or pronutrition PSAs. A fourth group of children watched the TV shows without ads. After each viewing session, children chose two snacks from a selection of two fruits and two candies that had appeared in the commercials. Gorn and Goldberg found that the children who saw the candy commercials consumed significantly more candy than children in the other three conditions.

In Resnik and Stern's (1977) experiment, children watched a television show either with or without a commercial for an unfamiliar brand of potato chips and were then invited to choose one of two brands of potato chips to take home with them. Children who had seen the potato chip commercial were significantly more likely to select the advertised brand of potato chips than children in the control group.

Evidence also suggests that food marketing influences children's regular dietary intake (Bolton 1983; Boynton-Jarrett et al. 2003; French et al. 2001; Gracey et al. 1996; Phillips et al. 2004; Utter et al. 2003; Wiecha et al. 2006; Woodward et al. 1997). With the exception of Bolton (1983), however, these studies correlated overall television viewing with indicators of diet. Thus, behaviors associated with television viewing, such as eating while watching TV (e.g., Matheson et al. 2004), or the influence of television content other than advertising may explain the observed relationship between television exposure and diet. Similarly, a large body of literature links television exposure to childhood overweight (e.g., Andersen et al. 1998; Dietz and Gortmaker 1985; Gortmaker et al. 1996; Hancox, Milne, and Poulton 2004), and exposure to food marketing is only one of several possible mechanisms that may explain the association (Henderson 2006; Kaiser Family Foundation 2004).

Rather than use overall television viewing as proxy for exposure to food marketing, Bolton (1983) combined TV diaries completed by parents and TV station broadcasting logs to create a measure of children's exposure to food commercials. Bolton found that exposure to food ads was positively associated with snacking and the consumption of low-nutrient, high-calorie foods (as captured by a seven-day food diary). Interestingly, Bolton's results indicated that parents' eating behavior had a much stronger influence on children's diets than advertising.[1]

Finally, numerous studies point to a link between children's exposure to food marketing and purchase requests directed at parents (Brody et al. 1981; Donkin, Neale, and Tilston 1993; Galst and White 1976; Isler, Popper, and Ward 1987; Stoneman and Brody 1982; Taras et al. 1989, 2000). Similar to the long-term dietary consumption studies, overall television exposure is often correlated with the number of children's requests for advertised foods (Donkin, Neale, and Tilston 1993; Isler, Popper, and Ward 1987). It is therefore possible (although unlikely) that depictions of characters eating and drinking, rather than advertising, led to children's purchase requests. It is also possible that a third variable, such as parenting style, accounted for both children's television viewing and the frequency of their purchase requests. The methods employed also make it difficult to establish a direct link between exposure to a commercial and requests for the specific product and brand featured in the ad.

Supporting the theory that food advertising—and not other forms of television content—drives children's purchase requests is Galst and White's (1976) study in which preschoolers and their parents were observed shopping in a supermarket. Galst and White identified a positive correlation between the number of purchase requests children directed to parents and the number of hours per week children spent watching commercial television at home (as reported by parents), while the correlation between the number of requests and overall television viewing (which included exposure to noncommercial programming such as PBS) was not statistically significant.

Perhaps the strongest evidence for an effect of food marketing on children's purchase requests comes from Stoneman and Brody's (1982) experiment conducted with preschoolers. Children watched a television show with or without food commercials and then participated in a simulated shopping trip with their mothers. Children exposed to the commercials requested significantly more products than children who did not see the commercials and requested a greater number of products that had been featured in the ads.

Moderating Effect of Age

While the literature generally shows a positive effect of food marketing on children's preferences and behavior, demographic factors may moderate the effects of advertising. Age is frequently cited as a moderator, and it is often assumed that younger children are more susceptible to advertising than older children because they lack knowledge of persuasive intent (American Academy of Pediatrics 1995; Federal Trade Commission 1978; Institute of Medicine 2005; Kunkel et al. 2004). While knowledge of persuasive intent generally increases with age (Blosser and Roberts 1985; Robertson and Rossiter 1974; Ward, Wackman, and Wartella 1977), there is little conclusive evidence to support the assertion that younger children are more vulnerable to advertisers' messages than older children (Christenson 1985; Livingstone and Helsper 2004, 2006).

While the literature generally shows a positive effect of food marketing on children's preferences and behavior, demographic factors may moderate the effects of advertising.

In the food marketing literature, most studies have been conducted with samples that cover very narrow age ranges (e.g., preschoolers, first-graders, etc.; Livingstone and Helsper 2004, 2006), making it impossible to test an interaction between ad exposure and age. As a result, the moderating effect of age has been largely inferred from comparisons between different studies conducted with separate populations of children. This is problematic because differences in study design, stimuli, and measures limit one's ability to make valid inferences. After reviewing the literature, Livingstone and Helsper (2004) tentatively concluded that *older* children and teenagers are more influenced by food advertising than younger children. Livingstone and Helsper justified this claim by noting that studies conducted with older children and teens consistently report significant effects of advertising exposure on product preference, while the results among samples of younger children are more mixed. The authors also acknowledged, however, that measures of food choice may be less valid and reliable when administered to younger children. The Institute of Medicine (2006, 294) adopted a more conservative stance, stating that "age has not been found to be a consistent moderator of advertising effects on precursors of diet." Given this lack of evidence, it is somewhat surprising that scholars continue to argue that younger children are more vulnerable to advertising than older children.

Moderating Effects of Gender

Gender has also been proposed as a potential moderator of advertising effects, although there is little theoretical justification for such a claim (Institute of

Medicine 2006).[2] Nonetheless, several researchers have sought to determine if boys and girls are differentially affected by food marketing. In Pine and Nash's (2003) observational study of preschoolers, girls expressed greater preferences for heavily advertised, branded products than boys; however, this does not conclusively demonstrate that girls were more persuaded by the advertising for the products than boys.

Jeffrey, McLellarn, and Fox (1982) randomly assigned four- and five-year-olds to watch a children's television show embedded with commercials for one of three types of products: foods low in nutritional value, foods high in nutritional value, or toys (control condition). Children were then invited to eat as much as they wanted of twelve foods that had been featured in the low- and high-nutrition commercials. While the main effect of the control condition on the amount and type of food consumed was not significant, Jeffrey, McLellarn, and Fox identified a significant interaction between gender and the control condition such that boys exposed to the low-nutrition ads consumed more low-nutrition food and more food overall than girls who had seen low nutrition ads, and boys and girls in the two other conditions.

Summary

A large body of literature indicates that exposure to food marketing affects children's food preferences, their short-term eating behavior, and purchase requests directed to parents. Food marketing also likely affects long-term dietary consumption and may contribute to childhood obesity. While it is frequently argued that younger children are inherently more susceptible to advertising than older children, surprisingly little research supports this claim. There is also minimal evidence that gender moderates the effects of marketing.

While it is frequently argued that younger children are inherently more susceptible to advertising than older children, surprisingly little research supports this claim. There is also minimal evidence that gender moderates the effects of marketing.

The present study examined the influence of two commercials—one for Sprinkle Spangles cereal, the other for Tang—on children's product preferences.

Sprinkle Spangles cereal was introduced by General Mills in 1994 and discontinued shortly thereafter. This product was selected because it was originally marketed to children but was unfamiliar to the participants. Tang is an orange-flavored, powdered drink mix first marketed in the 1950s by Kraft Foods. While Tang is currently available in stores, the commercial itself was likely unfamiliar to most of the participants because it aired during the mid-1990s.

Based on previous research, it was expected that exposure to the commercials would result in increased preferences for the advertised products.

> *Hypothesis 1:* Children exposed to a commercial will display greater preference for the advertised product than children who did not see the commercial.

While both commercials were expected to influence preferences, the study examined the relative persuasiveness of the Sprinkle Spangles and Tang commercials.

> *Research Question 1:* Is the effect of ad exposure on product preference similar for the Sprinkle Spangles and Tang commercials?

The present study also tested whether age and gender moderated the effects of ad exposure on product preference.

> *Research Question 2:* Does age moderate the effects of exposure to advertising on product preference?
> *Research Question 3:* Does gender moderate the effects of exposure to advertising on product preference?

Method

Sample[3]

Kindergarteners through fourth-graders were recruited from two elementary schools in suburban Philadelphia. Consent forms were distributed to all students in kindergarten through fourth grade at both schools. At the first school, 79 out of a possible 263 consent forms were returned, yielding a response rate of 30 percent. At the second school, 54 out of a possible 239 consent forms were returned, a 22.6 percent response rate. Each school received $10 for every child who returned a consent form.[4]

The total sample consisted of 133 children ranging in age from five to eleven years old ($M = 8.18$ years, $SD = 1.45$). Among the 132 children for whom age data was available, 6.8 percent were five years old, 20.5 percent six years old, 18.2 percent seven years old, 24.2 percent eight years old, 15.9 percent nine years old, and 14.4 percent ten or eleven years old.[5] The sample was 60.2 percent female. With regard to race, for the 98.5 percent ($n = 131$) of children for whom race data was available, 67.9 percent were white non-Hispanic, 13.7 percent black non-Hispanic, 8.4 percent Hispanic, and 9.9 percent "other."

The study protocol was approved by the University of Pennsylvania's institutional review board, and both parental consent (written) and child assent (verbal or written, depending on the age of the child) were obtained before testing began.

Design and Procedure

The study design was a single-factor between-subjects experiment.[6] Participants were randomly assigned, stratified by grade level and gender, to view either the Sprinkle Spangles commercial or the Tang commercial. After securing children's assent to participate in the study, an expressive vocabulary test was administered. Approximately two weeks later, participants watched a thirteen-minute segment of *Foster's Home for Imaginary Friends*, an animated television series airing on the Cartoon Network. The segment was embedded with one of the two experimental commercials, in addition to the ads that originally aired during the episode. The experimental commercial the child was assigned to was seen twice, once during the first commercial break and once during the second commercial break. Participants viewed the stimuli on individual laptops, wearing headphones. Participants then completed several measures related to the television show and the products featured in the ads. The final measure consisted of asking children if they had heard of Tang prior to participating in the study.

Parents completed a brief survey that requested information about family demographics, their child's television viewing and knowledge of advertising, and parent-child conversations about advertising. The present study makes use of only the demographic data. Parents returned 107 of 133 surveys, yielding a response rate of 80.5 percent. The likelihood of returning the survey did not vary as a function of the child's age or gender.

Measures

Expressive vocabulary

Children's expressive vocabulary was assessed with the Expressive One-Word Picture Vocabulary Test–2000 (EOWPVT-2000; Brownell 2000). Brownell (2000) reported a three-week test-retest correlation of .91, and EOWPVT scores are positively associated with other measures of expressive and receptive vocabulary (Beery and Taheri 1992). The EOWPVT can be used with children between the ages of two and eighteen, and raw scores have a possible range of 0 to 170 points. The mean expressive vocabulary score was 78.5 points ($SD = 21.2$), and the two experimental groups were not significantly different from one another with regard to vocabulary, $t(131) = -.47$, $p = .64$.

Distracter questions

Children were asked the following questions about *Foster's Home for Imaginary Friends*: Did you like the show? (Why or why not?) What do you think is going to happen next? Who was your favorite character or person on the show? These questions were used to distract children from the true purpose of the study and are not used in the present analyses.

Product preference

Two product preference measures were created, one for each of the advertised products. All participants completed both measures, one associated with the product they had seen in the experimental commercial, the other associated with the product they had not seen advertised. The responses associated with the nonviewed ad provided an estimate of baseline product preference, that is, preference absent the influence of advertising. The baseline, or control group, responses for a given product were compared to those provided by children who had seen the commercial for the product to estimate the effects of exposure to the ad on preference.

For each measure, the advertised product was compared to three alternatives in the same product category. Sprinkle Spangles was compared to three other sweetened cereals (Hidden Treasures,[7] Frosted Chex, and Golden Grahams), and Tang was compared to three other orange-flavored drink mixes (Richfood Orange Overload, Orange Gatorade, and Orange Kool-Aid). The products were evaluated using paired comparisons, a method where each item is matched with every other item and participants then choose one item in each pair (Thurstone 1927; Woodworth and Schlosberg 1955). In the present study, each measure consisted of four products being compared to one another (one of which was the advertised product), resulting in a total of six comparisons per measure.[8]

For each preference measure, children were presented with the six comparisons in random order. Each comparison featured color pictures of the two products being evaluated. The question wording for the Sprinkle Spangles measure was, "If you could eat one of these two cereals for breakfast tomorrow, which one would you choose?" The wording for the Tang measure was, "If you could have a glass of one of these two drinks, which one would you choose?"

The dependent variable in the analyses below captured the number of times the advertised product was chosen over a competitor. For each measure, the advertised product appeared in three of the six comparisons (i.e., the advertised product compared to each of the three alternatives). Thus, the scores for each advertised product had a possible range of 0 (product was not chosen over a competitor in any of the three comparisons in which it appeared) to 3 (product was chosen over a competitor in all three of the comparisons in which it appeared).

Prior familiarity with Tang

Children were shown a picture of Tang and asked, "Before today, had you ever heard of Tang?" There was no significant difference in Tang familiarity between the two conditions. Among children randomly assigned to view the Tang commercial, 31 percent of children had heard of Tang, while 29 percent of children assigned to the view the Sprinkle Spangles commercial had heard of Tang, $t(130) = -.26$, $p = .79$.[9]

Analytic Approach

To evaluate the hypotheses and research questions, the original data set was reshaped such that each child contributed two cases: one for the commercial to which he or she was exposed and one for the commercial to which he or she was not exposed. Or, put another way, each child contributed two observations: one associated with the Sprinkle Spangles commercial and one associated with the Tang commercial. Each case provided responses for three main variables (in addition to covariates): (1) the commercial to which the case referred, (2) whether the child had been exposed to that commercial, and (3) the child's preference for the product featured in that commercial. Ordinary least squares (OLS) regression was used to determine if exposure to advertising resulted in increased preferences for the advertised products (Hypothesis 1). Research Question 1, which compared the persuasiveness of the two commercials, was tested by adding a product term to the model (Ad Exposure × Ad). Research Questions 2 and 3, which addressed interactions between ad exposure and age and gender, respectively, were also examined by adding product terms to the regression model. For all analyses, standard errors were adjusted for nonindependence resulting from the fact that each child contributed two observations to the data set.

Results

Hypothesis 1, which predicted an overall positive effect of exposure to commercials on product preference, was supported. Exposure to the commercials was positively (and significantly) associated with preference for the advertised product (see Table 1). The main effect of age was not statistically significant. Thus, younger and older children exhibited similar preferences for the products. Gender was also largely uncorrelated with preference. The significant coefficient associated with the "ad" variable indicates that preference for Sprinkle Spangles (coded as 1) was greater than preference for Tang (coded as 0) irrespective of exposure to the commercials.

The relative persuasiveness of the two commercials (Research Question 1) was examined by testing an interaction between ad exposure and the ad variable. The product term was not statistically significant ($B = -.15$, robust $SE = .22$, $p = .51$), suggesting that the two commercials were equally persuasive.

Research Question 2 addressed an interaction between ad exposure and age. The product term was not statistically significant ($B = .07$, robust $SE = .07$, $p = .36$), indicating that younger and older children were equally persuaded by the commercials.[10] Research Question 3 examined the interaction between ad exposure and gender. The product term was statistically significant ($B = -.48$, robust $SE = .22$, $p = .03$), and the negative coefficient indicates that boys (coded as 0) were more influenced by the commercials than girls (coded as 1).[11] The interaction is displayed in Figure 1.

Discussion

Exposure to commercials significantly increased children's preferences for the advertised products, and these effects were comparable for the Sprinkle Spangles

TABLE 1
EFFECT OF EXPOSURE TO ADVERTISING ON PRODUCT PREFERENCE

Variable[a]	B	Robust SE
Exposure to advertising	.33**	.11
Ad (Tang = 0; Sprinkle Spangles = 1)	.45***	.11
Age	−.02	.05
Gender (boys = 0; girls = 1)	.06	.11
Race[b]		
Black	.02	.16
Hispanic	.02	.15
Other	−.001	.21
Vocabulary	−.002	.003
Ad Exposure × Ad	−.15	.22
Ad Exposure × Age	.07	.07
Ad Expo]sure × Gender	−.48*	.22
Adjusted R-squared = .10[c]		

a. Main effects calculated without interaction terms in model.
b. Reference category = white.
c. R-squared is for model without interactions.
*$p \leq .05$. **$p \leq .01$. ***$p \leq .001$.

and Tang commercials. The products appealed equally to younger and older children, and there was no evidence of an interaction between ad exposure and age on product preference. As a result, the present findings do not support the claim that younger children are inherently more persuasible than older children. It is frequently argued that younger children lack of knowledge of persuasive intent, a deficit that predisposes them to accept advertisers' messages. If, however, younger and older children are equally persuaded by food marketing, the importance of knowledge of persuasive intent in the persuasion process is called into question.

The present findings do not support the claim that younger children are inherently more persuasible than older children.

It has been suggested that children's affective responses to marketing may play a more important role in the persuasion process than cognitive factors such as knowledge of persuasive intent and skepticism toward advertising (Christenson

FIGURE 1
INTERACTION BETWEEN AD EXPOSURE AND GENDER
ON PRODUCT PREFERENCE

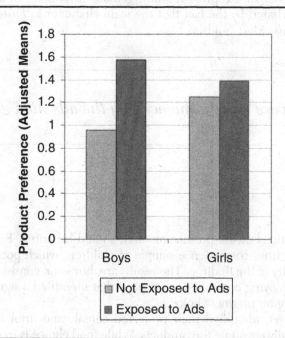

NOTE: The product preference measure captures the average number of times children selected the advertised product over one of the three competitors. Scores have a possible range of 0 to 3. Values are adjusted for demographic characteristics other than gender.

1985; Wartella 1984; Young 1990). Wartella (1984, 181) commented that "there is substantial reason to argue that for too long research on television advertising's influence on children has focused on rational cognitive-oriented approach to studying children's information processing of advertising messages." Future research should examine the relationship between children's emotional responses to advertising and their preferences for advertised products, as well as the relative contributions of affective and cognitive variables in explaining persuasion outcomes.

While age did not moderate the effects of ad exposure, a significant interaction between exposure to the commercials and gender was detected. Boys were more influenced by the ads than girls. This was somewhat surprising given that the products were not strongly gendered (as evidenced by the absence of a main effect of gender of product preference) and both boys and girls were featured in both commercials. One possible explanation for this result is that boys paid more attention to the commercials than girls and this increased attention resulted in greater receptivity to the persuasive appeals. While the present study did not assess children's attention to the ads, research suggests that boys allocate more visual attention to television than girls (Alvarez et al. 1988; Rolandelli et al. 1991; Wright et al. 1984). In the present study, gender differences in attention may have been exacerbated by the fact that the main character in *Foster's Home for Imaginary Friends*, Mac, is a boy.

Boys were more influenced by the ads than girls.

Limitations

Several limitations of the present research should be noted. First, the study was conducted with a convenience sample of children, which potentially limits the generalizability of the findings. The results are, however, consistent with prior studies (also employing convenience samples) that identified a significant effect of food marketing on product choice.

Second, children identified their preferred cereals and drinks from images and did not actually consume the products. While food choice is frequently operationalized as preference (e.g., Borzekowski and Robinson 2001; Goldberg, Gorn, and Gibson 1978; Gorn and Goldberg 1980), it is unclear if the opinions children expressed will persist and translate into behavior. The preference measures can potentially be viewed as indicators of intention to consume a product relative to other choices, and research testing the Theory of Reasoned Action (Ajzen and Fishbein 1980; Fishbein and Ajzen 1975) with children suggests that intention predicts subsequent behavior (Morrison et al. 2002, 1996; Norman and Tedeschi 1989; Otis et al. 1992). In contrast, however, Jeffrey, McLellarn, and Fox (1982) found that children's verbalized food preferences were only moderately correlated with behavioral measures of food consumption.

Third, it is potentially problematic that Tang was available in stores at the time the study was conducted. Prior familiarity with and preexisting attitudes toward Tang may have influenced children's choices; however, random assignment should have ensured that the groups exposed and not exposed to the ad were equivalent in these regards. In addition, analyses indicated that familiarity with Tang was not significantly different across the two commercial conditions.

Finally, it should be noted that the regression model explained only a small amount of variance in product preference. The model likely omitted variables that could have contributed additional explanatory power. This again points to the need to examine children's affective responses to advertising.

Conclusion

Consistent with prior research, the present study found that exposure to food marketing significantly increased children's preferences for advertised products. While it is often argued that younger children are more persuasible than older children, the results indicated that age did not moderate the effects of ad exposure on product preference. This suggests that knowledge of persuasive intent did not influence children's responses to the commercials. Future research should explicitly test the moderating role of knowledge of persuasive intent in the persuasion process and examine how children's affective responses to commercials influence their preferences for advertised products.

Public policy in the area of food marketing to children should be based on strong empirical evidence. While efforts to restrict advertising to young children are well intentioned (e.g., Kunkel et al. 2004), it has yet to be conclusively demonstrated that younger children are inherently more persuasible than older children. In fact, given that older children have more control over their diets than younger children, perhaps older children's responses to food marketing should be of greater concern. Media literacy education is a possible avenue for intervention that can be tailored to children of different ages.

Notes

1. As both Hastings et al. (2003) and Livingstone and Helsper (2004) noted, the magnitude of the effect of food marketing relative to other potential influences on children's preferences and behavior has yet to be conclusively determined.

2. Commercials for products that appeal strongly to one gender will likely be more persuasive among children of that gender; however, this is a function of the product itself and not the result of differential advertising effects.

3. Demographic information was obtained from the parent survey. For cases where the parent survey was not returned, the child's date of birth was obtained from the consent form and gender and race were observed by the interviewer. One child's (0.8 percent) age was coded as missing (the date of birth entered on the consent form was incorrect). For two participants (1.5 percent), race was coded as missing because it could not easily be inferred by observation.

4. Schools were asked to use the stipends to advance the education of students.

5. Only one child was eleven years old at pretest.

6. The study had a second experimental factor that was excluded from the analyses. Children were also randomly assigned to view either a brief media literacy video or a control video of equal length. Inclusion of the second factor as a control variable did not change the present results; it was therefore omitted to simplify the presentation of the study design. Results pertaining to the effects of exposure to the media literacy video are detailed elsewhere (Chernin 2007).

7. This cereal, like Sprinkle Spangles, was introduced in the mid-1990s and discontinued shortly thereafter.

8. Product A vs. product B; product A vs. product C; product A vs. product D; product B vs. product C; product B vs. product D; product C vs. product D.

9. It is possible that children falsely claimed to have heard of Tang, but there was no way to confirm this. In hindsight, it would have been useful to have asked the same familiarity question in reference to Sprinkle Spangles (an unfamiliar product) to assess children's tendency to respond affirmatively regardless of the question.

10. A three-way interaction between ad exposure, age, and ad was tested, but the coefficient was not statistically significant ($p = .28$).

11. A three-way interaction between ad exposure, gender, and ad was tested, but the coefficient was not statistically significant ($p = .14$). The Ad Exposure × Gender interaction was somewhat more pronounced for the Tang ad, but it was not a statistically significant difference.

References

Ajzen, Icek, and Martin Fishbein. 1980. *Understanding attitudes and predicting social behavior.* Englewood Cliffs, NJ: Prentice Hall.

Alvarez, Mildred M., Aletha C. Huston, John C. Wright, and Dennis D. Kerkman. 1988. Gender differences in visual attention to television form and content. *Journal of Applied Developmental Psychology* 9:459-75.

American Academy of Pediatrics, Committee on Communications. 1995. Children, adolescents, and advertising. *Pediatrics* 95:295-97.

Andersen, Ross E., Carlos J. Crespo, Susan J. Bartlett, Lawrence J. Cheskin, and Michael Pratt. 1998. Relationship of physical activity and television watching with bodyweight and level of fatness among children. *Journal of the American Medical Association* 279:938-42.

Auty, Susan, and Charlie Lewis. 2004. Exploring children's choice: The reminder effect of product placement. *Psychology and Marketing* 21:697–714.

Beery, Keith E., and Colleen M. Taheri. 1992. *Beery Picture Vocabulary Test.* Odessa, FL: Psychological Assessment Resources.

Blosser, Betsy J., and Donald F. Roberts. 1985. Age differences in children's perceptions of message intent. *Communication Research* 12:455-84.

Bolton, Ruth N. 1983. Modeling the impact of television food advertising on children's diets. *Current Issues and Research in Advertising* 6:173-99.

Borzekowski, Dina L. G., and Thomas N. Robinson. 2001. The 30-second effect: An experiment revealing the impact of television commercials on food preferences of preschoolers. *Journal of the American Dietetic Association* 101:42-46.

Boynton-Jarrett, Renee, Tracy N. Thomas, Karen E. Peterson, Jean Wiecha, Arthur M. Sobol, and Steven L. Gortmaker. 2003. Impact of television viewing patterns on fruit and vegetable consumption among adolescents. *Pediatrics* 112:1321-26.

Brody, Gene H., Zolinda Stoneman, T. Scott Lane, and Alice K. Sanders. 1981. Television food commercials aimed at children, family grocery shopping, and mother-child interactions. *Family Relations* 30:435-39.

Brownell, Rick. 2000. *Expressive One-Word Picture Vocabulary Test.* Novato, CA: Academic Therapy.

Chernin, Ariel. 2007. The relationship between children's knowledge of persuasive intent and persuasion: The case of televised food marketing. Ph.D. diss., University of Pennsylvania, Philadelphia.

Christenson, Peter G. 1985. Children and commercials: The relationship between general trust and specific influence. *Communication Research Reports* 2:41-45.

Dietz, William H., and Steven L. Gortmaker. 1985. Do we fatten our children at the television set? Obesity and television viewing in children and adolescents. *Pediatrics* 75:807-12.

Donkin, Angela J. M., R. J. Neale, and C. Tilston. 1993. Children's food purchase requests. *Appetite* 21:291-94.

Federal Trade Commission. 1978. *FTC staff report on television advertising to children.* Washington, DC: Federal Trade Commission.

Fishbein, Martin, and Icek Ajzen. 1975. *Belief, attitude, intention and behavior: An introduction to theory and research.* Reading, MA: Addison-Wesley.

French, S. A., M. Story, D. Neumark-Sztainer, J. A. Fulkerson, and P. Hannan. 2001. Fast food restaurant use among adolescents: Associations with nutrient intake, food choices and behavioral and psychosocial variables. *International Journal of Obesity* 25:1823-33.

Galst, Joann Paley. 1980. Television commercials and pronutritional public service announcements as determinants of young children's snack choices. *Child Development* 51:935-38.

Galst, Joann Paley, and Mary Alice White. 1976. The unhealthy persuader: The reinforcing value of television and children's purchase-influencing attempts at the supermarket. *Child Development* 47:1089-96.

Goldberg, Marvin E., Gerald J. Gorn, and Wendy Gibson. 1978. TV messages for snack and breakfast foods: Do they influence children's preferences? *Journal of Consumer Research* 5:73-81.

Gorn, Gerald J., and Marvin E. Goldberg. 1980. Children's responses to repetitive TV commercials. *Journal of Consumer Research* 6:421-24.

————. 1982. Behavioral evidence of the effects of televised food messages on children. *Journal of Consumer Research* 9:200-205.

Gortmaker, Steven L., A. Must, A. M. Sobol, K. Peterson, G. A. Colditz, and W. H. Dietz. 1996. Television viewing as a cause of increasing obesity among children in the United States, 1986-1990. *Archives of Pediatrics and Adolescent Medicine* 150:356-62.

Gracey, D., N. Stanley, V. Burke, B. Corti, and L. J. Beilin. 1996. Nutritional knowledge, beliefs and behaviours in teenage school students. *Health Education Research* 11:187-204.

Hancox, Robert J., Barry J. Milne, and Richie Poulton. 2004. Association between child and adolescent television viewing and adult health: A longitudinal birth cohort study. *The Lancet* 364:257-62.

Hastings, Gerard, Martine Stead, Laura McDermott, Alasdair Forsyth, Anne Marie MacKintosh, Mike Rayner, Christine Godfrey, Martin Caraher, and Kathryn Angus. 2003. *Review of research on the effects of food promotion to children: Final report*. Glasgow, UK: Centre for Social Marketing.

Henderson, Vani R. 2006. Investigating TV viewing and overweight in pre-adolescent and adolescent girls. Ph.D. diss., University of Pennsylvania, Philadelphia.

Institute of Medicine. 2005. *Preventing childhood obesity: Health in the balance*. Washington, DC: National Academies Press.

————. 2006. *Food marketing to children and youth: Threat or opportunity?* Washington, DC: National Academies Press.

Isler, Leslie, Edward T. Popper, and Scott Ward. 1987. Children's purchase requests and parental responses: Results from a diary study. *Journal of Advertising Research* 27:28-39.

Jeffrey, D. Balfour, Robert W. McLellarn, and Daniel T. Fox. 1982. The development of children's eating habits: The role of television commercials. *Health Education Quarterly* 9:78-93.

Kaiser Family Foundation. 2004. *The role of media in childhood obesity*. Menlo Park, CA: Kaiser Family Foundation.

Kunkel, Dale, Brian L. Wilcox, Joanne Cantor, Edward Palmer, Susan Linn, and Peter Dowrick. 2004. *Report of the APA task force on advertising and children: Psychological issues in the increasing commercialization of childhood*. Available at http://www.apa.org/releases/childrenads/pdf#search=%22FTC%20report%201978&20advertising%22.

Livingstone, Sonia, and Ellen Helsper. 2004. *Advertising "unhealthy" foods to children: Understanding promotion in the context of children's daily lives*. London: Ofcom.

————. 2006. Does advertising literacy mediate the effects of advertising on children? A critical examination of two linked research literatures in relation to obesity and food choice. *Journal of Communication* 56:560-84.

Matheson, Donna M., Joel D. Killen, Yun Wang, Ann Varady, and Thomas N. Robinson. 2004. Children's food consumption during television viewing. *American Journal of Clinical Nutrition* 79:1088-94.

Morrison, Diane M., Corinne M. Mar, Elizabeth A. Wells, Mary Rogers Gillmore, Marilyn J. Hoppe, Anthony Wildson, Elise Murowchick, and Matthew E. Archibald. 2002. The Theory of Reasoned Action as a model of children's health behavior. *Journal of Applied Social Psychology* 32:2266-95.

Morrison, Diane M., Edith E. Simpson, Mary Rogers Gillmore, Elizabeth A. Wells, and Marilyn J. Hoppe. 1996. Children's decisions about substance use: An application and extension of the Theory of Reasoned Action. *Journal of Applied Social Psychology* 26:1658-79.

Norman, Nancy M., and James T. Tedeschi. 1989. Self-presentation, reasoned action and adolescents' decisions to smoke cigarettes. *Journal of Applied Social Psychology* 19:543-58.

Office of Communications (Ofcom). 2004. *Childhood obesity: Food advertising in context*. London: Ofcom.

Otis, Joanne, Dominique Lesage, Gaston Godin, Bruce Brown, Celine Farley, and Jean Lambert. 1992. Predicting and reinforcing children's intentions to wear protective helmets while cycling. *Public Health Reports* 107:283-89.

Paliwoda, Stan, and Ian Crawford. 2003. An analysis of the Hastings review: "The effects of food promotion on children." London: Food Advertising Unit.

Phillips, Sarah M., Linda G. Bandini, Elena N. Naumova, Helene Cyr, Skye Colclough, William H. Dietz, and Aviva Must. 2004. Energy-dense snack food intake in adolescence: Longitudinal relationship to weight and fatness. *Obesity Research* 12:461-72.

Pine, Karen J., and Avril Nash. 2003. Barbie or Betty? Preschool children's preference for branded products and evidence for gender-linked differences. *Developmental and Behavioral Pediatrics* 24:219-24.

Resnik, Alan, and Bruce L. Stern. 1977. Children's television advertising and brand choice: A laboratory experiment. *Journal of Advertising* 6:11-17.

Robertson, Thomas S., and John R. Rossiter. 1974. Children and commercial persuasion: An attribution theory analysis. *Journal of Consumer Research* 1:13-20.

Rolandelli, David R., John C. Wright, Aletha C. Huston, and Darwin Eakins. 1991. Children's auditory and visual processing of narrated and nonnarrated television programming. *Journal of Experimental Child Psychology* 51:90-122.

Stoneman, Zolinda, and Gene H. Brody. 1982. The indirect impact of child-oriented advertisements on mother-child interactions. *Journal of Applied Developmental Psychology* 2:369-76.

Taras, Howard L., James F. Sallis, Thomas L. Patterson, Philip R. Nader, and Julie A. Nelson. 1989. Television's influence on children's diet and physical activity. *Developmental and Behavioral Pediatrics* 10:176-80.

Taras, Howard, Michelle Zive, Philip Nader, Charles C. Berry, Tricia Hoy, and Christy Boyd. 2000. Television advertising and classes of food products consumed in a paediatric population. *International Journal of Advertising* 19:487-93.

Thurstone, L. L. 1927. A law of comparative judgment. *Psychological Review* 34:273-86.

Utter, Jennifer, Dianne Neumark-Sztainer, Robert Jeffery, and Mary Story. 2003. Couch potatoes or french fries: Are sedentary behaviors associated with body mass index, physical activity, and dietary behaviors among adolescents? *Journal of the American Dietetic Association* 103:1298-1305.

Ward, Scott, Daniel B. Wackman, and Ellen Wartella. 1977. *How children learn to buy: The development of consumer information-processing skills.* Beverly Hills, CA: Sage.

Wartella, Ellen. 1984. Cognitive and affective factors of TV advertising's influence on children. *Western Journal of Speech Communication* 48:171-83.

Wiecha, Jean L., Karen E. Peterson, David S. Ludwig, Juhee Kim, Arthur Sobol, and Steven L. Gortmaker. 2006. When children eat what they watch: Impact of television viewing on dietary intake in youth. *Archives of Pediatrics and Adolescent Medicine* 160:436-42.

Woodward, D. R., F. J. Cumming, P. J. Ball, H. M. Williams, H. Hornsby, and J. A. Boon. 1997. Does television affect teenagers' food choices? *Journal of Human Nutrition and Dietetics* 10:229-35.

Woodworth, Robert S., and Harold Schlosberg. 1955. *Experimental psychology.* New York: Henry Holt.

World Health Organization (WHO). 2003. *Diet, nutrition, and the prevention of chronic disease* (WHO Technical Report Series no. 916). Geneva, Switzerland: WHO.

Wright, John C., Aletha C. Huston, Rhonda P. Ross, Sandra L. Calvert, David Rolandelli, Lee Ann Weeks, Pouran Raeissi, and Richard Potts. 1984. Pace and continuity of television programs: Effects on children's attention and comprehension. *Developmental Psychology* 20:653-66.

Young, Brian. 1990. *Television advertising and children.* Oxford, UK: Clarendon.

———. 2003. Does food advertising influence children's food choices? A critical review of some of the recent literature. *International Journal of Advertising* 22:441-59.

Children, Television Viewing, and Weight Status: Summary and Recommendations from an Expert Panel Meeting

By
AMY B. JORDAN
and
THOMAS N. ROBINSON

Overweight and obesity among American children has reached epidemic proportions. More than 9 million youth between the ages of six and nineteen years are considered overweight, and more than 80 percent of overweight adolescents will go on to become obese adults. Research has indicated a wide range of factors believed to contribute to obesity among children, but of growing concern is the potential contribution made by children's media use. In April 2006, an expert panel meeting was convened to meet and address children, television viewing, and weight status. This article reviews the evidence discussed at this meeting about the role that media, specifically television, play in the prevalence of overweight among children. It lays out the panel member's conclusions about the most promising strategies for reducing the negative effects of television on children's weight status and makes recommendations for future research that is needed to fully understand the relationship.

Keywords: television; mass media; childhood overweight; childhood obesity

A lthough much has been written over the decades about the possible deleterious effects of television viewing on children's imagination, academic performance, and aggressive behavior, researchers in the social and medical sciences and public health fields have only recently begun to explore the physical consequences of children's television viewing. In April

Amy B. Jordan, PhD, is director of the Media and the Developing Mind sector of the Annenberg Public Policy Center of the University of Pennsylvania.

Thomas N. Robinson, MD, MPH, is an associate professor of pediatrics and medicine in the division of General Pediatrics and the Stanford Prevention Research Center at Stanford University School of Medicine and director of the Center for Healthy Weight at Lucile Packard Children's Hospital at Stanford.

NOTE: Drs. Jordan and Robinson served as cochairs of the Expert Panel on Children, Television Viewing and Weight Status. The findings and conclusions in this article are those of the authors and do not necessarily represent the views of the Centers for Disease Control and Prevention.

DOI: 10.1177/0002716207308681

2006, under a contract between the Division of Nutrition, Physical Activity, and Obesity of the Centers for Disease Control and Prevention and Educational Services, Inc., an expert panel[1] was convened to address the topic of children, television, and weight status. The multidisciplinary nature of the topic was acknowledged in the diversity of backgrounds of panelists participating in the meeting: pediatricians, public health professionals, psychologists, communications researchers, and dietitians. The charge to the panel was (1) to examine the evidence for and mechanisms underlying the television viewing/childhood weight connection, (2) to identify the most promising public health strategies based on current knowledge and expert opinion to diminish the negative effects of television viewing and other screen media behaviors on childhood obesity, and (3) to develop a research agenda that will best inform strategies to diminish the negative effects of television viewing and other screen media behaviors on childhood overweight. The panel's charge specifically excluded the topics of using media as an intervention to improve physical activity and eating behaviors or changing media content, including advertising.

Children, Television, and Weight Status: The Research Evidence

The first goal of the expert panel meeting was to systematically examine the evidence for and mechanisms underlying the television (TV) viewing/childhood weight connection. We did this by examining the uses of media by children and families and by laying out four potential explanations for the observed correlation.

Patterns of media use

As childhood obesity has dramatically increased, so too has the ubiquity of television and other screen media in children's lives. National surveys of U.S. families have found that patterns of viewing start very young: 75 percent of babies, toddlers, and preschoolers watch TV for an average of more than an hour per day (despite American Academy of Pediatrics [AAP; 2001] recommendations discouraging any screen media use before the age of two). Moreover, nearly a third live in households where the television set is on all or most of the time, and an additional 30 percent live in homes where the television is on during meals (Rideout and Hamel 2006). Older children spend substantially more time with television than the two hours per day or less recommended by the AAP.[2] Recent surveys find that school-age children spend, on average, three hours per day watching television, and when computers and video games are accounted for, children's time with screen media exceeds five hours per day. The average family owns four working television sets and the vast majority subscribe to cable or satellite TV, more than two-thirds of children have a bedroom television, and four in ten families have a television set in a room where they eat (Roberts et al. 1999; Rideout, Roberts, and Foehr 2005; Jordan et al. 2006).

Recent surveys find that school-age children spend, on average, three hours per day watching television, and when computers and video games are accounted for, children's time with screen media exceeds five hours per day.

The evidence for a connection

Many scholars would agree on the persuasive evidence for a relationship between heavy television viewing and childhood overweight. Cross-sectional surveys indicate that as the number of hours spent viewing rises, so too does body fat percentage and the risk of overweight, in a dose-response fashion (e.g., Andersen et al. 1998; Hernandez et al. 1999; Gortmaker et al. 1996; Hancox and Poulton 2006). Prospective studies suggest childhood television viewing is a risk factor for subsequent weight gain and overweight (Dietz and Gortmaker 1985; Hancox and Poulton 2006). Finally, several randomized controlled trials, often cited as the gold standard by which to judge causality, have linked reducing television and other screen media use to decreased body mass index (BMI), waist circumferences, and triceps skinfold thicknesses in elementary school children (Robinson 1999); decreased overweight in middle school girls (Gortmaker et al. 1999); and weight loss among overweight eight- to twelve-year-old children (Epstein et al. 2000, 1995).

Potential causal mechanisms

Four hypothesized mechanisms through which television viewing may lead to childhood overweight (Robinson 2001) are as follows:

1. *Lower resting energy expenditure.* Some experimental data have suggested that watching television reduces resting energy expenditure (Klesges, Shelton, and Klesges 1993), but others have found no differences in metabolic rate compared to reading (Dietz et al. 1994).

2. *Displacement of physical activity.* Another hypothesis is that television viewing, generally a sedentary activity, displaces more energy-burning pursuits.

Some early ecological studies of the initial introduction of television into small communities supported this hypothesis (Williams and Handford 1986; Brown and Cramond 1974), although the results of more recent epidemiological studies have been mixed (Grund et al. 2001; Sallis, Prochaska, and Taylor 2000; Robinson 2001). Several studies have found only a weak negative association between viewing time and physical activity (Neumark-Sztainer et al. 2003; Robinson et al. 1993; Hernandez et al. 1999; Durant et al. 1994) or no significant relationship. Experimental research has also failed to demonstrate increases in physical activity in response to decreased television viewing and other sedentary behaviors (Epstein et al. 2002; Robinson 1999). These studies are unable to exclude the possibility that screen viewing reduces energy expenditure by displacing low-intensity activity over long periods. However, the sum of these studies suggest that TV viewing may be only weakly related to physical activity and that sedentary behaviors may produce their effects on children's adiposity independent of physical activity levels.

3. *Food advertising leading to greater energy intake.* Content analyses of U.S. television programming directed at children (Harrison and Marske 2005; Connor 2006) and general audiences (Henderson and Kelly 2005) indicate a preponderance of food advertising, of which the vast majority is for foods high in calories and low in nutritional content. A 2006 Institute of Medicine (IOM) report that reviewed published reports spanning three decades concluded, "Food and beverage marketing influences the preferences and purchase requests of children, influences consumption at least in the short term, is a likely contributor to less healthful diets, and may contribute to negative diet-related health outcomes and risks" (p. 307).

4. *Eating while viewing leading to greater energy intake.* Some epidemiological and experimental evidence suggests that television may affect weight status by interrupting normal satiety cues or encouraging consumption of additional calories or more calorie-dense, nutritionally poor foods while viewing TV. A recent study found that college students consumed significantly more pizza or macaroni & cheese while eating with a television program on than eating with the TV off (Blass et al. 2006). Studies in a diversity of samples have shown that elementary school children consume a large proportion (17 to 35 percent) of their total daily calories while watching television, with some evidence for eating fewer fruits and vegetables than when eating without the TV on (Matheson, Killen, et al. 2004; Matheson, Wang, et al. 2004).

Intervention Strategies

The second goal of the meeting was to identify the most promising public health strategies based on current knowledge and expert opinion to diminish the negative effects of television viewing and other screen media behaviors on childhood obesity.

Drawing from evidence addressing potential mechanisms and the existing experimental research, the panel was asked to propose and prioritize strategies to limit the negative effects of television viewing on children that, in their opinions, were most promising for use in public health campaigns and programs, clinical practice, and/or individual households. Although the panel found that the evidence base was insufficient to lead to a consensus ordering of specific strategies, panel members identified a number of strategies that they considered priority candidates for feasibility studies, implementation, and/or evaluation research.

Eliminate TV from children's bedrooms

Nationally, two-thirds of children over the age of eight years have TVs in their bedrooms (Rideout, Roberts, and Foehr 2005). Several studies suggest children with bedroom TVs watch significantly more television than those without (Rideout, Roberts, and Foehr 2005; Dennison et al. 2002). The panel recommends that TVs be eliminated completely from children's bedrooms, either by removing them if they are currently present or by never putting them into bedrooms from the start. In addition, it must be recognized that proliferation of new media—as well as the growing convergence of media platforms—means that parents must beware that children do not simply substitute one screen medium for another.

Encourage mindful viewing by monitoring screen media watched, budgeting TV time, fostering media literacy, and deliberately choosing programs to be viewed

This recommendation is supported by evidence from successful experimental trials of reducing television viewing (Gortmaker et al. 1999; Dennison et al. 2004; Robinson 1999; Robinson et al. 2003). The committee terms this "mindful" viewing, a process that assists parents in taking control of children's viewing by allowing input from the child and encouraging clear parent-child communication on the topic of how much time and what kinds of content are appropriate.

The panel recommends that parents begin by monitoring the screen media their children use before they make a decision on budgeting, as many parents are not aware of the full extent of children's time with television and other screen media (Jordan et al. 2006). After monitoring, parents, in collaboration with their children, should establish a budget of time the children are allowed to watch. For example, a family could start with ten hours of TV per week. Successful goal budgets in experimental studies have ranged from one to two hours per day or less (Gortmaker et al. 1999; Robinson 1999; Robinson et al. 2003), an amount consistent with recommendations from the AAP and the IOM Committee on Prevention of Obesity in Children and Youth (IOM 2005). However, the committee noted that the experimental and observational associations between television viewing and obesity appear to be dose-response in nature with no clearly evident lower- or upper-time thresholds. Finally, the budget should be "spent" on programs that are chosen in advance, for example, by looking at a TV program listing and planning the subsequent week's viewing to remain within the agreed budget (a process that has been called "intelligent viewing" in some studies) (Robinson 1999; Robinson et al. 2003).

Turn off the TV while eating

Four in ten families have a television set in the dining room or kitchen (Jordan et al. 2006), and several studies have suggested that television is often on while the family is eating meals together and when children are consuming snacks (Boutelle et al. 2003; Gore et al. 2003; Jordan et al. 2006). This may increase the amount of time children spend viewing, and it may undermine healthy eating habits. Matheson, Killen, et al. (2004) and Matheson, Wang, et al. (2004) reported that one-quarter to two-thirds of children's snacking and one-third to one-half of their dinners are eaten while watching television. Moreover, children in households that consume their family meals with the TV on report eating more red meat, pizza, snack foods, and soft drinks, and fewer fruits and vegetables (Coon et al. 2001). In one experimental screen time reduction study that found reduced weight gain, the children in the treatment group reduced the number of meals eaten with TV on compared to controls, but reported high-fat food intake was not significantly different (Robinson 1999). Based on testimonial evidence from this and other past experimental studies, it was suggested that disconnecting food from TV viewing may increase awareness of food consumption, while also increasing family communication, and decreasing total TV watching time. In other words, it might not just be what is consumed but how much is consumed and how the family develops patterns around television that are reflected during mealtimes.

Disconnecting food from TV viewing may increase awareness of food consumption, while also increasing family communication, and decreasing total TV watching time.

Use school-based curricula to reduce children's screen time

Delivering a classroom-based television reduction curriculum represents one of the few strategies supported by evidence of efficacy for reducing the effects of television viewing on children's weight. The panel noted schools are an excellent forum for efficiently and effectively reaching a large number of youth with a focused curriculum. Several curricula with evidence of efficacy for reducing television viewing and, in some cases, reducing obesity and/or weight gain, exist and are available for preschools (Dennison et al. 2004), elementary schools (Robinson 1999), and middle schools (Gortmaker et al. 1999).

Provide training for health care professionals to counsel on reducing children's media use

About three-quarters of U.S. newborn to eighteen-year-old youth are seen regularly (once a year or more) by a medical care provider (Dey, Schiller, and Tai 2004). As a result, medical care visits represent a potential opportunity for health care professionals to provide guidance to parents and youth on children's media use. To take advantage of this opportunity, the panel recommended training and support for health care professionals on issues related to reducing children's use of media (which would include television viewing but might also address other recreational screen time such as video game playing and computer/internet use). Training can even include making media "the fifth vital sign" during a health care provider office visit. Because media use accounts for such a substantial part of most children's lives, the panel suggested that training on children and media should be included in curricula at all stages and made a required content area for child health professional accreditation, certification, and continuing education (Rich and Bar-on 2001).

Research Agenda

The third goal of the meeting was to develop a research agenda that will best inform strategies (including home-based, public health, educational, and regulatory policies and practices) to diminish the negative effects of television viewing and other screen media behaviors on childhood obesity.

This goal was selected to emphasize informative, solution-oriented research (Robinson and Sirard 2005), to result in answers to the questions, "What works?" and "How do we implement or deliver 'it' to produce an impact on the public's health?" In developing priorities for research, it was noted that nonexperimental research (i.e., informal and systematic clinical observations, theory, and cross-sectional and longitudinal correlational and risk factor studies) already have generated a large number of hypothesized strategies for reducing screen media exposures, hypothesized mechanisms for the effects of screen media exposure on weight gain and/or obesity, and hypothesized high-risk groups that might be more or less responsive to screen time reduction interventions. Because nonexperimental studies are unable to confirm causal relationships and, by themselves, may not directly inform specific policies and practices, it was recommended that the highest priority be placed on experimental, intervention research including feasibility and pilot studies, efficacy studies, and effectiveness studies. Further nonexperimental studies are considered a lower priority. In order of priority, the panel recommended pursuit of the following research agenda, which suggests a combination of foci, from individual child/family studies to environmental change explorations to policy-oriented research.

Feasibility/pilot studies

Pilot studies are needed to assess the feasibility of hypothesized screen media reduction strategies and interventions to reduce weight gain and/or obesity. As outlined above and including those prioritized by the expert panel, a large number of potential intervention strategies and implementation approaches have been suggested as promising by past research. However, little research is available to provide guidance on how to implement these strategies and whether they can be brought to scale in a cost-effective manner.

Efficacy studies

Interventions that are demonstrated to be feasible and promising are suitable to evaluate in experimental efficacy studies. Efficacy studies are generally randomized controlled trials with high levels of internal validity, to be able to infer causality and estimate effect sizes with a high degree of confidence. When choosing among hypothesized interventions for evaluation in efficacy studies, priority should go to those interventions with the greatest potential for effectiveness (based on theory, feasibility, and pilot studies) and/or the greatest potential population impact, as well as considerations of anticipated sustainability, effects on equity, side effects, and acceptability to stakeholders, as suggested by Swinburn, Gill, and Kumanyika (2005).

A second purpose of efficacy studies is to identify and explore mechanisms leading to reduced screen time and/or reduced weight gain or obesity. Studies are designed in which specific elements of interventions (e.g., targeting child behaviors versus parent behaviors, targeting media environment factors, varying doses of interventions or varying screen time exposures) or types of screen time exposure (e.g., advertising versus total screen time, contrasts of different media hardware, content, and format) are manipulated. This allows the researcher to identify the intervention mechanisms responsible for the greatest effect on the outcome of interest (i.e., child weight status) and intervention dose responsiveness (e.g., the maximum number of hours of viewing). In earlier stages of efficacy testing, outcomes may include hypothesized behavioral and physiological mediators (e.g., components of dietary intake, physical activity, resting metabolism, and sleep). Those studies may lead to future efficacy trials in which these potential mediating variables are directly manipulated to assess their effects on weight gain or obesity.

A third purpose for efficacy trials is to identify individual or group characteristics that define subpopulations that respond more or less to various interventions (moderators) (Kraemer et al. 2002). The panel identified a number of potential moderators to consider when designing efficacy studies, including sociodemographic characteristics (e.g., age, gender, race and ethnicity, socioeconomic status, acculturation status and cultural characteristics, and family structure), cognitive and behavioral factors (e.g., other media/marketing exposure, child and parental attitudes regarding screen media, prior media use/exposure, parenting practices, diet, activity, sleep behaviors, and cognitive development) and physiological characteristics (e.g., child and parental weight status and genetics).

Effectiveness and diffusion studies

Similar to criteria for efficacy trials, when choosing interventions for effectiveness and diffusion studies, priority should go to those interventions with the greatest potential for effectiveness and/or the greatest potential population impact. One must also consider their potential feasibility, sustainability, side effects, and acceptability to stakeholders (Swinburn, Gill, and Kumanyika 2005). As noted previously, several existing interventions based in school settings have demonstrated efficacy in reducing screen time and, in some cases, reducing BMI or the rates of weight gain. These existing interventions are suitable for effectiveness trials and diffusion research. Effectiveness and diffusion evaluations may include "natural experiments," as these interventions are delivered in different settings. They may also be designed as true experimental studies, in which children and families are randomly assigned to experimental and control groups.

Several existing interventions based
in school settings have demonstrated efficacy
in reducing screen time and, in some cases,
reducing BMI or the rates of weight gain.

True experimental studies in which the interventions and methods of diffusion and implementation are tested in different settings may offer greater internal validity and thus stronger evidence. These studies also allow one to estimate the magnitudes of effects likely to result when the interventions are replicated. In addition to questions of effectiveness in reducing screen time and reducing weight gain and/or obesity and effect sizes achieved, effectiveness studies also provide an opportunity to identify mediators and moderators of intervention response. They provide insight into the resources needed and cost-effectiveness of the interventions as well. Assessing mediators, moderators, costs, and cost-effectiveness of various clinical and population-based intervention strategies is of particular relevance for guiding policy regarding how and to whom interventions should be delivered to produce the greatest benefits when resources are finite.

Measurement development studies

In addition to the types of studies noted above, another priority research area identified by the panel is developing better measures of screen media use and/or exposure. Reliable and valid measures are necessary to be able to accurately assess the promise, efficacy, and effectiveness of hypothesized strategies for reducing screen media exposure and its effects on weight gain and/or obesity. The panel thought this was particularly important as children's media use and exposures evolve with new media-related technologies.

Additional types of research, generally classified as etiological or mechanistic studies, may advance understandings of screen media behaviors and the effects of screen media exposure on weight gain and/or obesity, but were not judged to be a high priority because they would not connect directly to specific policies and practices. They are, however, important for gaining new insights that may inform future feasibility/pilot and efficacy studies and even more effective policies and practices in the future.[3]

Establish a priority for funding research on children's television and other media use and weight

The panel recognized that its recommendations will all depend on the availability of funding. Research funding is particularly needed for early-stage feasibility and pilot studies, efficacy and effectiveness studies, the high-priority studies in the research agenda. These are the studies with the best chances of answering questions of most relevance to parents, health professionals, schools, public health professionals and agencies, and public policy makers. Thus, long-term funding is needed to establish a coherent research program on television and other forms of electronic media and children's weight status, specifically, and child development, health and behavior, more broadly.

Notes

1. Expert panel members: The panel consisted of eleven experts in public health, public policy, pediatrics, nutrition, psychology, sociology, and communication. **Amy B. Jordan, PhD**, and **Thomas N. Robinson, MD, MPH**, served as cochairs of the meeting. Dr. Jordan is a senior research investigator for media and the developing child sector at the University of Pennsylvania's Annenberg Public Policy Center. Dr. Robinson is an associate professor of pediatrics and medicine at the Stanford University School of Medicine. In addition to the cochairs, the panel included the following experts:

Dimitri A. Christakis, MD, MPH
Professor of Pediatrics
Director, Child Health Institute
General Pediatrics
University of Washington

Barbara A. Dennison, MD
Director, Bureau of Health Risk Reduction
Division of Chronic Disease Prevention and Adult Health
New York State Department of Health

Nancy A. Gelbard, MS, RD
Chief, School Health Connections/California
Obesity Prevention
Chronic Disease and Injury Control
California Department of Health Services

Steven L. Gortmaker, PhD
Professor of the Practice of Health Sociology
Department of Society, Human Development, and Health
Harvard School of Public Health

Kristen S. Harrison, PhD
Associate Professor
Department of Speech Communication & Division of Nutritional Sciences
University of Illinois

Leonard Jason, PhD
Professor
Psychology Department
Center for Community Research
DePaul University

Donna B. Johnson, RD, PhD
Associate Director
Center for Public Health Nutrition
Nutritional Sciences Program
School of Public Health and Community Medicine
University of Washington

Michael Rich, MD, MPH
Director, Center on Media and Child Health
Assistant Professor of Pediatrics
Children's Hospital Boston/Harvard Medical School

Donald F. Roberts Jr., PhD
Thomas More Storke Professor
Department of Communication
Stanford University

2. The American Academy of Pediatrics recommends that children two years and older spend no more than one to two hours per day with screen media, and that a significant proportion of that time be spent with educational content.

3. These types of studies include (1) case studies, case-control, cross-sectional and prospective epidemiological studies of associations between exposure to screen media types, amount, content, patterns of use and context with physical activity, eating behaviors, metabolism and energy balance, and weight and/or

body fat, including exploring for possible moderators and mediators; and (2) experimental animal and human laboratory studies manipulating screen media types, amount, content, patterns of use, context and observing the resulting effects on physical activity, eating behaviors, metabolism and energy balance, and weight and body fat. The panel also noted the need for further research on the effects of changing television and other screen media behaviors on other physical, psychological, and social outcomes for individual children, families, and populations.

References

American Academy of Pediatrics (AAP). 2001. Children, adolescents, and television. Pediatrics 107:423-26.

Andersen, R. E., C. J. Crespo, S. J. Bartlett, L. J. Cheskin, and M. Pratt. 1998. Relationship of physical activity and television watching with body weight and level of fatness among children: results from the Third National Health and Nutrition Examination Survey. *Journal of the American Medical Association* 279:938-42.

Blass, E. M., D. R. Anderson, H. L. Kirkorian, T. A. Pempek, I. Price, and M. F. Koleini. 2006. On the road to obesity: Television viewing increases intake of high-density foods. *Physiology and Behavior* 88:597-604.

Boutelle, K. N., A. S. Birnbaum, L. A. Lytle, D. M. Murray, and M. Story. 2003. Associations between perceived family meal environment and parent intake of fruit, vegetables, and fat. *Journal of Nutrition Education and Behavior* 35:24-29.

Brown, J. R., and J. K. Cramond. 1974. Displacement effects of television and the child's functional orientation to media. In *The uses of mass communications: Current perspectives on gratification research*, ed. Jay G. Blumler and Elihu Katz, 93-112. Beverly Hills, CA: Sage.

Connor, S. M. 2006. Food-related advertising on preschool television: Building brand recognition in young audiences. *Pediatrics* 118 (4): 1478-85.

Coon, K. A., J. Goldberg, B. L. Rogers, and K. L. Tucker. 2001. Relationships between use of television during meals and children's food consumption patterns. *Pediatrics* 107:E7.

Dennison, Barbara A., Tara A. Erb, and Paul L. Jenkins. 2002. Television viewing and television in bedroom associated with overweight risk among low-income preschool children. *Pediatrics* 109:1028-35.

Dennison, B. A., T. J. Russo, P. A. Burdick, and P. L. Jenkins. 2004. An intervention to reduce television viewing by preschool children. *Archives of Pediatrics and Adolescent Medicine* 158:170-76.

Dey, A. N., J. S. Schiller, and D. A. Tai. 2004. Summary health statistics for U.S. children: National Health Interview Survey, 2002. *Vital Health Statistics* 10:1-78.

Dietz, W. H., L. G. Bandini, J. A. Morelli, K. F. Peers, and P. L. Ching. 1994. Effect of sedentary activities on resting metabolic rate. *American Journal of Clinical Nutrition* 59:556-59.

Dietz, W. H., and S. L. Gortmaker. 1985. Do we fatten our children at the television set? *Pediatrics* 75 (5): 807-11.

Durant, R. H., T. Baranowski, M. Johnson, and W. O. Thompson. 1994. The relationship among television watching, physical activity, and body composition of young children. *Pediatrics* 94:449-55.

Epstein, L. H., R. A. Paluch, A. Consalvi, K. Riordan, and T. Scholl. 2002. Effects of manipulating sedentary behavior on physical activity and food intake. *Journal of Pediatrics* 140:334-39.

Epstein, L. H., R. A. Paluch, C. C. Gordy, and J. Dorn. 2000. Decreasing sedentary behaviors in treating pediatric obesity. *Archives of Pediatrics and Adolescent Medicine* 154:220-26.

Epstein, L. H., A. M. Valoski, L. S. Vara, J. McCurley, L. Wisniewski, M. A. Kalarchian, K. R. Klein, and L. R. Shrager. 1995. Effects of decreasing sedentary behavior and increasing activity on weight change in obese children. *Health Psychology* 14:109-15.

Gore, S. A, J. A. Foster, V. G. DiLillo, K. Kirk, and D. Smith West. 2003. Television viewing and snacking. *Eating Behaviors* 3:399-405.

Gortmaker, S. L., A. Must, A. M. Sobol, K. Peterson, G. A. Colditz, and W. H. Dietz. 1996. Television viewing as a cause of increasing obesity among children in the United States, 1986-1990. *Archives of Pediatrics and Adolescent Medicine* 150:356-62.

Gortmaker, S. L., K. Peterson, J. Wiecha, A. M. Sobol, S. Dixit, M. K. Fox, and N. Laird. 1999. Reducing obesity via a school-based interdisciplinary intervention among youth: Planet Health. *Archives of Pediatrics and Adolescent Medicine* 153:409-18.

Grund, A., H. Krause, M. Siewers, H. Rieckert, and M. J. Muller. 2001. Is TV viewing an index of physical activity and fitness in overweight and normal weight children? *Public Health Nutrition* 4:1245-51.

Hancox, R. J., and R. Poulton. 2006. Watching television is associated with childhood obesity: But is it clinically important? *International Journal of Obesity* (London) 30:171-75.

Harrison, K., and A. L. Marske. 2005. Nutritional content of foods advertised during the television programs children watch most. *American Journal of Public Health* 95:1568-74.

Henderson, V. R., and B. Kelly. 2005. Food advertising in the age of obesity: Content analysis of food advertising on general market and African American television. *Journal of Nutrition Education and Behavior* 37:191-96.

Hernandez, B., S. L. Gortmaker, G. A. Colditz, K. E. Peterson, N. M. Laird, and S. Parra-Cabrera. 1999. Association of obesity with physical activity, television programs and other forms of video viewing among children in Mexico City. *International Journal of Obesity and Related Metabolic Disorders* 23:845-54.

Institute of Medicine (IOM), Committee on Food Marketing and the Diets of Children and Youth, and Food and Nutrition Board. 2006. *Food marketing to children and youth: Threat or opportunity?* Washington, DC: National Academies Press.

Institute of Medicine (IOM), Committee on Prevention of Obesity in Children and Youth, and Food and Nutrition Board. 2005. *Preventing childhood obesity: Health in the balance.* Washington, DC: National Academies Press.

Jordan, A. B., J. C. Hersey, J. A. McDivitt, and C. D. Heitzler. 2006. Reducing children's television-viewing time: A qualitative study of parents and their children. *Pediatrics* 118 (5): e1303-10.

Klesges, R. C., M. L. Shelton, and L. M. Klesges. 1993. Effects of television on metabolic rate: Potential implications for childhood obesity. *Pediatrics* 91:281-86.

Kraemer, H. C., G. T. Wilson, C. G. Fairburn, and W. S. Agras. 2002. Mediators and moderators of treatment effects in randomized clinical trials. *Archives of General Psychiatry* 59:877-83.

Matheson, D. M., J. D. Killen, Y. Wang, A. Varady, and T. N. Robinson. 2004. Children's food consumption during television viewing. *American Journal of Clinical Nutrition* 79:1088-94.

Matheson, D. M., Y. Wang, L. M. Klesges, B. M. Beech., H. C. Kraemer, and T. N. Robinson. 2004. African-American girls' dietary intake while watching television. *Obesity Research* 12 (Suppl. 1): 32S-37S.

Neumark-Sztainer, D., M. Story, P. J. Hannan, T. Tharp, and J. Rex. 2003. Factors associated with changes in physical activity: A cohort study of inactive adolescent girls. *Archives of Pediatrics and Adolescent Medicine* 157:803-10.

Rich, M., and M. Bar-on, 2001. Child health in the information age: Media education of pediatricians. *Pediatrics* 107 (1): 156-62.

Rideout, V. J., and E. Hamel. 2006. *The media family: Electronic media in the lives of infants, toddlers, preschoolers and their parents.* Rep. no. 7500. Menlo Park, CA: Henry J. Kaiser Family Foundation.

Rideout, V. J., D. F. Roberts, and U. G. Foehr. 2005. *Generation M: Media in the lives of 8-18 year-olds: Executive summary.* Menlo Park, CA: Henry J. Kaiser Family Foundation.

Roberts, D. F., U. G. Foehr, V. J. Rideout, and M. Brodie. 1999. *Kids and media at the new millennium: A comprehensive national analysis of children's media use.* Menlo Park, CA: Henry J. Kaiser Family Foundation.

Robinson, T. N. 1999. Reducing children's television viewing to prevent obesity: A randomized controlled trial. *Journal of American Medical Association* 282:1561-67.

———. 2001. Television viewing and childhood obesity. *Pediatric Clinics of North America* 48:1017-25.

Robinson, T. N., L. D. Hammer, D. M. Wilson, J. D. Killen, H. C. Kraemer, C. Hayward, and C. Barr Taylor. 1993. Does television viewing increase obesity and reduce physical activity? Cross-sectional and longitudinal analyses among adolescent girls. *Pediatrics* 91:273-80.

Robinson, T. N., J. D. Killen, H. C. Kraemer, D. M. Wilson, D. M. Matheson, W. L. Haskell, L. A. Pruitt, T. M. Powell, A. S. Owens, N. S. Thompson, N. M. Flint-Moore, G. J. Davis, K. A. Emig, R. T. Brown, J. Rochon, S. Green, and A. Varady. 2003. Dance and reducing television viewing to prevent weight gain in African-American girls: The Stanford GEMS pilot study. *Ethnicity and Disease* 13:S65-S77.

Robinson, T. N., and J. R. Sirard. 2005. Preventing childhood obesity: A solution-oriented research paradigm. *American Journal of Preventive Medicine* 28:194-201.

Sallis, J. F., J. J. Prochaska, and W. C. Taylor. 2000. A review of correlates of physical activity of children and adolescents. *Medicine and Science in Sports and Exercise* 32:963-75.

Swinburn, B., T. Gill, and S. Kumanyika. 2005. Obesity prevention: A proposed framework for translating evidence into action. *Obesity Reviews* 6:23-33.

Williams, T. M., and A. G. Handford. 1986. Television and other leisure activities. In *The impact of television: A natural experiment in three communities*, ed. Tanus MacBeth Williams, 143-213. New York: Academic Press.

Calories for Sale: Food Marketing to Children in the Twenty-First Century

By
SUSAN LINN
and
COURTNEY L. NOVOSAT

Budgets for marketing to children have spiked well into the billions, an escalation that mirrors the rise in childhood obesity rates. Children are targets for a maelstrom of marketing for all sorts of products enabled by sophisticated technology and minimal government regulation. Despite the fact that recent studies document links between food advertising and childhood obesity, a significant proportion of marketing that targets children is for energy-dense, low-nutrient food. Moreover, advances in digital technology allow marketers to find more direct, personalized gateways to reach young audiences that sidestep parental authority and bank as much on the unknowing parent as the gullible child. Cataloguing the depth and breadth of child-centered food marketing while discussing grassroots strategies for instituting change, the authors argue that parents can no longer keep pace either with innovations in advertising or increased spending, suggesting the need for more stringent government regulations on food marketing to children.

Keywords: food marketing; food advertising; childhood obesity; marketing to children; advertising to children; advertising regulation

Obesity Rates Mirror Rise in Marketing; History of Television Deregulation Complicit

Childhood obesity is a serious and escalating public health concern, yet children are targeted as never before by marketing for high-calorie, nutritionally deficient foods.

Overweight children are at risk for a number of medical problems, including hypertension, asthma (American Academy of Pediatrics 2003, 424), and type 2 diabetes, a disease previously found primarily in adults (Sinha et al. 2002, 802). Since 1980, the proportion of overweight children ages six to eleven has doubled to 15.3 percent; for adolescents, the rate has tripled to 15.5 percent (Ogden, Carroll, and Johnson 2002, 1728). The most recent studies suggest that "over 30% of American children are overweight

DOI: 10.1177/0002716207308487

or obese" while "only 2% eat a diet consistent with United States Department of Agriculture (USDA) guidelines" (Batada and Wootan 2007, 1). This unprecedented escalation of childhood obesity mirrors the equally unprecedented escalation of largely unregulated marketing that targets children. In 1983, corporations were spending $100 million on television advertising to children, which was essentially the only avenue available (Schor 2004, 21). By 2000, Burger King spent $80 million on advertising to children (Cebryznski and Zuber 2001) and Quaker Oats had allocated $15 million just to market Cap'n Crunch cereal (Thompson 1999). Today, food and beverage advertisers alone spend between $10 billion to $15 billion a year targeting youth (Eggerton 2007). Given the exponential rise in dollars spent on marketing to children, there is little doubt that the food industry believes that marketing is a critical factor in children's food choices—and research bears that out.

In recent years, the World Health Organization (WHO 2003), the Institute of Medicine (McGinnis, Goodman, and Kraak 2006), and the British Food Commission (Dalmeny, Hanna, and Lobstein 2004) conducted reviews of academic research pointing to a link between child-targeted marketing and childhood obesity. The 2006 report released by the Institute of Medicine (IOM) found that "for younger and older children, the evidence clearly supports the finding that television advertising influences their food and beverage purchase requests" (McGinnis, Goodman, and Kraak 2006, 21). Moreover, of the $200 billion spent by children and youth consumers, the four categories leading in sales are candy and snack foods, soft drinks, fast food, and cereal (McGinnis, Goodman, and Kraak 2006, 22). The IOM's findings underscore the important results of the 2003 review conducted by the WHO, which concluded that "the heavy marketing of high-calorie and low-nutrient foods and fast food outlets represents a probable increased risk for childhood obesity" (McGinnis, Goodman, and Kraak 2006, 301-2). Confirming the barrage of advertisements, a subsequent study published by the *American Journal of Public Health* of food commercials aired during the most popular shows for children ages six to eleven found that 83 percent were for snacks, fast foods, or sweets (Harrison and Marske 2005, 1568). Furthermore, the researchers found that a diet based on foods advertised on these programs would exceed U.S. Department of Agriculture Recommended Daily Values of

Susan Linn is associate director of the Media Center of Judge Baker Children's Center and Instructor in Psychiatry, Harvard Medical School. She has written extensively about the effects of media and commercial marketing on children. Her book Consuming Kids: The Hostile Takeover of Childhood *was praised in publications as diverse as the* Wall Street Journal *and* Mother Jones. *She is director and cofounder of the national coalition Campaign for a Commercial-Free Childhood.*

Courtney L. Novosat is the program coordinator at the Campaign for Commercial-Free Childhood in Boston. Approaching the social sciences by way of the humanities, she is particularly interested in the historical rise of commercialized consumer culture and the effects of commercialism on self-definition and language use among children and adolescents. She has also been published in MP: An International Feminist Journal Online.

fat, saturated fat, and sodium (Harrison and Marske 2005, 1568). Most recently, researchers at Stanford University found that when offered identical food including chicken nuggets, French fries, milk, and carrots in both McDonald's-branded wrapping and unbranded wrapping, 54 to 77 percent of the three- to five-year-old participants preferred the taste of the food they believed was from McDonald's. In fact, all the offerings were from the fast food giant, suggesting that the influence of market branding is so strong among preschoolers that it even trumps sensory input (Robinson et al. 2007, 796).

The current food marketing environment has its roots in the history of the Federal Communications Commission (FCC) and the Federal Trade Commission (FTC), which share most of the authority to regulate advertising and marketing to children. During the 1970s, Action for Children's Television (ACT), a public interest organization, criticized broadcasting networks for their failure to provide enough valuable educational programming to children and for failing to "protect children who are too young to effectively recognize and defend against commercial persuasion" (Kunkel 2001, 385). Citing several landmark studies[1] confirming that children younger than seven or eight cannot differentiate between program content and advertisements, ACT petitioned the FCC to devise protective regulatory policies, a petition that led to the first federal policies restricting advertisements during children's television (Kunkel 2001, 385). The FCC regulations limited commercial time, required a "clear separation" between program and commercial content, and restricted "host selling," or sales by program characters within program content (Kunkel 2001, 385).

The FTC attempted to reify and strengthen the former decision in 1978 by ruling that "advertising directed to children too young to understand a message's persuasive intent was inherently unfair and deceptive" (Kunkel 2001, 387). Amid a general climate of government deregulation in the late 1970s and early 1980s, the FTC's decision was met with shock from the advertising industry and from the government. Congress responded in 1980 by rescinding the FTC's authority to regulate advertising deemed "unfair" and, subsequently, abated policies for advertising to children (Kunkel 2001, 387). Although the FTC maintains authority to regulate advertising deemed "deceptive," the restriction of its authority crippled the potential for any broad-spectrum regulation in advertising to children for nearly three decades. As a result of the restriction placed on the FTC, today it is easier to regulate advertising targeted to adults than advertising targeted to children. Since the FTC Improvements Act of 1980 removed the FTC's power to regulate advertising to children that is deemed unfair, advertising to children is only regulated on the basis of practices deemed deceptive (Kunkel 2001, 387). In contrast, advertising to adults continues to be regulated on the basis of unfairness and deception (FTC.gov 2007).

In 1984, a watershed moment for advertisers, the FCC "rescinded all restrictions on the amount of commercial content" in favor of a self-regulatory policy that remains in effect today; it maintained that the advertising industry could better establish appropriate commercial levels (Kunkel 2001, 387). The Children's Advertising Review Unit (CARU), created in 1974 and funded by the advertising

industry, establishes and encourages the self-regulatory guidelines for the industry. The disempowerment of the FTC and the FCC's recanting of its previous
policy enabled CARU's rise to prominence; an era of industry self-regulation was
born and continues today. Although the Children's Television Act of 1990 rein-
stated commercial time limits, restricting the time to 10.5 minutes per hour on
weekends and 12 minutes per hour on weekdays during children's programming,
restrictions were not placed on the content within those advertising windows,
which have become gateways for an onslaught of food marketing to children
(Kunkel 2001, 386).

---

*As a result of the restriction placed
on the FTC, today it is easier to regulate
advertising targeted to adults than advertising
targeted to children.*

Food Marketing Tactics and Parental Authority

Under industry self-regulation, child-targeted marketing has become so ubiquitous and sophisticated that it presents a challenge to parental influence over
children's food choices, particularly when companies frequently work with huge
budgets and employ child psychologists to exploit children's developmental vulnerabilities. A study recently released by the Center for Digital Democracy cites
several advertising conglomerates relying on social scientists, including the
Gepetto Group, a marketing firm whose chief strategic officer claims to have pio-
neered the use of psychology and anthropology to understand what makes young
consumers tick (Gepetto Group n.d.). Past clients have included Coca-Cola,
McDonald's, Frito-Lay, and Kraft (Chester and Montgomery 2007, 19). This type
of predation in tandem with the sheer ubiquity of print, screen, and digital advertisement, as well as marketing in schools, makes it nearly impossible for parents
to intercede and limit children's exposure to food marketing and, subsequently,
to control their children's food choices—especially outside the home. Food marketing, which takes place in a maelstrom of other marketing, now goes well
beyond the thirty-second commercial and makes use of such marketing techniques as brand licensing, product placement, contests, promotions, cross-brand-
ing, and in-school marketing.

By pairing high-calorie, low-nutrient foods with beloved media characters or
favorite media programs, marketing methods pose problems for parents attempting

to make healthy food choices since their children are attracted to the characters on less healthful ones. For example, the 2007 film *Shrek the Third* had licensing agreements with McDonald's, M&Ms, and Kellogg's, permitting several of the film's most popular characters to adorn packages and advertisements. Research conducted as early as the 1970s suggests a correlation between media viewing and children's purchase requests. After researching parent-child interaction in the supermarket, Charles K. Atkin (1978, 41) reported that one-third of parent participants responded that children "often" ask for cereals after seeing television commercials, while an additional two-fifths report that children "sometimes" ask. In fact, researchers from Stanford University found that one 30-second food commercial can affect the brand choices of children as young as two, and repeated exposure has even more impact (Borzekowski and Robinson 2001, 42-46).

In general, techniques that partner characters with products are designed to lure children into selecting foods associated with favorite media programs. They are also designed to remind children of brands continually throughout the day. As one marketing expert noted, corporations are "trying to establish a situation where kids are exposed to their brand in as many different places as possible throughout the course of the day or the week, or almost anywhere they turn in the course of their daily rituals" (Bob Brown, MarketResearch.com, as cited in Kjos 2002, 1).

Brand Licensing

Brand licensing is particularly prevalent in children's television programming and is used to fund programs aimed at children, even on public television (Linn 2004, 41-60); it has also become an increasingly pervasive tactic for marketing blockbuster animated and family films like *Shrek the Third* and *Pirates of the Caribbean: At World's End*. Once a program or its characters are associated with a particular brand, the program itself becomes an ad for that food. Supermarket shelves are filled with examples of the links between media programs and food manufacturers.

A review by the Campaign for a Commercial-Free Childhood (CCFC) found the recently released *Shrek the Third* characters licensed to a variety of products marketed to children, including Kellogg's Marshmallow Froot Loops cereal, Keebler E.L. Fudge Double Stuffed cookies, "ogre-sized" Peanut Butter M&M's, Cheetos, and Kellogg's Frosted S'Mores Pop Tarts. The film's release also inspired a line of promotional glasses at McDonald's that entice children to such nutritionally remiss "ogre-fied" foods as the "ogre-tastic" Minty Mudd Bath Triple Thick Shake (McDonald's 2007). Tempting an audience of older children, *Pirates of the Caribbean: At World's End* also partnered with Kellogg's products through a send-away promotion for a Pirate Projection Alarm Clock, which, along with a shipping and handling fee, requires five "pirate tokens" from their products to order.

Although it seems logical to conclude that popular, recognizable characters like Shrek or Johnny Depp's "Captain Jack Sparrow" influence children's choices, the effect of licensed characters on product recognition and requests among children is hotly contested by marketing and academic researchers alike. However, most researchers do agree that children's recognition of spokes-characters is high. In fact, a 2004 study published in the *Journal of Advertising* suggested that spokes-characters elicit attention, recognition, and liking as well as product recognition and liking. While researchers Sabrina M. Neeley and David W. Schumann (2004, 18) refrained from concluding that spokes-characters influence children's choices, they did find that two- to five-year-olds could correctly partner a spokes-character to its product at "relatively high rates." Moreover, the use of spokes-characters to advertise commercial products to children is further complicated by their use in public service announcements (PSAs); the overlap may present conflicting messages to children. For instance, while Shrek appeared in advertising campaigns for McDonald's, he was simultaneously featured in PSAs for the U.S. Department of Health and Human Services healthy lifestyles and childhood obesity campaigns (CCFC 2007a).

While blockbuster films have frequently taken center stage as unhealthy vehicles for marketing to children, television show–linked products have been mainstays on store shelves. Nickelodeon's hit program *SpongeBob SquarePants* was Kraft's top selling macaroni and cheese in 2002 and the number one "face"-shaped Good Humor Ice Cream Bar (Nevius 2003, 37). Kraft has also recently featured Spiderman- and Shrek-shaped macaroni noodles alongside Scooby-Doo and Nickelodeon's *Fairly OddParents* shapes. Nickelodeon and Cartoon Network each have their own lines of Kellogg's fruit-flavored snacks (Saunders 2005, 2E). Along with *Blue's Clues*– and *Dora the Explorer*–shaped snacks, *Go Diego Go!* and the popular toy brand, Lego, join the company's list of commercially linked food products. Recognizing the popularity of media-linked, fruit-flavored snacks, General Mills's Betty Crocker line has licensing agreements with popular toys like My Little Pony, Polly Pocket, and Tonka trucks, and with the cable television station Animal Planet.

In response to growing concerns about childhood obesity and food marketing, Nickelodeon announced that *SpongeBob SquarePants*, *Dora the Explorer*, and other characters would appear on packages of spinach, carrots, and other vegetables (Hill 2005, 1C). Nickelodeon will continue, however, to license these same characters to products of questionable nutritional value. While it is possible that branding vegetables with cartoon characters will lead to a rise in sales, no evidence indicates that it will lead to a decrease in children's desire for, or consumption of, branded junk food. In fact, a more recent study of Nickelodeon television programming suggests that its "healthier" in-store marketing efforts are undercut by its television marketing. Of the 652 ads witnessed during twenty-eight hours of viewing, 168 were food ads, which account for 26 percent of the total ads viewed; the foods most commonly advertised were sugary cereals (25 percent of all food ads), fast-food restaurants (19 percent), and pastries (12 percent) (Batada and Wootan 2007, 2). In any case, the use of licensed characters to sell even healthy food to children is problematic. In addition to selling products, marketing to children promotes habits and behaviors. We have to ask ourselves if it is in children's best interest to be trained to select food based on what is decorating its packaging rather than on its nutrition or even its taste, particularly when packaging seems a leading determinant for children. Sesame Workshop, endowed with a grant from the Dr. Robert C. Atkins Foundation in 2005 to replicate and expand its research conducted a study titled "The Effectiveness of Characters on Children's Food Choices," which found that appending a sticker of a recognizable Sesame Street character to food's packaging strongly affected children's food selection. Most striking, the study found that when given an unbranded choice between a chocolate bar and broccoli, 78 percent of children participating chose the chocolate bar while only 22 percent selected the broccoli. When an Elmo sticker was added to the broccoli and an unknown character placed on the chocolate, the results changed drastically—50 percent of children chose the Elmo-branded broccoli (Sesame Workshop 2005). What remains unexamined, however, is what a child would choose if offered both vegetables and sweets featuring the same favorite media character—a possibility likely found at the supermarket.

Product Placement

Product placement in children's television programming is technically prohibited by law (FTC 1974) but is rampant in the prime-time programs that are children's favorites. According to *Business Week*, Coca-Cola paid $20 million for product placement in *American Idol*, which is consistently rated among the top ten shows for children ages two to eleven and is frequently among the top three (Foust and Grow 2004, 77). From April 23 to May 20, 2007, each episode of *American Idol* exposed between 1.93 million to 2.4 million two- to eleven-year-old children to Coca Cola's product placement (Nielsen Media Research 2007).

Product placement in children's television programming is technically prohibited by law but is rampant in the prime-time programs that are children's favorites.

Nor is product placement limited to television programs. No regulation exists for placing brands within the context of films, video games, or the Internet. Reaching beyond the television, *American Idol*'s 2007 Live Tour is being sponsored by Pop Tarts, which will offer "exclusive tour webisodes" on its Web site. McDonald's food products were embedded in the hit children's film *Spy Kids*, while Burger King used product placement in the film *Scooby Doo 2* (Minnow 2004). Mountain Dew pushed product placement to its logical conclusion—a high-budget feature film doubling as an advertisement—by producing *First Descent* (Lawton 2005, B4). The film, documenting five snowboarders' "first descent" down a previously unridden mountainside, features snowboards and helmets emblazoned with Mountain Dew's logo (firstdescentmovie.com 2005). Continuing to pad its on-screen resume, product placement for Mountain Dew also appeared in the *Transformers* movie released on July 3, 2007 (Reuters 2007).

Product placement in video and online games is a booming business expected to reach $1 billion by the end of the decade (Gentile 2005). Burger King ads, for instance, appear in video sports games, and in the online game *Everquest* it is possible to click on a Pizza Hut icon and have a pizza delivered in thirty minutes (Gentile 2005). The popular children's Web site, *Neopets*, now owned by Nickelodeon, trademarked the term "Immersive Advertising," a description of the way that brands such as McDonald's, General Mills, Disney, and others have been incorporated into children's use of the site (Winding 2002, 17). As part of the game, for instance, children are encouraged to send their friends a Reese's Puffs Cereal screen saver and to watch commercials for sugary cereals (Neopets.com 2005). After placing EZ squirt ketchup in the *Neopets* Web site, a Heinz executive commented that product awareness "just went through the roof. . . . Trials of the product increased by 18 percent" (Winding 2002, 17).

Another kind of product placement that targets children is called "advergaming" in which computer games are totally built around products in order to keep children's attention focused on specific brands much longer than traditional commercials (Powell 2003, 11). One site, called *Candystand*, consists of games featuring products from the confectioner Wrigley, such as Lifesavers, Gummie Savers, and Wrigley's Extra (Wrigley's Candystand 2007). Many advergames give an advantage to players who have purchased specific foods. For example, at Kraft's Lunchables Web site, visitors can access only two of the eight puzzle games promoting the July 2007 *Tranformers* movie without promotional codes found within the products (Kraftsbrands.com 2007b). Likewise, the SpongeBob SquarePants Bubble Trouble Cereal Game does not allow children to play more than once unless they can answer questions about the cereal's packaging (SpongeBob SquarePants Bubble Trouble Cereal Game 2005).

Even music is not exempt from product placement. McDonald's attempt to pay hip-hop artists to incorporate Big Macs into their lyrics has stalled, but there is every reason to expect that they and other food companies will keep trying (Grasser 2005).

Contests

Contests or sweepstakes targeting children are frequently partnered with films or foods. In the summer of 2007, Sunny D's "Sunmobile" toured seventeen states featuring games, prizes, and giveaways spotlighting the sugary beverage. While the drink does contain 100 percent of a child's RDA of vitamin C, that benefit comes with a high caloric price. An eight-ounce serving of the original Sunny D has 120 calories and a whopping 29 grams of sugar (SunnyD.com 2007b), while beverages in its "Baja" line, only available in twelve-ounce bottles, spike to 190 calories and 43 grams of sugar (SunnyD.com 2007a). Warner Brothers, owners of Hanna-Barbara, partnered with Post Cereal's Fruity and Cocoa Pebbles to offer a prize a week for a year in its "52 Weeks . . . 52 Winners!" promotion (Warnerbros.com 2007). Kraft Macaroni & Cheese promoted its "Mac & Cheese-a-palooza" contest, which required entering product UPC codes for entry. The winners are flown to Los Angeles as VIP guests with backstage access to a Cheetah Girls concert (Kraftsbrands.com 2007a)—the Cheetah Girls, a Radio Disney phenomenon, also inspired several CDs, DVDs, and a line of books (The Cheetah Girls Official Site 2007).

Promotions

Promotions and tie-ins that target children also frequently accompany films that are designed for a more general audience. *Star Wars: Episode III—Revenge of the Sith*, released in May 2005, had sixteen food promotions featuring twenty-five different products. Many of these promotions encouraged young children to consume large portions of food that is high in calories, fat, and sugar. To collect all seventy-two *Star Wars* M&M wrappers, children would need to buy forty-five pounds of M&Ms (containing more than 10,000 grams of sugar). To collect all thirty-one *Star Wars* Super D toys "for free," kids would need to buy more than five Burger King children's meals; a typical children's meal of a cheeseburger, small fries, and kid's Coke contains 690 calories, 28 grams of fat, and 35 grams of sugar. The prizes in many of these promotions—toys, puzzles, the Lego Star Wars Video Game—were clearly chosen for their appeal to very young children, despite the fact that *Revenge of the Sith* was rated PG-13 (CCFC 2005b). In 2007, Burger King enticed children to collect eight toys promoting the release of the *Transformers* movie and Kraft's Lunchables include one of six *Transformer* toys with purchase (Kraftsbrands.com 2007b).

Food and beverage promotions are used to market films weeks before they premiere. More than a month before the release of the 2005 blockbuster film *King Kong*, the giant gorilla appeared on 18 million boxes of Apple Jacks and Corn Pops, 10 million packages of Butterfinger and Baby Ruth Bars, as well as in Burger King promotions (Feeny 2005, C3). However, the results of CCFC's (2007c) review of *Shrek the Third* certainly suggests an ogre's appetite is as hearty as a gorilla's—the film, the target audience of which is children, inspired more than seventeen separate food promotions linked to more than seventy nutrition-poor foods.

In-School Marketing

Marketing to children is not limited to time spent using media. In 2000, a report from the federal government's General Accounting Office (GAO) called marketing in schools a "growth industry" (U.S. GAO 2000). Companies find marketing in schools to be especially effective because students constitute a captive audience unable to avoid commercial messages (Consumers Union 1998).

Corporate-sponsored newscasts, exclusive beverage contracts, corporate-sponsored teaching materials, and book covers featuring ads are just a few of the ways that food marketing infiltrates educational settings.

Corporate-sponsored newscasts,
exclusive beverage contracts,
corporate-sponsored teaching materials,
and book covers featuring ads are just a few
of the ways that food marketing infiltrates
educational settings.

Channel One. According to its Web site, the corporate sponsored news program Channel One is shown in nearly twelve thousand schools to almost eight million students (Channel One 2005). In exchange for free video equipment, schools agree to a show a Channel One program every day to their students, consisting of ten minutes of news and approximately two minutes of commercials. Food advertising has been quite popular on Channel One. Regular advertisers on Channel One have included Pepsi, Mountain Dew, Snickers, and Kellogg's Pop Tarts. It should be noted that Channel One was facing serious financial difficulties until its April 23, 2007, sale to Alloy Inc., a major teen and 'tween marketing company (Fung 2007). These difficulties were due, in part, to growing public pressure to curtail junk food marketing—Kellogg's and Kraft no longer advertise on Channel One (Atkinson 2005, 3). However, in July 2007, Alloy-owned Channel One announced a new partnership with NBC, which will now provide news content for the station (Miller 2007, C5). Although Channel One's future in schools is still in doubt, the new partnership—which includes ties to a youth marketing company—is worrisome for those concerned about the extensive commercial content formerly seen on the station.

Vending machines, direct sales, and exclusive agreements. In 2000, a national survey found that 94 percent of high schools, 84 percent of middle schools, and 58 percent of elementary schools allowed the sale of soda or other sugar-laden soft drinks on their premises. The same survey also found nearly two-thirds of all schools allowed the sale of salty snacks with high fat content; more than half of all schools allowed the sale of candy (Centers for Disease Control and Prevention [CDC] 2001). In addition, more than 20 percent of schools sell brand-name fast food such as McDonald's and Taco Bell on their premises (CDC 2001). While several states and a number of school districts have instituted new policies to restrict the sale of unhealthy foods in schools, an August 2005 report by the GAO reported that junk food was still available in nearly nine out of ten schools.

Many school districts sign pouring rights contracts with Coca-Cola or Pepsico. These contracts give beverage companies exclusive rights to sell their products at school events and place vending machines on school property. The amount of money a school receives is often tied to the sale of beverages, thus giving schools an incentive to encourage the consumption of soft drinks. While both Coke and Pepsi claim that they no longer insist that schools sign a pouring rights contract, nearly half of all schools in 2003-2004 had an exclusive beverage agreement and the percentage of middle schools with an exclusive beverage contract more than doubled between 1998-1999 and 2003-2004 (U.S. GAO 2005, 20). In one-third of these schools, the agreement covers five years or more (U.S. GAO 2005, 15).

Incentive programs. Many schools now use corporate-sponsored incentive programs as rewards for students. For example, Pizza Hut's Book-It program offers free pizzas to students who read a certain number of books. The program has involved millions of students and has expanded into preschools (Schlosser 2001, 56). Similarly, Papa John's gives students who earn at least a C in all of their classes a "Winner's Card" that can be exchanged for prizes including pizza, ice cream, and donuts ("School News" 2004).

Direct advertising on school space. Advertising frequently appears on interior and exterior school walls, gymnasiums, scoreboards, and at school athletic events. A 2004 report found a significant increase in advertising on school buses (Molnar 2004, 35). Much of this advertising is for soft drinks and snack foods. Cover Concepts, a company that distributes free textbook covers, posters, and other sponsored materials in schools, claims to reach 30 million schoolchildren in more than half of the nation's schools (Cover Concepts 2005). Cover Concepts includes McDonald's, Pepsi, Frito Lay, M&M's, and General Mills among its clients (Story and French 2004, 3).

Sponsored educational materials and programs. Many corporations produce educational materials for use in the classroom. A Consumers Union review of seventy-seven corporate-sponsored classroom kits, however, found nearly 80 percent to be biased or incomplete, "promoting a viewpoint that favors consumption of the sponsor's product or service or a position that favors the company or its economic agenda" (Consumers Union 1998, 3). Analyses of teaching materials produced by the food industry support this conclusion. For instance, according to a Kellogg's nutrition curriculum, students should be concerned only about fat content when choosing breakfast. Sugar, a prominent ingredient in many cereals, is not mentioned (Schor 2004, 93). A poster on nutrition put out by Frito-Lay exhorted kids to "Snack for Power, Snack for Fun!" "Did you know," the poster asked, "Cheetos, Doritos, and other Frito-Snacks give you the bread/brain power that the food guide pyramid says you need?" (Linn 2004, 89).

Coca-Cola partners with Reading Is Fundamental (Reading Is Fundamental 2001) and also provides elementary schools with a reading program called The Coca-Cola Story Chasers Mobile (Hacket 2005, BV4). In recent years, McDonald's has been particularly aggressive in pursuing in-school marketing opportunities. The fast-food chain sends Ronald McDonald into schools to promote, among other things, literacy (Meyers 2004), character education (Townville Elementary School Web site 2005), and first aid (Save a Life Foundation 2005).

In September 2005, McDonald's unveiled "Passport to Play" teaching materials and giveaways featuring the McDonald's logo that suggest ways to encourage children to be more active. In this, they joined several other food companies producing physical education materials for schools, which serve the dual purpose of promoting their brand to children and shifting the focus away from the role that their food products play in the obesity epidemic by emphasizing exercise as the key to a healthy lifestyle. McDonald's expects the program to be in at least thirty-one thousand schools nationwide (Hellmich 2005, 7D).

Similarly, Coca-Cola's "Live It" program features Lance Armstrong and other popular athletes who encourage kids to be active. "Live It" is expected to reach more than 2 million sixth-graders (Warner 2005). Meanwhile, Pepsi plans to reach 3 million elementary school students with its "Balance First" fitness program (Simon 2005, B9).

Fund-raising. Scarce funding for public education has provided new opportunities for companies to market in schools under the guise of fund-raising. Programs such as Campbell's Labels for Education and General Mills Box Tops for Education (Linn 2004, 89) encourage children to put pressure on parents to buy particular brands to raise money for their school, even if they may be more expensive or less desirable than brands a family would normally buy. Students are also encouraged to sell candy, such as M&M's, to raise money (School Fund-Raisers.com 2005).

Unfortunately, evidence suggests that schools—unlike advertisers—fail to profit from in-school marketing, making the partnership a deceptively unilateral pairing. In a study released in 2007, Arizona State University's Commercialism in Education Research Unit (CERU) reported that of the schools participating in income-generating advertising activities, 73.4 percent did not receive any income in the 2003-2004 academic year through activities with corporations that sell foods of minimal nutritional value. An additional 12.6 percent of schools received $2,500 or less, while only 0.4 percent of schools that participated in income-generating advertising activities received more than $50,000 from corporations that sell foods high in fat and sugar (Molnar et al. 2006, 4).

New Technologies: Increased Access

The vast array of new technologies makes it possible for companies to target children without parental knowledge or consent and presents another challenge to parents' authority over their children's food choices. With children's ever-increasing access to and use of computers, the Internet is rife with marketing opportunities; given documented trends in Internet usage during the early 2000s, "a recent estimate suggests that more than 34 million children and youth ages 3 to 17 years in the United States use the internet" (Rubin 2004, as quoted in McGinnis, Goodman, and Kraak 2006, 177). The Internet, home to a myriad of commercialized networking sites like Facebook, MySpace, and Yahoo! Messenger, is replete with sidebar ads and pop-ups advertising the latest products, films, and video games. While the sites' home pages act as billboards, marketers also use the sites' potential for word-of-mouth and "click-of-mouse" advertisement. Social networking sites, which rely on interpersonal dialogues amid preextent social networks, are hotbeds for viral marketing. In addition to the Internet, cell phones and iPods provide intimate, personalized spaces for marketers to target children; for example, in 2006, Kellogg's Pop-Tarts offered codes for free music downloads in specially marked packages (Kellogg Company Press Releases 2006).

Scarce funding for public education has provided new opportunities for companies to market in schools under the guise of fund-raising. . . . Unfortunately, evidence suggests that schools—unlike advertisers—fail to profit from in-school marketing, making the partnership a deceptively unilateral pairing.

Video Games

While food marketing is frequently seen in product placement within games released for sale, Burger King has taken the partnership of food marketing and gaming to a new level. In 2006, Burger King released three video games for multiple platforms featuring its King character. Prominently bedecked in Burger King–emblazoned accoutrements of royalty, *Sneak King* players "step into the royal shoes of the King himself" and "silently unleash hot sandwiches on the hungry citizens of [the game's] famished world" (Xbox Games 2007, "Sneak King"). Despite releasing its own game, Burger King—like many other food-related Web sites—still participates in online advergaming, recently featuring a game on its Web site promoting the 2007 release of *Fantastic Four: Rise of the Silver Surfer* (Burger King and Dr. Pepper Seek the Silver Surfer Game 2007). Partnering with a cartoon or release of a film to offer an online video game seems a common practice; in a minisurvey of food and beverage Web sites, we found twelve sites featuring online games, including McDonald's, Burger King, Taco Bell, Mountain Dew, Dr. Pepper, Coca-Cola, Skittles, Starburst, M&Ms, Cheetos, Doritos, and Pringles. Many of these sites feature their products as game characters; for example, different variety Doritos' bags "duke it out" in the site's online "Fight for Flavor" game (Doritos.com 2007).

Cell Phones and iPods: Mobile Marketing

Between 2002 and 2004, the number of twelve- to fourteen-year-olds with cell phones jumped from 13 to 40 percent; phones are now being marketed to children as young as six (Pereca 2005). As companies market cell phones and video iPods to younger and younger children, they are providing food marketers with a new way to target youth. Frito Lay, for instance, created an integrated marketing approach to promote Black Pepper Jack Doritos that incorporated text messaging, billboards, and the Internet alongside television and radio commercials (Frito-Lay.com 2005). Cell phone-based contests, such as Pepsico's "Call upon Yoda" sweepstakes (CCFC 2005b) and Nestle's "Grab. Gulp. Win!" are increasingly common, and Coca-Cola plans to launch a line of mobile advergames for phones (Cuneo 2005). Like cell phones, iPods with video allow users to purchase and download content like films, television shows, or YouTube videos—complete with commercials.

Social Networking Sites

On July 25, 2007, Alloy Media & Marketing, which specializes in marketing to children and teens, released a white paper reporting that "96% of online tweens and teens connect to a social network at least once a week," bespeaking the overwhelming popularity of sites like MySpace (Klaassen 2007). With the plethora of ever-changing pop-ups and sidebars, food ads are certainly among those featured while a user navigates the site. Additionally, changing on a daily basis, the MySpace home page generally acts as a billboard for a single advertiser. In one visit to the site, the MySpace home page cast a magenta hue with an advertisement for Cherry Coke, which linked to its own networking page and information about its "Cherry Coke MySpace Page Design Contest" (MySpace.com 2007). To enter the contest, one is immediately prompted to add "Cherry Coke" to her or his friends list, allowing Coca-Cola to communicate directly with its list of "friends"—or, rather, potential consumers—talk about personalized and instantaneous marketing! However, we find Burger King again at the fore of digital innovation when in 2006 it launched a page for its King character—he had more than 120,000 "friends" by September of that year (King 2006). With an eye toward partnering the popularity of social networking sites and cell phones, in June 2007 Coca-Cola introduced Sprite Yard, which allows users to set up profiles and network via cell phones as one would on an online site. Additionally, users can redeem cap codes online for downloadable content like ring tones and video clips (Story 2007).

Marketing and Family Stress

Food comprises a significant portion of what is marketed to children, but it takes place in the context of a myriad of marketing ventures for other products. Toys, clothing, accessories, movies, television programs, video games, and countless other consumer goods are all marketed extensively to children, as are products traditionally purchased by adults such as automobiles and air travel (Linn 2004, 31-44).

The sheer volume of marketing targeted at children is stressful for families. As most parents struggle to set limits, corporations often undermine parental authority by encouraging children to nag (Linn 2004, 31-44). They also inundate children with images that tend to portray adults as incompetent, mean, or absent and encourage children to engage in behaviors that are troublesome to parents (Linn 2004, 189-90). A 1999 article in *Advertising Age* begins, "Mothers are known for instructing children not to play with their food. But increasingly marketers are encouraging them to" (Pollack 1999). Instead of acquiescing to parents' concerns, the marketing industry often sees parental disapproval as a strong selling point with kids (Linn 2004, 31-40). When discussing the strategy for selling Kraft Lunchables, a marketing expert put it this way: "Parents do not fully approve—they would rather their child ate a more traditional lunch—but this adds to the brand's appeal among children because it reinforces their need to feel in control" (Neville 2001, 17).

Government Regulation versus Self-Regulation

The United States currently regulates marketing to children less than most other industrialized democratic nations. Sweden and Norway ban marketing to children younger than twelve (Briggs 2003, A1). The Canadian Province of Quebec bans marketing to children younger than thirteen (Riverd and LeBlanc 2000, B10). Greece prohibits ads for toys on television between 7 a.m. and 10 p.m., while ads for toy guns and tanks are not allowed at any time (Hawkes 2004, 19). In Flemish-speaking areas of Belgium, no advertising is allowed within five minutes of a children's television program shown on a local station (Rowan 2002, 6). Finland bans advertisements that are delivered by children or by familiar cartoon characters (Hawkes 2004, 19). The French parliament banned all vending machines in middle and secondary schools (Taylor 2004, A11). Moreover, advertising regulations proposed by the European Union would ban commercials that imply that children's acceptance by peers is dependent on use of a product (Metherell 2002, 3), while New Zealand is considering a wholesale ban on junk food marketing to kids (Metherell 2002, 3). In recent years, Britain has begun to take steps to curb marketing to children. In 2004, the British Broadcasting Corporation severed marketing connections between their children's programming and junk food companies ("BBC to Limit Ties to Junk Food" 2004, D5). In addition, a bill in Parliament to ban all junk food marketing on television until after 9:00 p.m. currently has significant support (Brown 2007).

In the United States, the escalation of marketing to children and the rise of childhood obesity have occurred while the CARU—the advertising industry's self-appointed watchdog—has served as the primary self-regulatory agency responsible for monitoring child-directed advertising. This problematic internal monitoring has led advocates to call for increased government regulation of food marketing to children (CCFC 2005a). However, the current administration is philosophically opposed to regulation. Corporations are quick to exploit what has become a national zeitgeist of individual responsibility. The food industry has been a powerful lobby and food marketing to children is a profitable endeavor; it is naïve to think that companies are going to completely stop marketing their products to children without external regulations or that such regulations are going to come about without significant grassroots pressure from advocacy groups.

In June 2007, for instance, Kellogg's agreed to curtail its marketing to children younger than twelve and to stop marketing using media-licensed characters by 2008—but only as the result of negotiations following the threat of a potential lawsuit. The CCFC, the Center for Science in the Public Interest (CSPI), and two Massachusetts parents filed an "intent to file suit" in the Commonwealth of Massachusetts Superior Court (CCFC 2007b). If the agreement is faithfully implemented, this means that many of the Kellogg's-linked products described earlier in this article will no longer target children, with or without media characters.

A lawsuit, or the threat of one, is not an efficient way to establish national policy. Addressing the problem on a company-by-company basis drains valuable time and already scarce resources from advocacy groups.

While the extent of Kellogg's agreement to adopt stricter nutrition and marketing standards that reduce sugar and fat in their products, and advertising to children is unprecedented in the food industry, the agreement is still flawed. The negotiated standard for sodium is less stringent than that recommended by the IOM (2007) for foods acceptable in schools, and there is concern that the standard for sugar is too high ("Adult-Only Froot Loops" 2007, A12). More than that, the shortcomings of the agreement underscore an important point: a lawsuit, or the threat of one, is not an efficient way to establish national policy. Addressing the problem on a company-by-company basis drains valuable time and already scarce resources from advocacy groups.

Nevertheless, the formalized threat of a lawsuit heightened awareness and escalated pressure on food companies to curtail their child-targeted marketing. On July 18, 2007, to stave off threats of government regulation, eleven major food companies announced details of their own voluntary pledges to restrict marketing to children and, for the first time, to open their marketing plans to the Better Business Bureau and CARU (Zuill and Vorman 2007). How effective these pledges will be in actually restricting junk food marketing to children remains to be seen. Taken as a whole, however, these pledges represent many of the flaws inherent in self-regulation. Companies are not adhering to any uniform standard; rather, each company sets its own standard, which means that monitoring compliance is going to be quite difficult. More problematic, at no point has the entire food industry agreed to restrict marketing to children. As this article is written, Burger King, Nestle, ConAgra, and Chuck E. Cheese have publicly refused to participate (Tienowitz 2007). Finally, history suggests that because these pledges are voluntary and not legally binding, they can be broken, sidestepped, or even remain unimplemented with little or no consequence.

In June 2007, a month before the food companies' pledges were released, Representative Edward Markey (D-Mass.) ended a meeting of the House Committee on Energy and Commerce Subcommittee on Telecommunications with a promising warning: "The First Amendment is precious, but children are just as precious. We need a healthy balance to make sure our children aren't bombarded with these messages." He continued, "Most parents are not in the position to control what kids see—they are both working. While these kids have all these unhealthy choices presented to them in the media, if there is not a proper response from industry, I'm prepared to press the FCC to put on the books rules to protect kids from unhealthy messages" (as quoted in Greenberg 2007). Markey's warning echoes that of Senator Tom Harkin (D-Iowa), who made a similar comment about the FTC at a 2005 workshop on food marketing and self-regulation (Dobson and Knightly 2005). He and Senator Sam Brownback (R-Kansas) have formed an advisory committee to work with the FCC on issues of food marketing to children (Brownback.senate.gov 2007). In addition, as of this writing, the FTC is readying subpoenas to forty-four food companies and fast-food restaurants for a congressionally mandated study on food marketing to children (Tienowitz 2007). At this time, it is hard to know what the results of this government activity will be, but these efforts are significant. They occasion the federal government's first movements toward adopting a strong stance to curb marketing unhealthy food to children since 1980, when Congress restricted the FTC's ability to regulate marketing to children.

Conclusion

The rise of childhood obesity mirrors the unprecedented increase of food marketing aimed at children. Companies bypass parents and target children directly in a myriad of ways through the media, through toys, and even in schools. While food companies and the marketing industry tout self-regulation as a solution to the problem, current levels of child-targeted food marketing and the rise in childhood obesity strongly suggest that self-regulation has failed.

From a public-health perspective, what makes the most sense is to prohibit marketing brands of food to children altogether. When childhood obesity is a major public health problem, certainly there is no moral, ethical, or social justification for marketing low-nutrient, energy-dense foods to children. Even marketing healthier brands to children through media-linked spokes-characters or ads on television and the Web seems problematic. Do we want to encourage our children to make food requests or purchases based on commercials whose marketing implicitly or explicitly suggests a product will enhance their social life, make them happier, or increase their power—messages routinely embedded in advertising?

We should also question the wisdom of depending on the food and media industries to promote healthy eating to children. The partnership between the producers of *Shrek the Third* and the Department of Health and Human Services is emblematic of the inherent conflict of interest between encouraging healthy lifestyles and promoting the consumption of unhealthy food. It does not seem wise to depend on corporations, bound by law to promote profits, to be the guardians of public health. Instead, on both the state and federal level, the government should take steps to restrict the current onslaught of food marketing that targets children. The reality of drafting and bringing to fruition such legislation is both complex and cumbersome, but that should not prevent a creative and rigorous exploration of a wide range of options for restricting food marketing to children. The following are suggestions for changes in policy that would limit the amount of child-targeted junk food marketing:

- Congress should restore to the FTC its full capacity to regulate marketing to children.
- The marketing and sale of brands associated with unhealthy food products in schools should be prohibited, including corporate-sponsored teaching materials.
- Corporate tax deductions for advertising and marketing junk food to children could be eliminated.
- Product placement of food brands could be discouraged in movies, video and computer games, and television programs popular with children and adolescents by requiring that such embedded advertising be identified when it occurs.
- Food companies should be prohibited from using advertising techniques that exploit children's developmental vulnerabilities, such as commercials that encourage kids to turn to food for empowerment, or to be popular, or for fun.
- The use of licensed media characters to market food products to young children should be prohibited, as should child-targeted sweepstakes and contests.
- We should prohibit links between toy and food companies that lead to food-branded toys and toy giveaways by fast-food companies such as McDonald's and Burger King.
- We should support a truly commercial-free public broadcasting system that would provide programming for children free of any marketing, including brand licensing.

It is not in children's best interest to depend on the food industry to be the guardians of public health. Only an across-the-board set of policies—designed and enforced by a body from outside the food and marketing industries—can both protect children's health and maintain a level playing field between companies.

Note

1. For a catalogue of those studies, see Kunkel (2001).

References

Adult-only Froot Loops. 2007. Editorial. *New York Times*, June 16, sec. A16.

American Academy of Pediatrics. 2003. Policy statement: Prevention of pediatric overweight and obesity. *Pediatrics* 112 (2): 424–30.

Atkin, Charles. 1978. Observation of parent-child interaction in supermarket decision-making. *Journal of Marketing* 42 (4): 41–45.

Atkinson, Claire. 2005. Channel One hits bump, losing ads and top exec. *Advertising Age*, March 14, p. 3.

Batada, Ameena, and Margo G. Wootan. 2007. Nickelodeon markets nutrition-poor foods to children. *American Journal of Preventative Medicine* 33 (1): 1-3.

BBC to limit ties to junk food. 2004. *Wall Street Journal*, April 6, sec. D5.

Borzekowski, Dina L. G., and Thomas N. Robinson. 2001. The 30-second effect: An experiment revealing the impact of television commercials on food preferences of preschoolers. *Journal of the American Dietetic Association* 101 (1): 42-46.

Briggs, Billy. 2003. Wallace hints at ban on junk food adverts as the best way to fight obesity among young. *The Herald*, February 1, sec. A1.

Brown, Amanda. 2007. 9PM watershed bid for junk TV food ads. *Press Association National Newswire*, February 6, 2007. global.factiva.com (accessed July 27, 2007).

Brownback.senate.gov. 2007. Brownback, FCC announce media task force participants. Press Release, January 23. [cited 27 July 2007]. Available from http://brownback.senate.gov/pressapp/record.cfm?id=267849 (accessed July 27, 2007).

Burger King and Dr. Pepper Seek the Silver Surfer Game. 2007. http://www.seekthesilversurfer.com/index.html (accessed June 25, 2007).

Campaign for a Commercial-Free Childhood (CFCC). 2005a. Comments for the Federal Trade Commission Workshop on Marketing, Self-Regulation, and Childhood Obesity. June 7. http://www.ftc.gov/os/comments/FoodMarketingtoKids/516960-00053.pdf (accessed June 15, 2007).

———. 2005b. New Star Wars food lures children to the fat side: Revenge of the Sith rife with junk food promotions. Press Release, May 17. http://www.commercialfreechildhood.org/pressreleases/starwarsfood.htm (accessed July 2, 2007).

———. 2007a. CCFC to Health and Human Services: Fire Shrek. Press Release, April 26. 2007. http://www.commercialfreechildhood.org/pressreleases/fireshrek.htm (accessed July 26, 2007).

———. 2007b. Kellogg Company makes historic commitment, adopting nutrition standards for marketing to children. Press Release, June 14. http://www.commercialfreechildhood.org/pressreleases/jointpressrelease.pdf (accessed June 25, 2007).

———. 2007c. *Shrek the Third* food promotions. http://www.commercialfreechildhood.org/shrekfood.htm (accessed June 25, 2007).

Cebryznski, Gregg, and Amy Zuber. 2001. Burger behemoths shake up menu mix, marketing tactics. *Nation's Restaurant News*, February 5, p. 1.

Centers for Disease Control (CDC) School Health Policies and Program Study. 2001. Fact sheet on foods and beverages sold outside of the school meal programs. http://www.cdc.gov/HealthyYouth/shpps/factsheets/pdf/outside_food.pdf (accessed September 15, 2005).

Channel One. 2005. About Channel One. http://www.channelone.com/ (accessed September 14, 2005).

The Cheetah Girls Official Site. 2007. http://tv.disney.go.com/disneychannel/originalmovies/cheetahgirls/franchise/index.html (accessed June 25, 2007).

Chester, Jeff, and Kathryn Montgomery. 2007. Interactive food and beverage marketing: Targeting youth in a digital age. Center for Digital Democracy. http://digitalads.org/documents/digiMarketingFull.pdf (accessed June 25, 2007).

Consumers Union. 1998. *Captive kids: A report on commercial pressures on kids at school.* Washington, DC: Consumers Union. www.consumersunion.org/other/captivekids/ (accessed September 15, 2005).

Cover Concepts. 2005. http://www.coverconcepts.com/ (accessed September 3, 2005).

Cuneo, Alice Z. 2005. More big marketers turn to mobile phone ads. *AdAge.com*, July 11. http://www .commercialfreechildhood.org/news/marketersmovetophones.htm (accessed July 15, 2007).

Dalmeny, Kathy, Elizabeth Hanna, and Tim Lobstein. 2004. *Broadcasting bad health: Why food marketing to children needs to be controlled*. London: International Association of Consumer Food Organizations for the World Health Organization Consultation on a Global Strategy for Diet and Health. http://www.foodcomm.org.uk/Broadcasting_bad_health.pdf (accessed September 29, 2006).

Dobson, Allison, and Maureen Knightly. 2005. Remarks by Senator Tom Harkin (D-IA) at the FTC/HHS Workshop on Marketing, Self-Regulation, and Childhood Obesity. Press Release, July 14. http://www.commercialfreechildhood.org/ftcworkshop/harkincomments.htm (accessed July 27, 2006).

Doritos.com. 2007. Fight for flavor. Available from http://www.doritos.com/ (accessed June 25, 2007)

Eggerton, John. 2007. Food-marketing debate heats up; Congress to join FCC and FTC in pressing for action. *Broadcasting & Cable*, May 21. http://www.broadcastingcable.com/article/CA6444875.html (accessed June 22, 2007).

Federal Trade Commission (FTC). 1974. *Children's television programs: Report and policy statement*. 39 Fed. Reg. 39,396. Washington, DC: FTC.

Feeny, Mark. 2005. Gorilla marketing. *Boston Globe*, September 20, sec. C3.

FTC.gov. 2007. Facts for businesses: Frequently asked advertising questions: A guide for small business general advertising policies. http://www.ftc.gov/bcp/conline/pubs/buspubs/ad-faqs.shtm (accessed July 26, 2007).

Firstdescentmovie.com. 2005. Trailer. http://www.firstdescentmovie.com/ (accessed July 26, 2007).

Foust, Dean, and Brian Grow. 2004. Wooing the TiVo generation. *Business Week*, March 1, p. 77.

Frito-Lay.com. 2005. "If not now when?"—Doritos launches innovative campaign. http://www.fritolay .com/fl/flstore/cgi-bin/ProdDetEv_Cat_304_NavRoot_303_ProdID_390425.htm (accessed June 6, 2005).

Fung, Amanda. 2007. Alloy buys Channel One from Primedia. *New York Business.com*, April 23. http://www.newyorkbusiness.com/apps/pbcs.dll/article?AID=/20070423/FREE/70423007/1064 (accessed July 26, 2007).

Gentile, Gary. 2005. Products place liberally in video games. *Associated Press Business Wire*, May 21. http://sunherald.com/mld/ sunherald/bus iness/11700310 (accessed September 10, 2005).

Gepetto Group. n.d. The Gepetto Group: Bios. http://www.reveries.com/reverb/revolver/gepetto/gepetto_ bios.html.

Grasser, Marc. 2005. McDonald's rap song product placement stalls. *Advertising Age*, September 26. http://adage.com/abstract.php?article_id=46875 (accessed September 26, 2005).

Greenberg, Karl. 2007. Kids ad summit sets stage for new regulatory agenda. *Media Daily News*, June 25. http://publications.mediapost.com/index.cfm?fuseaction=Articles.showArticleHomePage&art_aid =62896 (accessed June 25, 2007).

Hacket, Kim. 2005. Coke's reading program can leave a funny taste. *Sarasota Herald-Tribune*, August 19, sec. BV4.

Harrison, Kristen H., and Amy L. Marske. 2005. Nutritional content of foods advertised during the television programs children watch most. *American Journal of Public Health* 9:1568-74.

Hawkes, Corinna. 2004. *Marketing food to children: The global regulatory environment*. Geneva, Switzerland: World Health Organization.

Hellmich, Nancy. 2005. McDonald's kicks off school PE program. *USA Today*, September 13, sec. 7D.

Hill, Michael. 2005. Hey Popeye! It's SpongeBob spinach. *San Diego Union Tribune*, July 19, sec. 1C. http://www.signonsandiego.com/uniontrib/20050719/news_1c19spongbob.html (accessed September 29, 2005).

Institute of Medicine (IOM). 2007. *Fact sheet for nutrition standards for foods in schools: Leading the way toward healthier youth*. http://www.iom.edu/CMS/3788/30181/42502.aspx (accessed July 2, 2007).

Kellogg Company Press Releases. 2006. Kellogg's Pop-Tarts and CONNECT Music, downloads powered by Sony, offer free song downloads. http://investor.kelloggs.com/releasedetail.cfm?releaseid=216649 (accessed June 25, 2007).

King, Rachael. 2006. Marketing to kids where they live. *Business Week*, September 11. http://www .businessweek.com/technology/content/sep2006/tc20060908_974400.htm?chan=technology_technology+ index+page_more+of+today's+top+stories (accessed September 24, 2005).

Kjos, Tiffany. 2002. Marketers compete fiercely for spending on kids. *Knight Ridder Tribune Business News*, April 15, p. 1.

Klaassen, Abbey. 2007. Social networking reaches near full penetration among teens and 'tweens. *Advertising Age*, June 25. http://adage.com/results?search_offset=0&search_order_by=score&search_phrase=Social+Networking+Reaches+Near+Full+Penetration+among+Teens+and+ (accessed June 25, 2007).

Kraftsbrands.com. 2007a. Kraft Mac & Cheese-a-palooza. http://www.kraftbrands.com/crex/cheese-a-palooza/index.html.

————. 2007b. Welcome to Lunchables.com. http://www.kraftbrands.com/lunchables/index.aspx ?area=TRANSFORMERS (accessed June 25, 2007).

Kunkel, Dale. 2001. Children and television advertising. In *Handbook of children and the media*, ed. Dorothy Singer and Jerome Singer, 375-93. Thousand Oaks, CA: Sage.

Lawton, Christopher. 2005. PepsiCo's Mountain Dew backs film. *Wall Street Journal*, September 12, sec. B4.

Linn, Susan. 2004. *Consuming kids: The hostile takeover of childhood*. New York: New Press.

McDonald's. 2007. Nutrition facts—Minty Mudd Bath Triple Thick Shake. http://app.mcdonalds.com/bagamcmeal?process=item &itemID=3889 (accessed June 15, 2007).

McGinnis, J. Michael, Jennifer Gootman, and Vivica I. Kraak, eds. 2006. *Food marketing to children and youth: Threat or opportunity?* Washington, DC: Institute of Medicine of the National Academies.

Metherell Mark. 2002. Doctors urged to look at TV's role in obesity. *Sydney Morning Herald*, December 9, p. 3.

————. 2003. EU Commission targets unfair businesses practices. *Sydney Morning Herald*, June 19, p. 3.

Meyers, Stephanie. 2004. Brookmeade Elem. named "MCS Reads" school of the month, students, faculty celebrate literacy with Ronald McDonald. http://www.mcsk12.net/admin/communications/newsreleases_dec_04.html (accessed June 25, 2007).

Miller, Lia. 2007. NBC News to provide content for Channel One. *New York Times*, July 9, sec. C5.

Minnow, Nell. 2004. Common sense review of Scooby Doo 2. http://commonsensemedia.org/reviews/review.php?id=2533&type=Video/DVD (accessed June 6, 2007).

Molnar, Alex. 2004. Virtually everywhere: Marketing to children in America's schools. http://epsl.asu.edu/ceru/CERU_2004_Annual_Report.htm (accessed August 28, 2005).

Molnar, A., David R. Garcia, Faith Boninger, and Burce Merrill. 2006. A national survey of the types and extent of the marketing of foods of minimal nutritional value in schools. Arizona State University: Commercialism in Education Research Unit (CERU). http://epsl.asu.edu/ceru/CERU_2006_Research_Writing.htm (accessed June 25, 2007).

MySpace.com. 2007. Cherry Coke. http://www.myspace.com/cherrycoke (accessed June 29, 2007).

Neeley, Sabrina M., and David W. Schumann. 2004. Using animated spokes-characters in advertising to young children. *Journal of Advertising* 33 (3): 7-23.

Neopets.com. 2005. General Mills cereal adventure. http://www.neopets.com/sponsors/cereal_adventure .phtml (accessed September 10, 2005).

Neville, Linda. 2001. Kids brands must exercise pest control. *Brand Strategy*, November, p. 17.

Nevius, C. W. 2003. One extremely absorbing cartoon: Nickelodeon's nutty "SpongeBob SquarePants" is a surprise runaway success. *San Francisco Chronicle*, March 9.

Nielsen Media Research. 2007. Cited in Cynthia Turner's *Cynopsis: Kids!* [E-mail Newsletter], May.

Ogden, Cythia L., Margaret D. Carroll, and C. L. Johnson, 2002. Prevalence and trends in overweight among US children and adolescents, 1999–2000. *Journal of the American Medical Association* 288:1728-32.

Pereca, Laura. 2005. Cell phone marketers calling all preteens. *USA Today*, September 5. http://www.usatoday .com/money/industries/technology/2005-09-05-preteen-cell-phones_x.htm (accessed September 15, 2005).

Pollack, Judann. 1999. Foods targeting children aren't just child's play: Shape-shifting foods, "interactive" products chase young consumers. *Advertising Age*, March 1.

Powell, Chris. 2003. Get in the game. *Marketing Magazine*, July 28, p. 11.

Reading Is Fundamental: Who We Are. 2001. Reading takes you places: A partnership between RIF and Coca-Cola. http://www.rif.org/about/partners/coca-cola.mspx (accessed July 2, 2007).

Reuters. 2007. "Transformers" director firing on all cylinders. http://www.reuters.com/article/filmNews/idUSN2724778820070627 (accessed July 2, 2007).

Rivard, N., and P. LeBlanc. 2000. Advertising to kids in Quebec no picnic. *Strategy*, May 8, sec. B10.

Robinson, Thomas N., Dina L. G. Borzekowski, Donna M. Matheson, and Helena C. Kramer. 2007. Effects of fast food branding on young children's taste. *Archives of Pediatric and Adolescent Medicine* 161 (8): 792-97.

Rowan, David. 2002. Hard sell, soft targets. *The Times* (London), October 18, p. 6.

Rubin, Ross. 2004. Kids vs. teens: Money and maturity guide online behavior. *eMarketer*. http://www.emarketer.com/Report.aspx?kids_may04 (accessed September 25, 2005).

Saunders, Kathy. 2005. SpongeBob snacks are fruity fun. *St. Petersburgh Times*, February 2, sec. 2E. http://www.sptimes.com/2005/02/02/Taste/SpongeBob_snacks_are_.shtml (accessed September 29, 2005).

Save a Life Foundation. 2005. Ronald McDonald joins SALF instructor Juan Sotomayor at Monroe Elementary. http://www.salf.org/media/news/2004_11/november_22_2004.aspx (accessed November 22, 2005).

Schlosser, Eric. 2001. *Fast food nation: The dark side of the all-American meal*. New York: Harper-Perennial.

School Fund-Raisers.com. 2005. Brand candy. http://www.school-fundraisers.com/brandcandy/index.html (accessed September 12, 2005).

School news. 2004. *The Times-Picayune*, March 14, 8.

Schor, Juliet. 2004. *Born to buy: The commercialized child and the new consumer culture*. New York: Scribner.

Sesame Workshop. 2005. "If Elmo eats broccoli, will kids eat it too?" Atkins Foundation Grant to fund further research. Press Release, September 20. http://www.sesameworkshop.org/aboutus/inside_press.php?contentId=15092302 (accessed July 27, 2007).

Simon, Michele. 2005. Big food's "health education." *San Francisco Chronicle*, June 7, sec. B9. http://www.sfgate.com/cgi-bin/article.cgi?file=/chronicle/archive/2005/09/07/EDGH4EJB7U1.DTL (accessed September 15, 2005).

Sinha, Ranjana, Gene Fisch, Barbara Teague, William V. Tamborlane, Bruna Banyas, Karin Allen, Mary Savoye, Vera Rieger, Sara Taksali, Gina Barbetta, Robert S. Sherwin, and Sonia Caprio. 2002. Prevalence of impaired glucose tolerance among children and adolescents with marked obesity. *New England Journal of Medicine* 346 (11): 802-10.

SpongeBob SquarePants Bubble Trouble Cereal Game. 2005. http://www.nick.com/ads/kelloggs/sbsp/ (accessed September 4, 2005).

Story, Louise. 2007. Promoting a thirst for Sprite in teenage cell phone users. *New York Times Online*, June 7. http://www.nytimes.com/2007/06/07/technology/07sprite.html?ex=1338868800&en=1968dd3faefca93b&ei=5089&partner=rssyahoo&emc=rss (accessed June 15, 2007).

Story, Mary, and Simone French. 2004. Food advertising and marketing directed at children and adolescents in the US. *International Journal of Behavioral Nutrition and Physical Activity* 1:3. http://www.ijbnpa.org/content/pdf/1479-5868-1-3.pdf (accessed September 15, 2005).

SunnyD.com. 2007a. Products—Nutritional information Sunny D Baja Orange-Pineapple. http://www.sunnyd.com/products/baja_orangepineapple.shtml (accessed June 25, 2007).

———. 2007b. Products—Nutritional information Sunny D Tangy Orange Original Style. http://www.sunnyd.com/products/original_tangy.shtml (accessed June 25, 2007).

Taylor, Paul. 2004. Liberty, equality, fraternity . . . obesity? *The Globe and Mail*, August 6, sec. A11.

Thompson, Stephanie. 1999. Cap'n goes AWOL as sales flatten; Quaker redirects cereal brand's marketing budget to focus on kids. *Advertising Age*, November 22, p. 8.

Tienowitz, Ira. 2007. Big food cuts $1B in kids ads; pols' hunger still not sated; critics call for media cos. to follow marketers' lead and reject junk-food spots. *Advertising Age*, July 23. (accessed July 27, 2007).

Townville Elementary School Web site. 2005. Townville, South Carolina. http://www.anderson4.k12.sc.us/schools/tes/Special%20Events.htm#Safe%20Kids%20Assembly (accessed September 20, 2005).

U.S. General Accounting Office (GAO). 2000. *Public education: Commercial activities in schools: Report to congressional requesters*. Washington, DC: GAO. http://www.gao.gov/archive/2000/he00156.pdf.

———. 2005. School meal programs: Competitive foods are widely available and generate substantial revenues for schools. http://www.gao.gov/new.items/d05563.pdf (accessed September 14, 2005).

Warner, Melanie. 2005. Coke is urging youths to get physical. *New York Times*, July 12. http://www
.nytimes.com/2005/07/12/business/media/12adco.html?ex=1278820800&en=f6e4aa955ed0bbdd&ei
=5088&partner=rssnyt&emc=rss (accessed June 25, 2007).

Warnerbros.com. 2007. Saturday morning forever: 52 Weeks . . . 52 Winners! Contest. Available from
http://www2.warnerbros.com/web/all/us/ sweepstakes/enter.jsp?sid=hbfreeprizeinsidesweeps&show
=SWEEPSTAKES (accessed June 25, 2007).

Winding, Elizabeth. 2002. Immersed in child's play: A website that offers virtual pets has found a successful way of advertising to children. *Financial Times*, June 10, p. 17.

World Health Organization (WHO). 2003. *Diet, nutrition, and the prevention of chronic diseases*. Geneva,
Switzerland: WHO. http://whqlibdoc.who.int/trs/WHO_TRS_916.pdf (accessed June 15, 2007).

Wrigley's Candystand. 2007. http://www.candystand.com/ (accessed June 29, 2007).

Xbox Games. 2007. Sneak King. http://www.xbox.com/en-US/ games/b/bksneakking/default.htm (accessed
June 25, 2007).

Zuill, Lilla, and Jolie Vorman. 2007. Food companies promise to limit ads for kids. *Reuters*, July 18. http://
www.reuters.com/article/technology-media-telco-SP-A/idUSN1841388520070718?pageNumber=1
(accessed July 27, 2007).

SECTION THREE

Public Policy Efforts

First Amendment Implications of Restricting Food and Beverage Marketing in Schools

By
SAMANTHA K. GRAFF

This article explores how the First Amendment bears upon a school district policy restricting junk food and soda marketing in public schools. The article highlights a clash between two fundamental American beliefs: that a public school should be a sheltered training ground for democratic citizenship and that the strength of the free market economy is dependent upon corporate access to consumers including children. The article begins by describing the "commercial speech doctrine," which explains why the First Amendment might be implicated in a school district advertising policy. The article then touches on actions a school district might take without involving the First Amendment. Next, the article distinguishes between two First Amendment standards of review that a court could apply to a school district advertising policy and argues that a "forum analysis" is the appropriate approach. The article identifies three types of advertising policies that should survive a forum analysis.

Keywords: First Amendment; commercial speech; in-school advertising; marketing to children; commercialization of childhood; obesity; nutrition; junk food and soda

In the American tradition, the U.S. public school system is the "cradle of our democracy."[1] As envisioned by the Supreme Court, the archetypal public school is a sheltered environment in which teachers are entrusted to prepare students "for participation as citizens" by "inculcating fundamental values necessary to the maintenance of a democratic political system."[2] Increasingly over the past few decades, however, K-12 public schools have thrown open their doors to commercial marketers seeking to inculcate a different set of values—those essential to the maintenance of a consumeristic society.

NOTE: Support for this research was provided by the Robert Wood Johnson Foundation's program, Healthy Eating Research: Building Evidence to Prevent Childhood Obesity. The author is grateful to Debora Pinkas, Randolph Kline, Leslie Zellers, Linda Lye, Susan Linn, and Professor Robert Post for their intellectual contributions to this article.

DOI: 10.1177/0002716207308398

School districts allow commercial messaging on school property for a variety of reasons, including the need to offset chronic underfunding with a non-tax-based revenue stream as well as the desire to enlist businesses as partners in the educational enterprise.[3] A less obvious but perhaps more insidious reason is that multi-billion-dollar corporate marketing campaigns are so elemental to our free market culture that some school districts fail to question whether an educational environment is an appropriate place for advertising to take place.[4]

For their part, corporations are more than eager to pay for access to a large, captive, demographically discrete, and impressionable audience of current and future loyal customers.[5] These corporations gain entry through many routes, which include obtaining the right to place logos or advertisements on school grounds or facilities, contributing electronic equipment in exchange for the ability to advertise to students, providing corporate-produced "educational" materials and activities, participating in fund-raising campaigns, initiating incentive programs that reward students who succeed in specified activities, sponsoring programs and activities, privatizing certain school programs, and selling and promoting a set of brands to the exclusion of all other brands in the school district.[6]

Candy, fast food, and soda manufacturers are leading the charge into the public schools.[7] It would not be unusual for a middle school student to ride a school bus covered with Burger King advertisements, start each day at school watching a Channel One newscast sprinkled with junk food and soda commercials, learn math with exercise books and candy provided by Jelly Belly, receive a Pizza Hut gift certificate as a reward for reading, play basketball in the school gym under a Pepsi billboard, lunch on Taco Bell nachos dispensed in the school cafeteria, and snack on junk food and soda products exclusively provided by a single manufacturer through branded vending machines scattered around the school.[8] Not even kindergarteners are immune from the onslaught of junk food and soda marketing at school. For example, the Coca-Cola Company has been known to "bring books to life" at elementary schools willing to host a visit by the Coca-Cola Story Chasers Reading Mobile,[9] and the McDonald's Corporation will send Ronald McDonald into elementary schools to be an "ambassador for an active, balanced lifestyle."[10]

Schools undoubtedly have a powerful influence on how students eat.[11] Studies have shown a direct correlation between the school food environment and the consumption of fruits, vegetables, and dietary fat as well as the body mass index of students.[12] Thus, the ubiquity on public school campuses of nonnutritious food and drinks, and of messages promoting their consumption, is of grave concern to many parents, teachers, administrators, and nutrition advocates. By allowing junk food and soda companies to saturate the school atmosphere with their products

Samantha K. Graff is a staff attorney with Public Health Law & Policy (PHLP), a project of the Public Health Institute, in Oakland, California. PHLP works with leaders in government and the nonprofit sector to create innovative policy solutions to critical public health challenges. She has published on law and public health topics in several law journals. She received a J.D. from the Yale Law School and an A.B. from Harvard University.

and messages, schools may not only be subverting their efforts to teach students about good nutrition but may also be helping to fuel the American childhood obesity epidemic.[13]

Across the country, there is a growing movement to urge public school districts to limit nonnutritious food and beverage marketing on campus.[14] A school district that wants to counteract the pervasiveness of junk food and soda manufacturers at school may be inhibited, however, not only by monetary and political pressures but also by legal questions relating to the First Amendment.[15]

This article seeks to demystify how the First Amendment bears upon efforts to restrict food and beverage marketing in public schools. The article begins by describing the origin of the "commercial speech doctrine," which explains why the First Amendment might be implicated in a school district policy to limit junk food and soda marketing on school grounds. The article then touches on actions a school district might take without involving the First Amendment. Next, the article distinguishes between two First Amendment standards of review that a court could apply to a school district advertising policy—a forum analysis and the commercial speech test—and argues that a forum analysis is the appropriate approach. The article determines that there are three types of advertising policies that should survive judicial review under a forum analysis: (1) a ban on all advertising on campus, (2) a ban on all food and beverage advertising on campus, or (3) a ban on advertising on campus for those foods and drinks that are not allowed to be sold on campus.

I. Origin of the Commercial Speech Doctrine

As recently as the 1970s, the Supreme Court found advertising to be entirely outside the scope of First Amendment protection.[16] The sanctuary of the First Amendment was reserved for "pure speech" relating to "truth, science, morality, and arts in general, in its diffusion of liberal sentiments on the administration of Government."[17] The Supreme Court had long held that a government ban on "pure speech" due to its content was subject to strict judicial scrutiny and was almost always per se invalid.[18]

Between the 1940s—when the question of constitutional protection for advertising first presented itself to the Supreme Court—and the 1970s, the Supreme Court generally analyzed advertising not as a form of free expression but rather as a standard business practice subject to government regulation.[19] The Court ruled that the profit motive driving advertising was trumped by a range of government interests, including enforcing a sanitary code provision forbidding the distribution of advertising leaflets in the street,[20] freeing the optical profession from the taint of commercialism associated with advertisements for eyeglass frames,[21] and sparing residents the annoyance of door-to-door solicitation.[22] The Court saw no First Amendment issue associated with a government body's decision to restrict certain advertising in order to advance the perceived health, safety, or welfare of the community.

In the 1976 case of *Virginia State Board of Pharmacy v. Virginia Citizens Consumer Council,*[23] however, the Supreme Court announced a new "commercial speech doctrine" that welcomed advertising into the protective domain of the First Amendment. The case involved a statewide ban on the advertisement of prescription drug prices.[24] Squarely before the Court was the question of whether speech that does "no more than propose a commercial transaction" is entitled to First Amendment protection.[25]

In the wake of Virginia Pharmacy, *courts treat a government advertising regulation as a First Amendment issue.*

The analysis in *Virginia Pharmacy* rested on the importance of the free flow of commercial information to the targeted consumer and society at large. The Court noted that a particular consumer's interest in an advertisement "may be as keen, if not keener by far, than his interest in the day's most urgent political debate."[26] This seemed especially true for the poor, sick, and elderly, who had scarce dollars to spend on medication and scarce resources to comparison shop among pharmacies. It also determined that "advertising, however tasteless and excessive it sometimes may seem," is essential to the smooth functioning of a free enterprise economy in a democracy.[27] In the Court's view, the free flow of commercial information is indispensable because it helps inform numerous private economic decisions that—in aggregate—determine the proper allocation of resources in a market system. In turn, it helps democratic decision makers form intelligent opinions about how this market system should be regulated. In striking down the prescription drug price advertising ban, the Court ruled that advertising, or "commercial speech," is entitled to some degree of protection under the First Amendment.[28]

Justice Rehnquist wrote a prescient dissent in *Virginia Pharmacy* in which he foresaw far-reaching implications of the Court's decision to "elevate . . . commercial intercourse between a seller hawking his wares and a buyer seeking to strike a bargain" to the plane of speech deserving of First Amendment protection.[29] He bemoaned that the path would now be open for advertising of such undesirable products as prescription drugs, liquor, and cigarettes.[30] Incredulous, he imagined a scenario in which a pharmacist would run an advertisement in a local newspaper—or even on television during family viewing time—saying, "Don't spend another sleepless night. Ask your doctor to prescribe Seconal without delay."[31]

In the wake of *Virginia Pharmacy*, courts treat a government advertising regulation as a First Amendment issue. This does not mean that courts will outlaw any government effort to limit advertising on specified topics, but it does mean that when such efforts are challenged, courts will subject them to close scrutiny. Even in the *Virginia Pharmacy* era, the Supreme Court has left school districts with a variety of options to limit nonnutritious food and beverage marketing on their campuses.

II. Avoiding First Amendment Scrutiny

Before addressing how a school district might design a policy to withstand a First Amendment challenge, it is worth noting that there are at least two ways the public schools could combat the rampant promotion of unhealthy food and drinks on their campuses without invoking First Amendment scrutiny at all: they could ban products without regulating speech, and they could draft individual contracts with vendors that do not permit certain sales and advertising practices. The downside of these approaches is that they would be significantly less comprehensive than a districtwide policy targeting all aspects of in-school food and beverage marketing.

A. Regulating Products

In envisioning the ways a school district might seek to reduce the promotion of junk food and sodas in schools, it is important to distinguish between policies that regulate products (e.g., by setting nutritional standards that eliminate categories of products) and those that regulate speech about the products. For example, a court will treat a ban on the sale of soda in schools very differently from a ban on soda advertising in schools.

When the government regulates a product directly, say by prohibiting the sale of a product or by restricting how or where a product is sold, the government generally does not implicate the First Amendment. If the regulation is challenged on constitutional grounds, a court is likely to apply the "rational basis test."[32] Under this test, a regulation will be upheld so long as it bears a rational relationship to a legitimate governmental purpose.[33] The rational basis test is very deferential to the government, and courts are quite reluctant to overturn regulations subject to the rational basis test.[34] A rational relationship need not be proven by scientific data but instead need only be supported by common sense.[35] Protecting public health and protecting children have long been accepted to be legitimate governmental purposes.[36]

If a school district decides to limit the types of food and beverage products that are allowed to be sold on campus, the policy should survive a constitutional challenge with ease under the rational basis test. (This article does not address the scientific and policy considerations involved in drawing the line around a set of food and beverage products that would be targeted by a particular policy. The article merely shows that courts will likely accept whatever line is drawn so long as the line is based on "rational speculation."[37] If, however, the school district also wants to restrict advertising for certain types of food and beverages on campus, the legal landscape becomes somewhat more complicated because the First Amendment is drawn in.

Sometimes it can be difficult to distinguish between a product regulation and an advertising regulation. For example, tobacco companies have alleged that a government prohibition on the distribution of free tobacco samples not only regulates products but also regulates commercial speech protected by the First Amendment.[38] Similarly, a food manufacturer might argue that a school district ban on the distribution of free candy samples is, in part, an advertising regulation subject to a First Amendment analysis. The case law is undeveloped regarding the distinction between product and advertising regulations, and it is beyond the scope of this article to imagine the range of product-based restrictions a school district might impose that could inadvertently sweep in commercial speech interests. Suffice it to say that when conceptualizing a school district policy limiting the distribution of specified food and beverage company products, it is worth considering whether commercial speech interests might be implicated and, if so, whether the policy could withstand a First Amendment challenge.

B. Restricting Advertising through Individual Contract Provisions

Often, an individual school is authorized to negotiate with outside vendors to provide food and food-related services and products to its campus. By limiting advertising through a contract provision with these vendors, a school might be able to ward off a First Amendment challenge.

A party may give up (i.e., "waive") its constitutional rights—including First Amendment free speech rights—in certain circumstances, including via a contract.[39] To be constitutional, the waiver must be done voluntarily and with full awareness of the legal consequences.[40] Courts are generally satisfied "where the parties to the contract have bargaining equality and have negotiated the terms of the contract, and where the waiving party is advised by competent counsel and has engaged in other contract negotiations."[41]

This means that during contract negotiations, a school can request that a vendor agree to any type of advertising prohibition envisioned by the school. If the vendor signs the contract with a provision containing an advertising prohibition, the vendor relinquishes any First Amendment rights it might have had to advertise in the school as long as the vendor entered into the contract voluntarily and with full awareness of the legal consequences. Given that competitive food and beverage vendors tend to be large companies with sophisticated business and legal savvy, they will be hard-pressed to argue after the fact that they did not sign the contract voluntarily and with full awareness of the legal consequences. Therefore, such a contract is almost certainly enforceable and invulnerable to a subsequent First Amendment challenge by the vendor.

[A] school can request that a vendor agree to any type of advertising prohibition envisioned by the school. If the vendor signs the contract with a provision containing an advertising prohibition, the vendor relinquishes any First Amendment rights it might have had to advertise in the school as long as the vendor entered into the contract voluntarily and with full awareness of the legal consequences.

Using contracts to restrict junk food and soda advertising on campus would be a particularly appealing strategy for a public school principal who cares about the issue and who has the authority to negotiate with vendors, but who cannot convince the governing body to tackle the problem at a districtwide level. If, however, many schools in a district start inserting the same advertising prohibition into their vending contracts, it may begin to appear that the district has a de facto policy (i.e., a policy that exists in fact if not on paper) of limiting food and beverage advertising.[42] As described above, a school district advertising policy will be treated by the courts as a First Amendment issue.

III. Two Possible First Amendment Standards of Review

From a First Amendment perspective, a limitation or ban on advertising nonnutritious food and beverages in public schools has two important attributes: it involves a content-based government regulation on *public property* and of *advertising*. As a result, if the regulation is challenged in court, one of two First Amendment standards of review could apply: a forum analysis or the commercial speech test.

A *forum analysis* focuses on the location of the speech regulation. Courts generally use a forum analysis when considering government restrictions on speech on *public property*. The *commercial speech test* focuses on the type of speech being regulated. Courts generally use the commercial speech test when considering government restrictions on *advertising*. This section describes the structure of a forum analysis and the commercial speech test and argues that a forum analysis should be the appropriate standard of review in a case involving a First Amendment challenge to a school district advertising policy.

A. Forum Analysis

A limitation or ban on advertising in public schools entails a content-based speech restriction on public property. A content-based speech restriction outlaws speech about a specified topic that the government deems to be inappropriate or offensive to the ears of a particular audience.[43] When a government body is subject to a First Amendment challenge for imposing a content-based speech restriction on public property, courts generally apply a standard of review called a "forum analysis." Under a forum analysis, the government's likelihood of victory depends largely on the nature of the public property targeted by the restriction.

The Supreme Court shaped the forum analysis in the case of *Perry Education Association v. Perry Local Educators' Association.*[44] *Perry* defines three categories of public property on which the government might seek to impose a content-based speech restriction:

- A *public forum* is public property, such as a street or park, which by long tradition or government fiat has been devoted to assembly and debate.[45]
- A *designated public forum* is public property that the government has opened for use by the public as a place for expressive activity.[46] Examples include a school board meeting or a municipal theater.[47]
- A *non–public forum* is public property that is neither by tradition or designation a forum for public communication.[48] Post offices and military installations are quintessential non–public forums.[49]

In public and designated public forums, content-based speech restrictions are subject to a strict test (i.e., "strict scrutiny") and are likely to be struck down by a court.[50] In non–public forums, however, such restrictions are subject to a much more lenient test and have a good chance of being upheld.[51] Specifically, in a non–public forum, a content-based speech restriction will be upheld as long as it is "reasonable and not an effort to suppress expression merely because public officials oppose the speaker's view."[52]

The Supreme Court presumes that all facilities in elementary, middle, and high schools are non–public forums subject to a lenient First Amendment test.[53] For example, in the important case of *Hazelwood School District v. Kuhlmeier,*[54] the Supreme Court held that a high school newspaper published as a part of a journalism class was a non–public forum.[55] The Court recognized that the "special characteristics of the school environment" justify giving school authorities a great deal of leeway to control speech in accord with their "basic educational mission."[56]

A school facility will be deemed a public forum or designated public forum subject to strict scrutiny "only if school authorities have by policy or by practice opened [it] for *indiscriminate use* by the general public or by some segment of the public, such as student organizations."[57] A court is unlikely to find a school facility to be a public forum even if it has been opened to the speech of select outside groups.[58] Nor will a court be inclined to name a school facility a public forum simply because it has been used for the purpose of raising money.[59] The case law precedent shows that a school district should be able to persuade a court easily that the facilities targeted by its advertising policy are non–public forums.

B. Commercial Speech Test

As described above, the *Virginia Pharmacy* case announced a new commercial speech doctrine that extended some First Amendment protection to advertising. In the 1980 case of *Central Hudson Gas & Electric Corporation v. Public Service Commission of New York*,[60] the Supreme Court shaped the commercial speech doctrine into a formal standard of review when it struck down a state regulation banning promotional advertising by electric utilities. The *Central Hudson* Court developed a special test to assess whether a government regulation of advertising passes First Amendment muster.[61] This test has four prongs:

1. The advertising must not promote illegal activity and must not be false or inherently misleading.
2. The government must declare a substantial interest that it intends to achieve with the advertising regulation.
3. The regulation must directly advance the government interest.
4. The regulation must be no more extensive than necessary to achieve the government interest.[62]

For the purpose of this article, it is less important to grasp the workings of the commercial speech test than it is to understand where the test stands in relation to the components of a forum analysis. The commercial speech test is an intermediate-level standard of review. It is easier for the government to pass than strict scrutiny but harder to pass than a lenient non–public forum analysis.[63]

C. Forum Analysis versus Commercial Speech Test

A thorough search of case law reveals no decision that directly addresses the issue of whether a forum analysis or the commercial speech test should apply to an advertising restriction on public school grounds. However, plain logic, Supreme Court precedent, and Ninth Circuit precedent provide three sources of support for the conclusion that, as long as the given school facilities have not opened themselves up to indiscriminate expressive use, a straightforward non–public forum analysis is the appropriate standard.

First, plain logic dictates that the commercial speech test can only be relevant in the context of a public or designated public forum. In a public or designated public forum, the default test is strict scrutiny. Since advertising is entitled to less protection than "pure" speech, however, the intermediate-level commercial speech test should substitute for strict scrutiny in a case involving advertising restrictions in a public or designated public forum.[64] In a non–public forum, the default test is more lenient than both strict scrutiny and the commercial speech test. Therefore, in a non–public forum, it should not matter whether the speech targeted by the restriction is "pure" or commercial because the government retains a great deal of discretion to curtail all kinds of speech. In fact, it would be nonsensical for the commercial speech test to apply because this would elevate commercial speech to a higher level of protection than "pure" speech in a non–public forum.

Second, Supreme Court precedent shows that the commercial speech test is specifically designed to secure adult access to advertising messages and that children do not enjoy the same rights as adults to receive information. In a string of commercial speech cases, the Supreme Court repeatedly has voiced its skepticism of "regulations that seek to keep people in the dark for what the government perceives to be their own good."[65] In contrast, the Court has applied lenient standards of review to government restrictions on speech aimed at audiences composed predominantly of children because their intellectual and emotional immaturity makes them particularly vulnerable to harm.[66]

[T]he Court has applied lenient standards of review to government restrictions on speech aimed at audiences composed predominantly of children because their intellectual and emotional immaturity makes them particularly vulnerable to harm.

As early as 1944, in the case of *Prince v. Massachusetts*,[67] the Supreme Court proclaimed: "The state's authority over children's activities is broader than over like actions of adults. . . . A democratic society rests, for its continuance, upon the healthy, well-rounded growth of young people into full maturity as citizens. . . . It may secure this against impeding restraints and dangers."[68] The Court reiterated this principle in the 1968 decision of *Ginsberg v. New York*, which involved a state law restricting youth access to sexual materials. The Court held that children do not have the same constitutional right as adults to receive pornographic magazines: "Because of the State's exigent interest in preventing distribution to children of objectionable material, it can exercise its power to protect the health, safety, welfare and morals of its community by barring the distribution to children of books recognized to be suitable for adults."[69] In the same spirit, the "special characteristics of the school environment" inspired the Court in the *Hazelwood* case to uphold a principal's decision to excise articles about pregnancy and divorce from the student newspaper.[70] The Supreme Court's inclination to extend differential treatment to adult and child audiences points toward the use of a lenient non–public forum analysis in place of the more stringent commercial speech test in a case involving an advertising restriction on public school grounds.

Third, the Ninth Circuit has applied a non–public forum analysis—without even pausing to consider whether the commercial speech test might pertain—to a case involving a public school district's decision to exclude certain advertisements from school newspapers.[71] In *Planned Parenthood v. Clark County School District*,[72] the Ninth Circuit relied on *Hazelwood* to determine that the school newspapers constituted a non–public forum because their advertising slots had not been opened to indiscriminate use by the public or some segment of the public.[73] After reaching this determination, the Ninth Circuit reflected on the degree of latitude it owed the school district under a non–public forum analysis in the context of the educational environment: " 'The education of the Nation's youth is primarily the responsibility of parents, teachers, and state and local officials, and not of federal judges.' We are not educators and curricular choices are not ours to make. We are not members of the Board of Education and it is not open to us as judges to decide this case as we might vote were we politicians."[74]

In sum, a court is very likely to apply a non–public forum analysis rather than the commercial speech test to a school district policy that restricts junk food and soda advertising on campus.

IV. Conceptualizing a Policy to Pass a Non–Public Forum Analysis

Under the First Amendment non–public forum analysis, a school district policy to limit or prohibit nonnutritious food and beverage advertising on campus must be both "reasonable" and "viewpoint neutral."[75] This section assesses whether four types of advertising policies are both reasonable and viewpoint neutral:

1. a ban on all advertising on campus,
2. a ban on all food and beverage advertising on campus,
3. a ban on advertising on campus for those foods and drinks that are not allowed to be sold on campus, and
4. a ban on the advertising on campus of unhealthy food and beverage products (however defined) while concurrently allowing the sale on campus of those same products.

The first three types of advertising policies should survive both the reasonableness and viewpoint neutrality prongs of a non–public forum analysis, but a school district will be in a riskier position if it implements a policy that forbids advertising on campus of products that are allowed to be sold on campus.

A. Reasonableness

A reasonableness determination turns on the question of whether the policy "is wholly consistent with the district's legitimate interest in preserving the property for the use to which it is lawfully dedicated."[76] The policy "need only be *reasonable*; it need not be the most reasonable or the only reasonable limitation."[77]

For example, in the *Planned Parenthood* case, the Ninth Circuit found that it was reasonable for a public school district to exclude advertisements for family-planning services from school newspapers. It did not matter that the schools accepted other advertisements, such as those for casinos, which might seem inappropriate for a teenage audience.[78] In assessing the reasonableness of the exclusion, the court acknowledged the right of educators to tailor the topics of advertising in public school to the emotional maturity of the audience. Moreover, given that a non–public forum "by definition is not dedicated to general debate or the free exchange of ideas," the court held that it was reasonable to forbid school newspaper advertisements that are "controversial, offensive to some groups of people, that cause tension and anxiety between teachers and parents, and between competing groups such as [Planned Parenthood] and pro-life forces."[79]

A school district policy most likely would be reasonable if it prohibited (1) all advertising on campus, (2) all food and beverage advertising on campus, or (3) all advertising on campus for those foods and drinks that are not allowed to be sold on campus. The district could assert a range of legitimate pedagogical interests backing each policy. For instance, the district could defend a total advertising ban by pointing to its efforts to promote an educational rather than a commercial atmosphere and to prevent corporate exploitation of students. The district could defend a ban on all food and beverage advertising on campus by showing it wants to avoid confusion by limiting messages about nutrition-related topics to the classroom. And the district could defend a ban on advertising for foods and drinks that it does not allow to be sold on campus by declaring a desire to be consistent in its wellness policy and to avoid the appearance of endorsing junk food and soda.[80]

If, however, a school district forbids advertising on campus for a category of food and drink products while simultaneously allowing the sale of those same products on campus, the district may be vulnerable to a reasonableness challenge. Common sense dictates that the district would greatly undercut its rationale for the advertising restriction if it concurrently allowed students to purchase products subject to the restriction. Moreover, the Supreme Court is more protective of commercial speech than it is of commercial sales, so courts will look very suspiciously on any prohibition that applies to speech about a product but not to the product itself.[81]

B. *Viewpoint Neutrality*[82]

A government body may impose reasonable content-based restrictions on third-party speech in a non–public forum as long as the restrictions are not "an effort to suppress the speaker's activity due to disagreement with the speaker's view."[83] "Viewpoint neutrality" is a difficult legal concept to grasp.[84] A policy is "viewpoint neutral" if it restricts all third-party speech relating to a given subject matter, including speech in favor of and against the subject matter.[85] In other words, if the government body allows third parties into the forum to speak on a topic that is deemed permissible, then it cannot exclude certain speakers on the topic just because it opposes their viewpoint.[86]

In the *Planned Parenthood* example, the Ninth Circuit found the school district's decision to exclude advertisements for family-planning services from school newspapers to be viewpoint neutral. The court recognized that the advertisements "were rejected, and schools enacted guidelines excluding advertising that pertains to 'birth control products and information,' in order to maintain a position of neutrality on the sensitive and controversial issue of family planning and to avoid being forced to open up their publications for advertisements on both sides of the 'pro-life'–'pro-choice' debate."[87]

A school district should succeed in arguing that its policy is viewpoint neutral if the policy prohibits (1) all advertising on campus, (2) all food and beverage advertising on campus, or (3) all advertising on campus for those foods and drinks that are not allowed to be sold on campus. In each instance, the policy would draw a clear line around an entire subject of impermissible speech for third parties in the forum:

Type of Policy	Viewpoint Neutrality of Policy
1. Forbids *all advertising* on campus	*Neutral* with regard to the messages of *all advertisers*
2. Forbids *all food and beverage advertising* on campus	*Neutral* with regard to the messages of *all food and beverage advertisers*
3. Forbids *all advertising* on campus *for those foods and drinks that are not allowed to be sold* on campus	*Neutral* with regard to the messages of *all advertisers who want to promote or oppose* the consumption of the *foods and drinks that are not allowed to be sold* on campus

On initial glance, the ban described in (3) may seem to express a viewpoint by showing a preference for advertising about those products that are allowed to be sold on campus. In other words, such a ban may appear to express a viewpoint that favors advertising about milk over advertising about soda. However, in legal terms, this ban should be considered viewpoint neutral as long as it allows advertising that promotes and criticizes milk. The viewpoint neutrality analysis first asks what topic of speech is permissible (e.g., advertising for food and beverage products that are allowed to be sold on campus) and second asks whether third-party speakers who espouse differing views of the permissible topic are given an opportunity to speak.[88]

V. Official School Speech and Incidental Student Speech on Campus

Although this article focuses on the constitutionality of policies regarding *third-party* advertising on campus, ancillary questions naturally arise of how the

First Amendment would treat *school officials* or *students* who want to express their views about food and beverage products within the school setting.

The First Amendment gives the government wide latitude to express a substantive position about a topic and to take steps consistent with that position without being viewpoint neutral. This means that a district or a school is free to express its own views about foods and drinks and has no obligation to provide a forum for others with differing views.

A. Official School Speech on Campus

A forum analysis does not apply when the government itself is speaking on its property. The First Amendment gives the government wide latitude to express a substantive position about a topic and to take steps consistent with that position without being viewpoint neutral.[89] This means that a district or a school is free to express its own views about foods and drinks and has no obligation to provide a forum for others with differing views.[90] So a district can implement a health curriculum or a teacher can use soda advertisements in a media studies class without any requirement that food and beverage companies be given a platform to communicate their perspectives on nutrition or marketing principles to students.

B. Incidental Student Speech on Campus

It is somewhat difficult to predict how a court would apply First Amendment precedent to a policy that prohibited students from wearing, carrying, or discussing materials promoting nonnutritious food and beverage products. The Supreme Court precedent relating to this issue is in flux.

The Court historically has been much more protective of the personal expression of students and teachers that incidentally takes place at school than of the expression of students, teachers, and others that occurs with the sanction, or under the guise, of school authorities.[91] For example, in *Tinker v. Des Moines Independent Community School District*,[92] the Court struck down a public high school policy prohibiting students from wearing black armbands to protest the Vietnam War.[93] The Court held school officials to an exacting standard: student expression may not be suppressed unless it will "materially and substantially disrupt the work and discipline of the school."[94]

However, the recent case of *Morse v. Frederick*[95] signals a departure from tradition, or at least carves out an exception. In *Morse*, the Court ruled that a high school principal did not violate the First Amendment when she suspended a student for displaying a banner reading "Bong Hits 4 Jesus" at a school-supervised event.[96] The Court declined to follow *Tinker* and instead crafted a more lenient and fact-specific standard: student expression that reasonably appears to promote illegal drug use may be suppressed in light of the special characteristics of the school environment and the principal's interest in preventing illegal drug use by students.[97]

It remains unclear what standard of review would apply to a case involving a public school campus ban on another kind of student expression, such as wearing T-shirts decorated with soda brands. But in this type of case, school officials are unlikely to receive the level of sympathy that the principal did in *Morse* because *Morse* addressed expression about illegal activity.[98]

VI. Conclusion

Marketing goods and services—including junk food and soda—to public school students results in a collision between two classic American ideals. On one hand, our society nurtures a long-standing belief that a public school should be a protected environment in which students learn wholesome information and skills in preparation for democratic citizenship. On the other hand, we believe in the free market, accepting that access to new groups of consumers, including our nation's youth, bolsters the strength of our economy. Often, the clash of such fundamental ideals finds expression in our legal system, where competing parties draw from the Constitution and judicial precedent to wrangle over which interests should prevail.

The specific issue of advertising regulations in schools has received scant attention from the Supreme Court and the lower courts. Open questions remain regarding which legal standards should apply to a given type of policy and what results those standards should produce. Nonetheless, a well-developed body of constitutional law suggests that while the First Amendment keeps a tight rein on government entities that want to restrict advertising intended for adult consumers, it gives public school districts significant leeway to curb advertising directed at their student bodies.

[A] well-developed body of constitutional law suggests that while the First Amendment keeps a tight rein on government entities that want to restrict advertising intended for adult consumers, it gives public school districts significant leeway to curb advertising directed at their student bodies.

A school district policy limiting junk food and soda marketing on its campuses has a good chance of avoiding First Amendment problems if it (1) bans all advertising on campus, (2) bans all food and beverage advertising on campus, or (3) bans advertising on campus for those foods and drinks that are not allowed to be sold on campus. A school district will be more vulnerable to a First Amendment challenge, however, if it restricts advertising for products that are allowed to be sold on campus or if it forbids students and teachers from wearing, carrying, or discussing materials promoting junk food and soda products.

Notes

1. *See Adler v. Bd. of Educ. of City of New York*, 342 U.S. 485, 508 (1952) (J. Douglas, dissenting); *James v. Bd. of Educ.*, 461 F.2d 566, 568 (2d Cir. 1972).

2. *Ambach v. Norwick*, 441 U.S. 68, 77-78 (1979).

3. *See* Public Health Institute, *Food Advertising to Children and Youth: Do They Influence Unhealthy Food Purchases?* (2004), available at http://www.californiaprojectlean.org/Assets/1019/files/Brief_2.pdf (accessed June 21, 2007); Council for Corporate and School Partnerships, *School Beverage Guidelines*, http://www.corpschoolpartners.org/bev_guidelines.shtml (accessed June 21, 2007).

4. MICHELE SIMON, APPETITE FOR PROFIT: HOW THE FOOD INDUSTRY UNDERMINES OUR HEALTH AND HOW TO FIGHT BACK 245-73 (2006).

5. *See* SUSAN LINN, CONSUMING KIDS: PROTECTING OUR CHILDREN FROM THE ONSLAUGHT OF MARKETING & ADVERTISING 77-78 (2004); Steven Manning, *Students for Sale*, THE NATION (Sept. 27, 1999); Lawrence Hardy, *The Lure of School Marketing*, AM. SCH. BOARD J. (Oct. 1999), available at http://www.asbj.com/199910/1099coverstory.html.

6. *See* Alex Molnar, *Commercialism in Education Research Unit*, NINTH ANNUAL REPORT ON SCHOOLHOUSE COMMERCIALISM TRENDS 6-27 (2006), available at http://epsl.asu.edu/ceru/Annual%20reports/EPSL-0611-220-CERU.pdf (accessed June 21, 2007).

7. *See* Alex Molnar et al., COMMERCIALISM IN EDUCATION RESEARCH UNIT, EXECUTIVE SUMMARY: A NATIONAL SURVEY OF THE TYPES AND EXTENT OF THE MARKETING OF FOODS OF MINIMAL NUTRITIONAL VALUE IN SCHOOLS 2-3 (2006), available at http://epsl.asu.edu/ceru/Documents/EPSL-0609-211-CERU-EXEC.doc (accessed June 17, 2007).

8. *See id.*; Linn, *supra* note 5, at 75-76.

9. *See* Kim Hacket, *Coke's Reading Program Can Leave a Funny Taste*, SARASOTA HERALD TRIBUNE (Aug. 19, 2003).

10. *See* Michelle Simon, *Junk Food's Health Crusade: How Ronald McDonald Became a Health Ambassador, and Other Stories*, 26 MULTINATIONAL MONITOR (2005), available at http://multinationalmonitor .org/mm2005/032005/simon.html (accessed June 18, 2007).

11. *See* Centers for Disease Control and Prevention, *Guidelines for School Health Programs to Promote Lifelong Healthy Eating*, 45(RR-9) MMWR 1 (June 14, 1996).

12. *See, e.g.*, Martha Y. Kubik et al., *The Association of the School Food Environment with Dietary Behaviors of Young Adolescents*, 93 AM. J. OF PUB. HEALTH 1168, 1168 (2003); Martha Y. Kubik et al., *Schoolwide Food Practices Are Associated with Body Mass Index in Middle School Students*, 159 ARCHIVES OF PEDIATRICS & ADOLESCENT MED. 1111, 1111 (2005).

13. *See* ALEX MOLNAR, COMMERCIALISM IN EDUCATION RESEARCH UNIT, SCHOOL COMMERCIALISM, STUDENT HEALTH, AND THE PRESSURE TO DO MORE WITH LESS (2003), available at http://epsl.asu.edu/ceru/Documents/ EPSL-0307-105-CERU.doc (accessed June 18, 2007).

14. This article presumes that a school district will be the level of government targeted for policy intervention, but the analysis would apply equally to laws and regulations adopted at the state level.

15. This article focuses on First Amendment issues and does not analyze all of the causes of action that might be brought against a school district for attempting to control food and beverage marketing in schools.

16. *See Valentine v. Chrestensen*, 316 U.S. 52, 54 (1942) (setting a thirty-year precedent for the principle that the First Amendment does not protect commercial advertising).

17. *Roth v. United States*, 354 U.S. 476, 484 (1957). The Court had allowed clear and narrow content-based restrictions on specified categories of speech that are considered to trigger immediate danger or to be of a low social value. *See, e.g.*, *Brandenburg v. Ohio*, 395 U.S. 444 (1969) (announcing a test for judging laws that restrict speech inciting imminent lawless action); *New York Times Co. v. Sullivan*, 376 U.S. 254 (1964) (setting forth a standard for recovery for an alleged defamatory falsehood relating to a public official); *Roth v. United States*, 354 U.S. 476 (1957) (finding obscenity to be outside the arena of constitutionally protected speech); *Chaplinsky v. New Hampshire*, 315 U.S. 568 (1942) (upholding a statute banning words that trigger an automatic violent response).

18. *See, e.g.*, *Regan v. Time, Inc.*, 468 U.S. 641, 648-49 (1984) ("Regulations which permit the Government to discriminate on the basis of the content of the message cannot be tolerated under the First Amendment."); *Street v. New York*, 394 U.S. 576, 592 (1969) ("It is firmly settled that under our Constitution the public expression of ideas may not be prohibited merely because the ideas are themselves offensive to some of their hearers.").

19. *See* Alex Kozinski & Stuart Banner, *The Anti-history and Pre-history of Commercial Speech*, 71 TEX. L. REV. 747 (1993) (arguing that prior to 1975, the Court construed advertising as a form of economic activity and did not consider or reject the notion that advertising might be speech subject to First Amendment protection).

20. *Valentine*, 316 U.S. at 54-55.

21. *Williamson v. Lee Optical Co.*, 348 U.S. 483 (1955).

22. *Breard v. Alexandria*, 341 U.S. 622 (1951).

23. 425 U.S. 748 (1976).

24. The Court first considered whether the plaintiffs had the right to assert a First Amendment claim when they were mere consumers seeking access to drug price information. The Court granted the plaintiffs standing, holding that "if there is a right to advertise, there is a reciprocal right to receive the advertising." *Id.* at 757.

25. *Id.* at 762 (quoting *Pittsburgh Press Co. v. Pittsburgh Comm'n on Human Relations*, 413 U.S. 376, 385 [1973]).

26. *Id.* at 763.

27. *Id.* at 765.

28. *Id.* at 770.

29. *Virginia State Bd. of Pharmacy v. Virginia Citizens Consumer Council*, 425 U.S. 748, 781 (1976) (J. Rehnquist, dissenting).

30. *Id.*

31. *Id.* at 788-89.

32. *See* Randolph Kline et al., *Beyond Advertising Controls: Influencing Junk-Food Marketing and Consumption with Policy Innovations Developed in Tobacco Control*, 39 LOY. L.A. L. REV. 603, 608-612 (2006).

33. *See, e.g., Minnesota v. Clover Leaf Creamery Co.*, 449 U.S. 456, 461 (1981).

34. *See Gregory v. Ashcroft*, 501 U.S. 452, 471 (1991).

35. *See FCC v. Beach Communications, Inc.*, 508 U.S. 307, 315 (1993).

36. *See Jacobson v. Massachusetts*, 197 U.S. 11, 29, 38 (1905); *Prince v. Massachusetts*, 321 U.S. 158, 168 (1944).

37. *FCC v. Beach Communications, Inc.*, 508 U.S. 307, 315 (1993).

38. *See Lorillard v. Reilly*, 533 U.S. 525, 570 (2001) (declining to rule on the issue because it was not sufficiently briefed and argued before the Court). In another example of the murky distinction between product and advertising regulation, the Supreme Court recognized in *Lorillard* that a regulation of the way products are displayed may involve a speech interest that triggers First Amendment review. *See id.* at 569-70.

39. *See Curtis Publishing Co. v. Butts*, 388 U.S. 130, 145 (1967) (addressing the waiver of First Amendment rights); *Erie Telecomm. Inc. v. City of Erie*, 853 F.2d 1084, 1094 (3d Cir. 1988) (listing Supreme Court cases recognizing that constitutional rights may be waived under particular circumstances); *Leonard v. Clark*, 12 F.3d 885 (9th Cir. 1993) (recognizing that First Amendment rights may be waived via contract).

40. *D.H. Overmyer Co., Inc. v. Frick Co.*, 405 U.S. 174, 187 (1972) (discussing requirements for waiver); *Fuentes v. Shevin*, 407 U.S. 67, 95 (1972) (discussing requirements for waiver).

41. *Erie Telecomm.*, 853 F.2d at 1096.

42. *See, e.g., Monell v. Dep't of Soc. Servs.*, 436 U.S. 658 (1978) (describing when individual government actions, taken together, become a government policy subject in and of itself to legal challenge); *Menotti v. City of Seattle*, 409 F.3d 1113, 1147 (9th Cir. 2005) (same).

43. *Boos v. Barry*, 485 U.S. 312, 321 (1988) (noting that a content-based speech restriction "focuses only on the content of the speech and the direct impact that speech has on its listeners").

44. 460 U.S. 37 (1983).

45. *Id.* at 45.

46. *Id.*

47. *Id.* (citing *City of Madison Joint Sch. Dist. v. Wisconsin Pub. Employment Relations Comm'n*, 429 U.S. 167 (1976); *Southeastern Promotions, Ltd. v. Conrad*, 420 U.S. 546 (1975)).

48. *Id.* at 46.

49. *See U.S. v. Kokinda*, 497 U.S. 720, 730 (1990) (holding that a post office is a non–public forum); *Greer v. Spock* 424 U.S. 828, 838 (1976) (finding an army post to be a non–public forum).

50. *Perry Educ. Ass'n v. Perry Local Educators' Ass'n*, 460 U.S. 37, 45 (1983). Note that the Supreme Court has allowed clear and narrow content-based restrictions on specified categories of speech that are considered to trigger immediate danger or to be of a low social value. *See* note 17, *supra*, for examples of such cases.

51. *Id.* at 46.

52. *Id.*

53. *See Hazelwood Sch. Dist. v. Kuhlmeier*, 484 U.S. 260, 267 (1988).

54. *Id.*

55. *Id.*

56. *Id.* at 266 (internal quotations marks, citations omitted).

57. *Id.* at 267 (internal quotations marks, citations omitted; emphasis added). *See also DiLoreto v. Downey Unified Sch. Dist. Bd. of Educ.*, 196 F.3d 958, 968 (9th Cir. 1999) (holding that advertising space on school's baseball field fence was a non–public forum); *Williams v. Vidmar*, 367 F. Supp. 2d 1265, 1273 (N.D. Cal. 2005) ("a K-12 classroom in a public elementary school is a nonpublic forum"); *Hedges v. Wauconda Cmty. Unit Sch. Dist.*, 9 F.3d 1295, 1302 (7th Cir. 1993) ("a junior high school is a nonpublic forum, which may forbid or regulate many kinds of speech").

58. *See Perry Educ. Ass'n v. Perry Local Educators' Ass'n*, 460 U.S. 37, 47 (1983) (holding that teacher mailboxes in an Indiana public school district were a non–public forum even though outside civic groups were allowed to place flyers in the boxes, since the school required permission to place the flyers and did not allow the public indiscriminate access to the boxes); *Planned Parenthood of S. Nev., Inc. v. Clark County Sch. Dist.*, 941 F.2d 817, 824 (9th Cir. 1991) (en banc) (finding that a school-sponsored publication was not a public forum even though the school solicited advertisements from certain businesses, including casinos, bars, churches, and political candidates, because the school did not open its publications, including advertising space, to "indiscriminate use").

59. *See Lehman v. City of Shaker Heights*, 418 U.S. 298, 303 (1974) (holding advertising space on a public transit system to be a non–public forum); *DiLoreto*, 196 F.3d at 966 ("where the government acts in a proprietary capacity to raise money or to facilitate the conduct of its internal business, the Supreme Court generally has found a nonpublic forum, subject only to the requirements of reasonableness and viewpoint neutrality").

60. 447 U.S. 557 (1980).

61. *Id*. at 563-64.

62. *Id*. at 564.

63. *Id*. at 562-63 (describing the commercial speech analysis as an intermediate standard of review).

64. *See, e.g., Bd. of Trs. of State Univ. v. Fox*, 492 U.S. 469, 474 n.2 (1989) (considering a public university's ban on Tupperware parties in student dorms and implying that the application of the commercial speech test in the case depended on the assumption that the dorms constituted a public forum).

65. *44 Liquormart, Inc. v. Rhode Island*, 517 U.S. 484, 503 (1996); *see, e.g., Lorillard v. Reilly*, 533 U.S. 525, 565 (2001) (discussing the importance of advertising to adults for retailers).

66. *See* Alan E. Garfield, *Protecting Children from Speech*, 57 FLA. L. REV. 565 (2005).

67. 321 U.S. 158 (1944)

68. *Id*. at 168.

69. *Ginsberg v. State of N.Y.*, 390 U.S. 629, 636 (1968) (internal quotations omitted).

70. *Hazelwood Sch. District v. Kuhlmeier*, 484 U.S. 260, 266 (1988); *cf. Bethel Sch. Dist. No. 403 v. Fraser*, 478 U.S. 675, 682 (1986) (holding that the First Amendment rights of students in public schools "are not automatically coextensive with the rights of adults in other settings").

71. *See Planned Parenthood of S. Nev., Inc. v. Clark County Sch. Dist.*, 941 F.2d 817 (9th Cir. 1991) (en banc). Note that the Ninth Circuit is the largest court of appeals in the country, and its decisions are binding in nine western states and the Territory of Guam.

72. 941 F.2d 817 (9th Cir. 1991) (en banc).

73. *Id*. at 828; *cf. DiLoreto v. Downey Unified Sch. Dist. Bd. of Educ.*, 196 F.3d 958, 964-65 (9th Cir. 1999) (applying a non–public forum analysis to a district's refusal to post a religious advertisement on the high school's baseball field).

74. *Planned Parenthood*, 941 F.2d at 819-20 (quoting *Hazelwood*, 484 U.S. at 273).

75. *Perry Educ. Ass'n v. Perry Local Educators' Ass'n*, 460 U.S. 37, 46 (1983).

76. *Id*. at 50-51 (internal quotations omitted). In assessing the reasonableness prong in non–public forum cases, the Supreme Court has also considered whether the policy leaves open alternative channels of communication to the target audience. *See id*. at 53-54; *Greer v. Spock*, 424 U.S. 828, 839 (1976); *Pell v. Procunier*, 417 U.S. 817, 827-28 (1974). However, it is questionable whether courts would apply this consideration when the target audience is children, who have lesser First Amendment rights to receive information than adults. *See, e.g., Ginsberg v. State of N.Y.*, 390 U.S. 629, 636 (1968).

77. *Int'l Soc'y for Krishna Consciousness, Inc. v. Lee*, 505 U.S. 672, 683 (1992) (internal quotations, citations omitted; emphasis in original).

78. *Planned Parenthood of S. Nev., Inc. v. Clark County Sch. Dist.*, 941 F.2d 817, 825-26 (9th Cir. 1991) (en banc).

79. *Id*. at 829.

80. *See id*. at 827 (finding a school district's decision to exclude particular advertisements to be reasonable in light of the school's pedagogical interests in "dissociating itself from speech inconsistent with its educational mission and avoiding the appearance of endorsing views"); *cf. Bd. of Trs. of State Univ. v. Fox*, 492 U.S. 468, 475 (1989) (applying the more rigorous commercial speech analysis and noting that a

university has a substantial interest in "promoting an educational rather than commercial atmosphere" and "preventing commercial exploitation of students").

81. *See, e.g., Lorillard v. Reilly*, 533 U.S. 525, 567-70 (2001) (upholding a government regulation requiring a vendor to place tobacco products behind the counter while presuming that the vendor still may communicate about the product by placing empty tobacco packaging on open display).

82. Note that in *Hazelwood School District v. Kuhlmeier*, the Supreme Court arguably dropped the viewpoint neutrality requirement for speech "that students, parents, and members of the public might reasonably perceive to bear the imprimatur of the school." 484 U.S. 260, 271, 273 (1988). The *Hazelwood* Court upheld a school's decision to censor certain newspaper articles, determining that "educators do not offend the First Amendment by exercising editorial control over the style and content of student speech in school-sponsored expressive activities so long as their actions are reasonably related to legitimate pedagogical concerns." *Id.* at 273. The Court did not address whether the decision was viewpoint neutral. In the wake of *Hazelwood*, the circuits are divided on whether a restriction on third-party speech that bears a school's "imprimatur" in a non–public forum must be viewpoint neutral. *See Fleming v. Jefferson County Sch. Dist.*, 298 F.3d 918 (10th Cir. 2002) (noting that the Third and Tenth Circuits interpret *Hazelwood* to eliminate the viewpoint neutrality requirement for "imprimatur" speech while the Ninth and Eleventh Circuits continue to require viewpoint neutrality for such speech).

83. *Int'l Soc'y for Krishna Consciousness, Inc. v. Lee*, 505 U.S. at 672, 679 (1992).

84. *See, e.g.*, Marjorie Heins, *Viewpoint Discrimination*, 24 HASTINGS CONST. L.Q. 99, 101 (1996) (noting that "the Supreme Court . . . has not been a model of clarity" with regard to defining "viewpoint neutrality").

85. See *Perry Educ. Ass'n v. Perry Local Educators' Ass'n*, 460 U.S. 37, 49 (1983).

86. See *Good News Club v. Milford Cent. Sch.*, 533 U.S. 98, 112 (2001).

87. See *Planned Parenthood of S. Nev., Inc. v. Clark County Sch. Dist.*, 941 F.2d 817, 829 (9th Cir. 1991).

88. *See, e.g., Hills v. Scottsdale Unified Sch. Dist.*, 329 F.3d 1044, 1053 (9th Cir. 2003) (finding that a school violated the viewpoint neutrality standard when it distributed literature about summer programs but excluded a brochure for a religious summer camp); *PMG Intern. Div. L.L.C. v. Rumsfeld*, 303 F.3d 1163, 1171 (9th Cir. 2002) (holding that a military base's ban on the sale of sexually explicit material was viewpoint neutral because it would eviscerate the line between content and viewpoint to characterize the ban as targeting the viewpoint that the human sexual response is positive and healthy).

89. *Legal Servs. Corp. v. Velazquez*, 531 U.S. 533, 541 (2001) ("Viewpoint-based funding decisions can be sustained in instances in which the government is itself the speaker."); *Rust v. Sullivan*, 500 U.S. 173, 192-93 (1991).

90. *See, e.g., Downs v. Los Angeles Unified Sch. Dist.*, 228 F.3d 1003, 1011-13 (9th Cir. 2000) (upholding the decision of school officials to remove a teacher's bulletin board that posted objections to the school's Gay and Lesbian Awareness Month bulletin board and listing cases holding that when the government is the speaker, it may advance a particular viewpoint).

91. *Compare Tinker v. Des Moines Indep. Cmty. Sch. Dist.*, 393 U.S. 503 (1969) *with Hazelwood Sch. District v. Kuhlmeier*, 484 U.S. 260, 270 (1988).

92. 383 U.S. 503 (1969).

93. *Id.* at 514.

94. *Id.* at 513.

95. No. 06-278 (U.S. June 25, 2007).

96. *Id.* at 15.

97. *Id.* at 14.

98. *See id.* (differentiating between student speech that is merely offensive and student speech that appears to promote illegal drug use).

Assessing the Feasibility and Impact of Federal Childhood Obesity Policies

By
VICTORIA L. BRESCOLL,
ROGAN KERSH,
and
KELLY D. BROWNELL

Research on childhood obesity has primarily been conducted by experts in nutrition, psychology, and medicine. Only recently have public policy scholars devoted serious work to this burgeoning public health crisis. Here the authors advance that research by surveying national experts in health/nutrition and health policy on the public health impact and the political feasibility of fifty-one federal policy options for addressing childhood obesity. Policies that were viewed as politically infeasible but having a great impact on childhood obesity emphasized outright bans on certain activities. In contrast, education and information dissemination policies were viewed as having the potential to receive a favorable hearing from national policy makers but little potential public health impact. Both nutrition and policy experts believed that increasing funding for research would be beneficial and politically feasible. A central need for the field is to develop the means to make high-impact policies more politically feasible.

Keywords: childhood obesity; obesity policy; obesity prevention; nutrition; public policy; school lunch

Public health experts and economists have recently converged on the idea that conditions should be created where behaviors that improve health and well-being become the default (Choi et al. 2003; Thaler and Sunstein 2003). For example, there is agreement that individuals, and the nation as a whole, would be best served if people enrolled in pension plans. Some employers do not enroll people unless employees actively choose to opt-in, while other employers enroll new employees automatically (while providing them the option to opt-out). Less than 50 percent of employees take part in pension plans in the first year if enrollment is optional, compared to almost 100 percent participation when enrollment is the default (Choi et al. 2004; Madrian and Shea 2001). Organ donation also illustrates this point. In European countries where people must opt-in to become a donor, only 15 percent are donors. In contrast, in European countries

DOI: 10.1177/0002716207309189

where donation is the default, 98 percent of the citizens are donors (Johnson and Goldstein 2003).

In the United States, the default conditions for children promote unhealthy eating and physical inactivity. Factors such as large portions, high consumption of soft drinks and high-calorie fast foods, low costs for high-calorie foods and higher costs for fruits and vegetables, limited access to healthy foods for the poor, and massive marketing campaigns targeting children are linked to poor diet, high risk for excess weight gain, and in some cases diseases such as diabetes (Brownell and Battle-Horgen 2003). Given these powerful forces in the environment, it is hard to imagine any outcome other than increasing rates of obesity. Today, more than 17 percent of American children and adolescents are overweight[1] or obese, with certain subgroups, such as African American youth, having even higher prevalence rates (18 to 26 percent) (Ogden et al. 2006). These trends have led to increased incidences of hypertension, diabetes, and even heart attacks among obese children (Komaroff 2003; Quattrin et al. 2005; Stephenson 2003).

In the United States, the default conditions for children promote unhealthy eating and physical inactivity.

Victoria L. Brescoll is a postdoctoral research associate at the Rudd Center for Food Policy and Obesity at Yale University. She received her Ph.D. in social psychology from Yale University, where she was supported by a graduate research fellowship from the National Science Foundation. She is interested in the applications of social psychology to public policy and law. She worked in the office of Senator Hillary Rodham Clinton under a congressional fellowship covering a variety of issues related to children and families from the Women's Research and Education Institute.

Rogan Kersh is an associate dean and professor of public service at NYU's Wagner School of Public Service, where he moved last year from Syracuse University's Maxwell School. He spent 1998 to 2000 at Yale as Robert Wood Johnson Fellow in Health Policy and 2006 as a fellow at Yale's Rudd Center. His scholarly publications include Dreams of a More Perfect Union *(Cornell, 2001);* Medical Malpractice and the U.S. Health Care System *(coeditor; Cambridge, 2006); and more than thirty scholarly articles/book chapters. He is currently completing two books, one on the politics of obesity and the other a study of interest-group lobbying.*

Kelly D. Brownell is a professor of psychology, professor of epidemiology and public health, and director of the Rudd Center for Food Policy and Obesity at Yale University, where he also served as chair of the Department of Psychology. He is in the Institute of Medicine, served as president of several national organizations, and in 2006 was listed by Time *magazine among "The World's 100 Most Influential People" in its special issue featuring those "whose power, talent or moral example is transforming the world."*

Overview

The aim of this article is to explore which childhood obesity policies are most likely to create optimal defaults for healthy eating and physical activity in children. To this end, we present the results of an empirical study with experts in public policy and nutrition. We first briefly review the nutrition environment for American children and provide examples of current and proposed federal policies aimed at combating childhood obesity. Then we present the results of our study and discuss them in light of the current political climate and the state of nutrition science.

The Nutrition Environment for American Children and Federal Policy

In recent years, the food landscape for children has been deteriorating. Between 1994 and 2004, 1,643 new types of candies were introduced and marketed specifically for children; only 52 fruit- and vegetable-related products were introduced (Institute of Medicine 2006). Food and beverage companies are keen to market products specifically to American youth: adolescents spend approximately $140 billion per year on food and beverages, while children younger than twelve spend another $25 billion—and may influence as much as an additional $200 billion of annual household food spending (Story and French 2004). In comparison, in 1997 McDonald's spent more than $571 million dollars on advertising while the National Institutes of Health spent a mere $1 million dollars on its "5 A Day" program to increase Americans' consumption of fruits and vegetables (French, Story, and Jeffery 2001).

Food marketers deliberately target children and adolescents, flooding them with advertising: researchers estimate that a child is exposed to twenty-one television advertisements for food every day, adding up to more than seventy-six hundred per year (Gantz et al. 2007). A recent review of these advertisements found that none of them promoted fruits or vegetables (Gantz et al. 2007). Anecdotal evidence suggests that parents find it difficult to compete not only with television ads, but also with product placements in video games, movies, and TV shows; sports, movie, and music stars endorsing foods; and ads on billboards, buses, taxicabs, bus shelters, trash receptacles, and more.

Food marketers have even infiltrated schools. Snack foods, desserts, pastries, candy, and soft drinks are part of the nation's school food landscape. Television in schools, via Channel One and other educational outlets, is filled with food advertising. The most recent example is "bus radio," where a marketing company supplies radio equipment for school buses claiming the service will reduce behavior problems, while filling the airwaves with content that contains advertising (National Public Radio 2006). Children are even exposed to food advertising when they walk by a soft drink machine in school. The typical American school today is an unhealthy and, thereby, *unsafe* nutrition environment (Brownell 2007).

School foods are a significant source of calories and nutrition for children and adolescents as they consume a significant portion of their daily caloric intake while at school (Institute of Medicine 2006). The nutritional quality of those calories varies widely. The National School Lunch Program (NSLP) requires schools to serve children foods that meet federal nutritional standards while excluding certain foods from sale (i.e., "Foods of Minimal Nutritional Value" or FMNV). Classifying some foods as FMNV is a good idea, but the definition of minimally healthful foods, established in 1979, is outdated for the modern school food environment. For example, under federal guidelines, foods such as French fries, ice cream, cookies, potato chips, and snack cakes can be served in school cafeterias during lunchtime, which may create damaging defaults for children.

American children and adolescents also get a significant percentage of their daily calories from foods sold in schools outside of the cafeteria. While foods that do not meet the FMNV standards are excluded from sale during lunch periods at schools participating in the NSLP, children are permitted access to them at other times throughout the day in vending machines, or school stores, which are not required to meet any nutrition standards (Harnack et al. 2000; Kann et al. 2004; Wechsler et al. 2001). One study found that 83 percent of elementary schools, 97 percent of middle schools, and 99 percent of high schools sell unhealthy foods inside and outside of the cafeteria (Government Accountability Office [GAO] 2005). Other research has found that the most frequently sold items are chips, candy, cookies, soft drinks, sports drinks, imitation fruit juices, and snack cakes (Wechsler et al. 2001).

Additional research has shown that the school food environment and food-related policies are associated with children's weight. Researchers in Minnesota studied school practices such as allowing students to have food in class, allowing food and beverages in the hallways, allowing beverages in class, using food as a reward or incentive, selling food for classroom fund-raising, and selling food for schoolwide fund-raising. They found that schools restricting such food-related activities had lower rates of obesity among their students (Kubik, Lytle, and Story 2006).

Policy makers, the lay public, and experts across many fields agree that child-hood obesity is a major public health problem in the United States (Kersh and Monroe 2002). One recent poll found that Americans view childhood obesity as the number one health issue facing the country today (Research America 2006) and that they support policy changes to fight this problem. A recent poll by the Robert Wood Johnson Foundation (2003) found that 90 percent of parents and teachers support replacing unhealthy items in school vending machines with healthy items. Another poll by the *Wall Street Journal*/Harris Interactive Health-Care (2005) revealed that 83 percent of adults believe that "public schools should do more to limit children's access to unhealthy foods like snack foods, sugary soft drinks, and fast food."

Given this consensus and rising fears about obesity's prevalence and medical toll, numerous federal, state, and local policies have been proposed to reduce and prevent obesity among children. On a federal level, there has been a flurry of rhetoric about the gravity of the problem and a number of bills introduced on both sides of the aisle, although actual passage of these bills has not occurred (Kersh and Monroe 2005). Former Senate Majority Leader William Frist's bill, which merely offered grants to encourage "healthy behavior" and "active lifestyles," did not even pass in the House. In contrast, the Personal Responsibility in Food Consumption Act (H.R. 339), which was introduced in July 2003 and would outlaw lawsuits against food and beverage companies, passed in the House (but was not brought to a vote in the Senate). This so-called "Cheeseburger Bill," however, was enacted by at least fourteen states, with at least eighteen others considering similar legislation (Kersh and Monroe 2005).

Congressional Democrats have proposed more progressive childhood obesity legislation, although as of July 2007, nothing has passed both chambers of Congress. For example, The Child Nutrition Promotion and School Lunch Protection Act—introduced by the current chair of the Senate's agriculture and nutrition committee (Senator Harkin), would require the U.S. Department of Agriculture (USDA) to update nutritional standards for foods sold outside of school lunch meals. This bill ultimately aims to create a better set of defaults and hence make progress in improving children's diets and preventing childhood obesity.

The most recently *enacted* federal legislation to address childhood obesity emphasizes local control over universal standards. However, many believe this approach is not a strong enough effort to reduce or prevent childhood obesity as local standards tend to be highly variable and in many cases weaker than universal standards. For example, the 2004 Child Nutrition and WIC Reauthorization Act required that all public and private schools participating in the USDA's Child Nutrition Programs (i.e., NSLP, School Breakfast Program, After-School Snack Program and Special Milk Program) create a local School Wellness Program (SWP) for the 2006-2007 school year. As a result, thousands of SWPs were written at the same time across the country. The law mandates that these policies address nutrition education, physical activity, nutrition guidelines for all foods available, compliance with national school meal nutrition regulations, and a plan for implementation of the policy as well as who must be on the School Health Team that develops the policy (e.g., parents, students, food service, school board members, administrators, and the public). Otherwise, the act allows each school district to exert local control over the specific language and guidelines.

Nutrition and Policy Experts Study

One problem facing policy makers and other opinion leaders is that there is little guidance to know which policy proposals would have greatest public health impact and which would be the most politically feasible (Wang and Brownell 2005). Scientific findings in childhood obesity cannot alone establish policy priorities. Data from fields such as tax policy, agricultural economics, trade policy, marketing, and political science need to be synthesized to help establish policy priorities. Given the gravity of the problem and the potential cost of implementing these policies, it is crucial to know two basic things about these policies: (1) their *political feasibility*—that is, the likelihood that they will receive a favorable hearing from policy makers; and (2) their *potential public health impact*—that is, the likelihood that they will help reduce and/or prevent childhood obesity.

To address this issue, we developed a methodological approach that asks policy and nutrition experts to assess the political feasibility and potential public health impact of a comprehensive list of childhood obesity policies. Our animating idea was to go to the "source"—leading figures in both nutritional science and health policy/politics—to gather valuable clues about how best to focus on and prioritize among specific childhood obesity policies.

Method

Participants

To develop our participant base of experts, we created two lists: one of the leading scientific experts on nutrition and physical activity and another comprising respected experts in federal obesity and related public health policies. We employed a "snowball" sampling technique wherein the experts we initially identified recommended additional sources of expertise. We contacted thirty-eight scientific experts in nutrition and physical activity, and thirty-three completed the survey.

For the sample of policy experts, we contacted forty-nine individuals, and twenty-eight completed the survey. We invited representative numbers of self-identified Democrats, Republicans, and Independents to participate in the survey. In the end, our policy experts consisted of six congressional legislative staff members (four Democrats, two Republicans), nine representatives of advocacy groups involved in federal health/nutrition policy, and eleven individuals from think tanks or the engaged academic community. Both the policy and nutrition experts completed the survey in the fall of 2006 (prior to the November 2006 elections), and both groups were assured complete anonymity to bolster our response rate and to generate more candid responses from our participants. The survey was administered over the Internet, and participants took, on average, fifteen minutes to complete it. Participants were not compensated for completing the survey.

Survey Instrument

We developed a comprehensive list of fifty-one federal obesity, nutrition, and physical activity policies relevant to children by reviewing all relevant federal legislation introduced between 2003 and 2005 and extracting every policy concerning childhood obesity prevention or treatment. We then reviewed state legislation that had been enacted or introduced and supplemented our list with policies that had been proposed in at least two states. We organized these fifty-one policies into five categories: Physical Activity Policies, Nutrition Education Policies, School Nutrition–Healthy School Environment Policies, Advertising Policies, and General/Miscellaneous Childhood Obesity Prevention Policies (see the appendix).

For each policy proposal, the nutrition experts rated its likely public health impact while the policy experts rated each policy's political feasibility. Specifically, the scientific experts in nutrition and physical activity were asked to "assess the likely impact of each policy item on improving nutrition and/or physical activity," using a 7-point Likert-type scale (1 = *none*, 2 = *minimal*, 3 = *minor*, 4 = *moderate*, 5 = *strong*, 6 = *major*, 7 = *maximal*). Our policy experts were asked to "assess the likelihood that each policy item on improving nutrition and/or physical activity will receive a favorable hearing from national policymakers," using a similar 7-point scale (ranging from 1 = *extremely unlikely*, 4 = *neutral*, to 7 = *extremely likely*).

Finally, both sets of experts had the opportunity to answer two open-ended questions asking them to (1) elaborate on and/or clarify their responses by specifying *why* they thought certain policies were more or less politically feasible or impactful and (2) suggest additional federal-level public policies that they believe would help prevent or reduce childhood obesity in the United States.

Analytic Approach

Because of the large number of policies that we asked participants to evaluate (and our necessarily small number of expert participants), we were unable to factor analyze the policies. However, upon visual inspection, there were no outliers or natural clusters of data among the policies. Additionally, all responses from participants were retained. To parsimoniously summarize these data, we took the median score of all policies for both policy experts' feasibility ratings (median = 3.71) and nutrition experts' public health ratings (median = 4.30). We then created a four-quadrant table wherein the fifty-one childhood obesity policies are ranked as "high impact, high feasibility," "high impact, low feasibility," "low impact, high feasibility," and "low impact, low feasibility." Policies were put in the high-impact quadrants if they were above the median score for impact (3.71) and in the high-feasibility quadrants if they were above the median score for feasibility (4.30). Table 1 displays these results in matrix form.

For the qualitative data analyses, we each examined the open-ended responses in light of the feasibility and impact ratings in the four-quadrant table. To summarize these qualitative data, we converged on a series of five themes (discussed below) through discussions with each other. To clarify the open-ended responses, we also conducted follow-up interviews with a sample of our participants.

Results and Discussion

Overall, the nutrition experts were more likely to think that the fifty-one childhood obesity policies would produce a significant public health impact ($M = 4.27$, $SD = 0.50$) than were the policy experts to believe that the same policies were politically feasible ($M = 3.58$, $SD = 0.88$). Although this difference was not statistically significant ($F < 1$, n.s.), it may be that nutrition experts are likely to view any policy as impactful because so few federal policies have passed that specifically aim to reduce childhood obesity. Or perhaps the policy experts were particularly pessimistic because most obesity-reduction policies are typically supported

TABLE 1
FEASIBILITY AND IMPACT RATINGS OF CHILDHOOD OBESITY POLICIES

	Feasibility	Impact	Total[a]
High feasibility, high impact			
Fund research on prevention and cost-effective interventions	4.96	5.19	10.2
Align federal programs with anti-obesity effort (National School Lunch Program [NSLP], food stamp, WIC [Women, Infants, and Children program])	4.39	5.03	9.42
Update federal law to include required fruit/ vegetable servings	4.64	4.7	9.34
Provide free/subsidized fruits and vegetables at school lunch	4.36	4.91	9.27
Fund public service advertising (PSA) campaigns: portion sizes, obesity's dangers	4.75	4.39	9.14
Implement programs to encourage breast-feeding	4.5	4.58	9.08
Fund impact assessment of interventions	4.39	4.55	8.94
Mandate/encourage reduced-fat (1 percent or skim) milk in schools	4.57	4.36	8.94
Earmark transportation funding to increase activity (bike and walking paths)	4.15	4.61	8.75
Establish federal standard for portion sizes in school cafeterias	4.21	4.45	8.67
Promote media literacy among children	4.11	4.38	8.48
Apply federal school-lunch standards to a la carte options	4	4.44	8.44
Fund indoor activity centers, especially in low-income neighborhoods	3.85	4.33	8.19
Low feasibility, high impact			
Ban advertising of unhealthful foods in schools and school venues	3.71	5	8.71
Require grade-schoolers to perform twenty minutes of phys-ed each school day	3.71	4.67	8.38
Extend Children's Television Act to cover nutritional messages	3.5	4.81	8.31
Return unfairness jurisdiction to FTC regarding children's advertising	3.25	4.91	8.16
Ban/restrict unhealthful-food advertising to children age six and younger	2.86	5.09	7.95
Increase per pupil/meal subsidy for school meals	3.54	4.3	7.84
Subsidize inclusion of milk and other healthy alternatives in vending machines	3.43	4.3	7.73
Prohibit sale of snacks with > 40 percent added sugar by weight and with > 6 grams of fat	3.32	4.39	7.72
Ban use of cartoon characters to sell unhealthy food to children	2.71	5	7.71
Mandate equal time for pronutrition and proactivity messages	2.82	4.78	7.6

(continued)

TABLE 1 (continued)

	Feasibility	Impact	Total[a]
Ban vending machines that sell Foods of Minimal Nutritional Value (FMNV)	3.04	4.42	7.46
Limit TV viewing in day care	2.64	4.75	7.39
Ban celebrity endorsement of junk foods	2	4.56	6.56
High feasibility, low impact			
Establish Leadership Commission to Prevent Childhood Obesity within the Centers for Disease Control and Prevention (CDC)	5.14	4.23	9.37
Assess physical education progress of school-age population	5.18	4.09	9.27
Provide nutritional information to parents about school lunches	5	3.81	8.81
Expand applicable FMNV regulations to all school food options	4.56	4.09	8.65
Research and promote walking and biking to school	4.54	4.09	8.63
Update the definition of FMNV to include wider range of school cafeteria foods	4.68	3.85	8.53
Increase federal funding for nutrition education	4.64	3.85	8.49
Require nutritional labeling for school-lunch options	4.29	4.03	8.32
Ban trans fats from all school-lunch options	3.86	4.24	8.1
Teach healthy meal preparation and cooking skills	3.82	4.13	7.95
Maintain minimum number of functioning water fountains per student	4	3.76	7.76
Post nutrition information for vending machine food purchase	3.82	3.91	7.73
Low feasibility, low impact			
Require nutritional labeling for a la carte foods in school cafeterias	3.64	4.13	7.77
Provide access to local foods and establishment of school gardens	3.43	3.97	7.4
Stock all beverage vending machines with water and 100 percent fruit juice	3.21	4	7.21
Require/promote corporate participation in PSAs	3.21	4	7.21
Rename "Foods of Minimal Nutritional Value" as "Foods of Poor Nutritional Value"	3.32	3.82	7.14
Ban fast-food corporations from school lunch programs	2.61	4.5	7.11
Limit school fund-raisers to healthy food or nonfood items	2.75	4.13	6.88
Stock 75 percent of beverage vending machines with water and 100 percent fruit juice	3.54	3.18	6.72
Eliminate sports drinks from school vending machines	2.68	3.52	6.19
Schedule all school lunches at midday	2.64	3.48	6.13
Increase length of school lunch period	2.39	3.55	5.94
Limit (or eliminate) school parties with high-sugar/high-fat foods	1.96	3.55	5.51
Tax sedentary activities: DVD/video game rentals, movie tickets	1.43	2.97	4.4

a. Policies are all sorted by total score.

by politically liberal members of Congress (i.e., Democrats) and the survey was conducted before the Democrats regained the majority in the House and Senate. Thus, feasibility ratings may be greater today than prior to the November 2006 elections; more on that speculative point below.

Looking across the policies as we initially grouped them revealed that the advertising category was the only one in which policy and nutrition experts had a statistically significant divergent opinion, $t(58) = 5.64$, $p < .001$. Nutrition experts were significantly more likely to assign high public health impact of advertising policies ($M = 4.81$, $SD = 1.33$) than policy experts were to indicate that these policies were politically feasible ($M = 3.07$, $SD = 1.00$).

Examining these data qualitatively reveals five major themes. First, policies that were viewed as being politically infeasible but having a great impact on childhood obesity emphasized outright bans on certain activities. For example, banning advertising in schools, prohibiting sales of unhealthy snacks, banning vending machines with unhealthy foods, banning the use of cartoon characters to sell unhealthy foods, banning fast-food corporations from school lunch programs, and banning celebrity endorsement of junk foods all fell into this category. Our nutrition experts evidently conclude that, given the gravity of the childhood obesity epidemic, more interventionary federal regulations are needed. But our policy experts indicate (and confirm, in open-ended comments) that since so little has been done on a federal level to deal with childhood obesity, only smaller steps (such as policies that do not involve strict mandates or outright bans) will have a reasonable chance of becoming U.S. law in the near term.

Second, nutrition labeling on menus in schools (including school vending machines and providing parents with nutritional information about school lunches) was seen as moderately feasible but *low* impact, relative to other policies. Our policy experts viewed labeling policies as moderately feasible because they have been implemented on both the state and local levels. Currently, fifteen states have introduced nutrition-labeling legislation, and New York City has passed a menu-labeling ordinance in conjunction with a ban on trans fats in foods. However, the nutrition experts we surveyed viewed these policies as potentially having little impact on childhood obesity. Judging from their accompanying comments, they did not think that most children would effectively use this information because they would either not seek it out, not understand it, or not change their eating behaviors as a result. Assessing the results of labeling laws on adult obesity patterns, researchers have found mixed results (e.g., Variyam and Cawley 2006).

Third, policies in which the federal government would impose mandates on schools were generally seen as politically infeasible. For example, requiring that schools schedule all school lunches at midday, increase the length of the school lunch period, ban or otherwise limit school parties involving unhealthy foods, have grade-school-aged children perform twenty minutes of physical education per day, and limit TV viewing in day care were judged among the least politically feasible policies. Our policy experts may hold this opinion in part because the current political climate favors local control of schools, particularly in the wake of the No Child Left Behind Act (NCLB), which became law in 2001. NCLB imposed intensive and unprecedented requirements on public schools in the

United States and has become a highly unpopular law (Hargrove and Stempel 2007), leaving little if any room for new mandates imposed on schools.

The fourth theme to emerge from these data involved education and information-dissemination policies, such as increasing federal funding for nutrition education, teaching healthy meal preparation and cooking skills to children, and providing nutritional information to parents about school lunches. The nutrition experts in our study viewed these policies as having little public health impact if they were enacted, while our policy experts believed that they would receive a favorable hearing from national policy makers. Nutrition experts, in dismissing the impact of education-based policies, cite research demonstrating that simply telling people (particularly children) what they should and should not eat or how much they should exercise does little to change people's eating and exercise behavior in the long term and therefore results in minimal, if any, weight loss or prevention of weight gain (Battle and Brownell 1996; Jeffery 2001; Kolata 2007; Mendoza 2007). However, individual-based education policies are popular among policy makers because, compared with large-scale environmental interventions, education policies are inexpensive, easier to implement, more in line with traditional American values that emphasize personal responsibility, and likely to be supported by the food industry. They also engender little political opposition, compared to new regulations or prohibitions.

Finally, the policy options that both nutrition and policy experts agreed would be impactful and politically feasible concerned funding for research. Both funding for research on prevention and cost-effective interventions and funding for impact assessments of childhood obesity interventions appeared in the five highest-rated policies. Since many of the nutrition experts we polled are researchers themselves, it is not surprising that they see research as important. As one of our experts pointed out in the open-ended section of the survey, "How can we have effective prevention strategies until we have better data on the causes?" Policy experts, on the other hand, cited different reasons for rating research funding policies as politically feasible. As with expanded educational resources, proposing policies that would fund research are generally less controversial and easier to pass than implementing regulations or additional taxes (Lowi 1972). Less political capital is necessary to appropriate additional funds for a program, as the process is common and even expected. Since we did not specify the amount of additional funding for research, it is possible that our policy experts had a specific funding ceiling in mind when considering these policy items in our survey. Perhaps our policy experts would not see increasing research funding for childhood obesity as politically viable if the question had asked whether funding could be tripled or quadrupled rather than just "increased."

In the open-ended questions, both nutrition and policy experts emphasized that to effectively combat childhood obesity, a wide array of these policies need to be enacted. As one nutrition expert put it, "Impact will only be achieved by a combination of these interventions along with many others. No individual intervention or policy will have a major or maximal impact." Nutrition experts we surveyed also repeatedly mentioned the need for increased funding for current childhood obesity programs and policies. Although this seems to be an obvious point, the lack of federal investment in childhood obesity is stark. Some estimate that the federal government spends approximately $4.30 per obese person on this issue—for both adults and children (Brescoll 2006; Trust for America's Health 2006). When compared with other public health problems, this is a very small investment. For example, spending on AIDS treatment and prevention hovers around $1,600 per HIV-positive individual and cancer prevention around $180 per person (Brescoll 2006).

Impact will only be achieved by a combination of these interventions along with many others. No individual intervention or policy will have a major or maximal impact.

The nutrition experts in our sample also repeatedly mentioned the need to involve parents in childhood obesity policies, although this was not included in the list of policies that they evaluated. For example, a number of respondents emphasized the need for research and education to encourage parents to modify their home environment in a way that develops healthy eating habits in children and the importance of engaging parents in school-based obesity prevention and treatment programs. Some of our nutrition experts noted that policy makers often talk about the role of parents in preventing obesity in their children but then do not reflect this rhetoric in the public policies they promote.

The policy experts we surveyed almost unanimously mentioned the need to reform school lunches, including revising the definition of FMNV and expanding the free fruit and vegetable program. Their consensus is that this is a promising policy change, but grassroots support for changing school foods remains crucial to gaining policy makers' support. As one policy expert wrote, "I believe that lawmakers will move decisively on this issue based on the groundswell felt back at home. Since Congress is facing enormous budget deficits, tight elections, and elevated partisan bickering, they are not as likely to move on very many things unless motivated by the voting public."

Conclusion

This study is a first step in outlining areas of childhood obesity legislation that seem politically plausible and genuinely significant if implemented. Future research should expand on this study by paring down the number of policies and performing structured interviews with a subset of nutrition and policy experts.

These interviews could supplement the quantitative data by supplying more detailed information as to *why* our experts rated certain policies as more or less impactful or feasible. Further investigation could also assess whether and how the political feasibility of these policies may have changed as a result of the Democrats taking control of Congress in the November 2006 elections.

In informal discussions with congressional staff members since we completed our survey, we learned that many of them believe that the overall feasibility of the childhood obesity policies would be rated higher now that Democrats are in control but that the order of the policies (i.e., the relative ranking) would remain generally similar. Although it is good that these policies may be more likely to be enacted with the new Congress, it remains troubling that a commitment toward a problem as serious as childhood obesity can change so rapidly with the political winds. To see any progress in preventing or reducing childhood obesity, Congress needs to put forth a consistent, and well-funded, commitment toward the problem. More grassroots lobbying and public awareness could persuade Congress to set aside a dedicated funding stream specifically for childhood obesity prevention and research at the Centers for Disease Control, the National Institutes of Health, and/or other government agencies.

The portfolio of obesity-related grants funded by the National Institutes of Health is dominated by biological and treatment research with a heavy emphasis on pharmacology and surgery. Relatively little work is being funded on economic and other social drivers of the obesity problem or on prevention.

It is noteworthy that funding more research on childhood obesity was ranked high by both policy and public health experts. We agree in principle, but it is important to look carefully at what gets funded. The portfolio of obesity-related grants funded by the National Institutes of Health is dominated by biological and treatment research with a heavy emphasis on pharmacology and surgery. Relatively little work is being funded on economic and other social drivers of the obesity problem or on prevention. The Centers for Disease Control supports such work, but its obesity budget is dwarfed by that of the National Institutes of Health. Research funds are needed to focus on factors that have created the epidemic and could be harnessed to reverse trends in prevalence; increased funding could be beneficial.

Once one places policies in a grid that crosses impact with feasibility, static or dynamic approaches might be taken. A static approach would accept where policies fall in the grid and argue for efforts in the high impact–high feasibility quadrant. Because we used median splits to place policies in the grid, one-fourth of the policies by definition will fall into the high impact–high feasibility quadrant. If one were to make absolute rather than relative placements of policies in the grid, relatively little would fall into the quadrant where both feasibility and impact are high.

This argues for a dynamic approach, one in which public health and policy experts work specifically to increase the political feasibility of high-impact policies. This will involve work on changing public opinion, creating a scientific foundation for policies, and examining novel legal and legislative approaches. Children are entitled to a nutrition environment that supports their becoming healthy adults, but currently unhealthy conditions are the default. It is not surprising that in the current environment, childhood obesity rates have skyrocketed. Given recent public interest in this issue and support for change, federal and state legislators are uniquely poised to make an important difference. Passing impactful legislation now, such as that which has been identified in this article, can prevent profound public health problems as the next generation of American citizens develops and matures.

Appendix
Childhood Obesity Policies Used in Survey

Physical Activity Policies

1. Fund indoor activity centers, especially in low-income neighborhoods
2. Assess physical education progress of school-age population
3. Require grade-schoolers to perform twenty minutes of phys-ed each school day
4. Tax sedentary activities: DVD/video game rentals, movie tickets
5. Research and promote walking and biking to school
6. Earmark transportation funding to increase activity (bike and walking paths)

Nutrition Education Policies

7. Increase federal funding for nutrition education
8. Teach healthy meal preparation and cooking skills
9. Align federal programs with antiobesity effort (National School Lunch Program [NSLP], food stamp, WIC [Women, Infants, and Children program])
10. Post nutrition information for vending machine food purchase

School Nutrition–Healthy School Environment

11. Stock all beverage vending machines with water and 100 percent fruit juice
12. Stock 75 percent of beverage vending machines with water and 100 percent fruit juice
13. Eliminate sports drinks from school vending machines
14. Subsidize inclusion of milk and other healthy alternatives in vending machines
15. Maintain minimum number of functioning water fountains per student
16. Update the definition of Foods of Minimal Nutritional Value (FMNV) to include much wider range of school cafeteria foods

(continued)

Appendix (continued)

17. Expand applicable FMNV regulations to all school food options
18. Rename "Foods of Minimal Nutritional Value" as "Foods of Poor Nutritional Value"
19. Ban vending machines that sell FMNV
20. Provide nutritional information to parents about school lunches
21. Require nutritional labeling for school-lunch options
22. Increase per pupil/meal subsidy for school meals
23. Increase length of school lunch period
24. Schedule all school lunches at midday
25. Provide free/subsidized fruits and vegetables at school lunch
26. Fund impact assessment of interventions
27. Provide access to local foods and establishment of school gardens
28. Apply federal school-lunch standards to a la carte options
29. Require nutritional labeling for a la carte foods in school cafeterias
30. Establish federal standard for portion sizes in school cafeterias
31. Mandate/encourage reduced-fat (1 percent or skim) milk in schools
32. Ban trans fats from all school-lunch options
33. Ban fast-food corporations from school lunch programs
34. Prohibit sale of snacks with > 40 percent added sugar by weight and with > 6 grams of fat
35. Limit school fund-raisers to healthy food or nonfood items
36. Limit (or eliminate) school parties with high-sugar/high-fat foods
37. Update federal law to include required fruit/vegetable servings

Advertising Policies

38. Ban/restrict unhealthful-food advertising to children age six and younger
39. Return unfairness jurisdiction to FTC regarding children's advertising
40. Ban advertising of unhealthful foods in schools and school venues
41. Ban use of cartoon characters to sell unhealthy food to children
42. Ban celebrity endorsement of junk foods
43. Mandate equal time for pronutrition and proactivity messages
44. Extend Children's Television Act to cover nutritional messages
45. Promote media literacy among children
46. Limit TV viewing in day care

General Childhood Obesity Prevention Policies

47. Fund public service advertising (PSA) campaigns: portion sizes, obesity's dangers
48. Require/promote corporate participation in PSAs
49. Fund research on prevention and cost-effective interventions
50. Establish Leadership Commission to Prevent Childhood Obesity within the Centers for Disease Control and Prevention
51. Implement programs to encourage breast-feeding

Note

1. Here, overweight is defined as being at or above the 95th percentile for body mass index (BMI) for sex-specific age growth charts.

References

Battle, E. K., and K. .D. Brownell. 1996. Confronting a rising tide of eating disorders and obesity: Treatment vs. prevention and policy. *Addictive Behavior* 21:755-65.

Brescoll, V. L. 2006. Federal spending on public health problems. Unpublished data, Yale University, New Haven, CT.

Brownell, K. D. 2007. *Congressional testimony before the Senate Agriculture, Nutrition and Forestry Committee hearing on Child Nutrition and the School Setting.* 110th Cong., 1st sess., March 6. Washington, DC: Government Printing Office.

Brownell, K. D., and K. Battle-Horgen. 2003. *Food fight: The inside story of the food industry, America's obesity crisis, and what we can do about it.* New York: McGraw-Hill.

Choi, J., D. Laibson, B. Madrian, and A. Metrick. 2003. Optimal defaults. *American Economic Review Papers and Proceeding* 93 (2): 180-85.

———. 2004. For better or for worse: Default effects and 401(k) savings behavior. In *Perspectives in the economics of aging,* ed. D. Wise, 81-121. Chicago: University of Chicago Press.

French, S. A., M. Story, and R. W. Jeffery. 2001. Environmental influences on eating and physical activity. *Annual Review of Public Health* 22:309-35.

Gantz, G., N. Schwartz, J. R. Angelini, and V. Rideout. 2007. *Food for thought: Television food advertising to children in the United States.* Washington, DC: Kaiser Family Foundation.

Government Accountability Office (GAO). 2005. *School meal programs: Competitive foods are widely available and generate substantial revenues for schools.* Washington, DC: GAO.

Hargrove, T., and G. H. Stempel III. 2007. Majority would like "no child" law left behind. *Scripps Howard News Service,* May 30.

Harnack, L., P. Snyder, M. Story, R. Holliday, L. Lytle, and D. Neumark-Sztainer. 2000. Availability of a la carte food items in junior and senior high schools: A needs assessment. *Journal of the American Dietetic Association* 100:701-03.

Institute of Medicine. 2006. *Food marketing to children: Threat or opportunity?* Washington, DC: National Academies of Science Press.

Jeffery, R. W. 2001. Public health strategies for obesity treatment and prevention. *American Journal of Health Behavior* 25:252-59.

Johnson, E. J., and D. Goldstein. 2003. Do defaults save lives? *Science* 302:1338-39.

Kann, L., J. Grunbaum, M. McKenna, H. Wechsler, and D. Galuska. 2004. Competitive foods and beverages available for purchase in secondary schools—Selected sites in the United States. *Journal of School Health* 75:370-74.

Kersh, R., and J. Monroe. 2002. How the personal becomes political: Prohibitions, public health, and obesity. *Studies in American Political Development* 16:162-175.

———. 2005. Obesity, courts, and the new politics of public health. *Journal of Health Politics, Policy, and Law* 30:840-68.

Kolata, G. 2007. *Rethinking thin: The new science of weight loss and the myths and realities of dieting.* New York: Farrar, Straus and Giroux.

Komaroff, A. L. 2003. An update on the obesity problem. *Journal Watch of the New England Journal of Medicine,* March 7. http://generalmedicine.jwatch.org/cgi/content/full/2003/307/8.

Kubik, M. Y., L. A. Lytle, and M. Story. 2006. School-wide food practices are associated with body mass index in middle school students. *Archives of Pediatric and Adolescent Medicine* 159:1111-14.

Lowi, T. 1972. Four systems of policy, politics and choice. *Public Administration Review* 33:298-310.

Madrian, B., and D. Shea. 2001. The power of suggestion: Inertia in 401(K) saving participation and saving behavior, *Quarterly Journal of Economics* 116:1149-87.

Mendoza, M. 2007. Anti-obesity initiatives failing to bear fruit. *Baltimore Sun,* July 5. http://www .baltimoresun.com/news/health/balte.obesity05ju105,0,245034.story?coll=bal-health-headlines.

National Public Radio. 2006. Radio rides along on the school bus. October 28. http://www.npr.org/ templates/story/story.php?storyId=6398889 (accessed June 30, 2007).

Ogden, C. L., M. Carroll, L. Curtin, et al. 2006. Prevalence of overweight and obesity in the United States, 1999-2004. *Journal of the American Medical Association* 295:1549-55.

Quattrin, T., E. Liu, N. Shaw, B. Shine, and E. Chiang. 2005. Obese children who are referred to the pediatric endocrinologist: Characteristics and outcome. *Pediatrics* 115:348-51.

Research America. 2006. Obesity poll. http://www.researchamerica.org/polldata/2006/endocrinepoll.pdf (accessed June 10, 2007).

Robert Wood Johnson Foundation. 2003. National polls show parents and teachers agree on solutions to childhood obesity. December 4. http://www.rwjf.org/newsroom/newsreleasesdetail.jsp?id=10166 (accessed May 31, 2007).

Stephenson, J. 2003. Obesity-hypertension link in children? *Journal of the American Medical Association* 289:1774-79.

Story, M., and S. French. 2004. Food advertising and marketing directed at children and adolescents. *International Journal of Behavioral Nutrition and Physical Activity* 1 (3): 1-17.

Thaler, R. H., and C. R. Sunstein. 2003. Libertarian paternalism. *American Economic Review* 93:175-79.

Trust for America's Health. 2006. *F as in fat: Why obesity policies are failing in America*. Washington, DC: Trust for America's Health.

Variyam, J. N., and J. Cawley. 2006. Nutrition labels and obesity. NBER Working Paper no. 11956, National Bureau of Economic Research, Cambridge, MA.

Wall Street Journal/Harris Interactive Health-Care. 2005. Most of the American public, including a majority of parents, believe that childhood obesity is a major problem. February 15. http://www.harrisinteractive.com/news/newsletters/wsjhealthnews/WSJOnline_HI Health-CareP0112005v014_iss03.pdf (accessed May 31, 2007).

Wang, S. S., and K. D. Brownell. 2005. Public policy and obesity: The need to marry science with advocacy. *Psychiatric Clinics of North America* 28:235-252.

Wechsler, H., N. Brener, S. Kuester, and C. Miller. 2001. Food service and foods and beverages available at school: Results from the School Health Policies and Programs Study 2000. *Journal of School Health* 71:313-24.

Generation O: Addressing Childhood Overweight before It's Too Late

Rates of overweight in children have more than tripled in the United States since 1980, putting the nation's children at risk for unprecedented levels of major diseases like diabetes and heart disease earlier in life. The American childhood overweight epidemic is a startling phenomenon. Because of the serious health consequences, there is an urgent need to make practical decisions to address the problem, based on common sense, the best prevailing research, and the advice of experts. This starts with addressing the contributing factors behind the real culprits—poor nutrition and inadequate physical activity. Over the past decade, experts have emphasized the need to develop overweight prevention and control strategies focused on instilling in children the importance of healthy behaviors that can help reduce their risk for obesity and related health issues throughout their lives. This article reviews policy recommendations and intervention strategies for addressing childhood overweight.

Keywords: childhood overweight policies; childhood overweight interventions

By
LAURA M. SEGAL
and
EMILY A. GADOLA

The American obesity epidemic is a startling phenomenon. Rates of overweight in children have more than tripled in the United States since 1980, putting the nation's children at risk for unprecedented levels of major diseases like diabetes and heart disease earlier in life (National Health and Nutrition Examination Survey [NHANES] 2005-2006). According to the National Institutes of Health (NIH) and the U.S. Centers for Disease Control and Prevention (CDC), being overweight or obese increases an individual's risk for a range of serious diseases, including type 2 diabetes, heart disease and stroke, and some forms of cancers (National Institutes of Diabetes and Digestive and Kidney Diseases [NDKKD] 2005).

Studies have documented that obesity and overweight in childhood and adolescence are often a path toward increased risk for and further development of a range of obesity-related

NOTE: Research for this article is based on a grant from the Robert Wood Johnson Foundation.

DOI: 10.1177/0002716207308177

diseases as children enter adulthood, leading to a lifetime of health problems. In addition, weight-related health problems, including type 2 diabetes, increased cholesterol levels, hypertension, and the danger of eating disorders are increasingly found in children (Dietz 1998). Being overweight as a child may lead to orthopedic ailments and premature onset of menstruation (Dietz 1998). Some studies show that obesity and overweight also negatively impact children's mental health and school performance (Datar and Sturm 2006). Overweight children have been found to engage in other unhealthy behaviors and tend to exhibit loneliness and nervousness (Hardy, Harrell, and Bell 2004).

Because of the serious health consequences related to overweight and obesity, there is an urgent need to make practical decisions to address the problem, based on common sense, the best prevailing research, and the advice of experts. This starts with addressing the contributing factors behind the real culprits—poor nutrition and inadequate physical activity.

A wide range of factors have contributed to the rise in both childhood and adult overweight and obesity. Most overweight and obesity management efforts have focused on encouraging individuals to "eat less and move more." However, people do not make decisions in a vacuum. There are numerous factors that influence how and what people eat and how much and what types of physical activity they get. Policies involving a range of issues—from the availability of sidewalks to the nutritional value of school lunches—impact the ability of individuals and communities to make healthier choices (see Leviton 2008 [this volume]).

Individuals live in a world influenced by their relationships with family, friends, neighbors, and colleagues; their home, workplace, and school environments; their neighborhoods; their economic limitations; and their genetics, physiology, psychology, and life stages. Efforts to combat the obesity crisis will not be successful until these social, economic, and physical influences are acknowledged and incorporated into future interventions. The fight against obesity and physical inactivity must also include well-funded, long-term approaches; a revitalized research agenda that emphasizes longitudinal studies; and a fresh look at what constitutes "success" and how it is measured.

Laura M. Segal oversees public affairs, communications, and policy research for Trust for America's Health (TFAH). Prior to joining TFAH, she directed corporate communications for Sigma Networks and Charitableway and worked for the Clinton/Gore campaigns and administration from 1992 to 2000 in a variety of capacities, including the 1992 and 1996 campaigns, in the White House, and in the Presidential Transition and Inaugural Offices. She graduated magna cum laude with distinction in communication from the University of Pennsylvania and received an M.A. from the Annenberg School for Communication.

Emily A. Gadola, as a public affairs research associate at Trust for America's Health, researches, analyzes, and writes about crucial public health policies. Prior to joining TFAH, she worked at the American Lung Association of Metropolitan Chicago (ALAMC) on the Smoke-Free Chicago campaign. She holds an M.P.P. from the Irving B. Harris School of Public Policy Studies at the University of Chicago and a B.S. in business economics and public policy from Indiana University.

There are numerous factors that
influence how and what people eat
and how much and what types of physical
activity they get. Policies involving a range
of issues—from the availability of sidewalks to
the nutritional value of school lunches—impact
the ability of individuals and communities
to make healthier choices.

Many Issues Influence Individual Decisions about Nutrition and Physical Activity

Over the past few decades, there have been many cultural changes that have impacted decisions people make about diet and exercise. People are eating more and less-nutritious food. The average American adult eats three hundred calories a day more than people ate in the 1980s (Putnam, Allshouse, and Kantor 2002). Portion sizes have grown and people eat more prepared or takeout foods and eat in restaurants more often (Nielsen and Popkin 2003). In addition, rural and urban neighborhoods often have limited access to supermarkets and nutritious foods like produce (Prevention Institute for the Center for Health Improvement 2003; Economic Research Service 1999; Cotterill and Franklin 1995). Low-income zip codes tend to have fewer and smaller grocery stores than higher-income zip codes (Potchuchuki 2003).

A range of studies have shown that habits of other family members influence health, eating and exercise patterns (Wadden, Brownell, and Foster 2004; Nelson, Carpenter, and Chiasson 2006; Johannsen, Johannsen, and Specker 2006; Wrotniak et al. 2004; Burdette and Whitaker 2006; Stice, Presnell, and Shaw 2005; Birch 2006; Myles et al. 2003; Fisher, Rolls, and Birch 2003). For example, mothers who are obese when pregnant can increase a child's risk for some birth defects, diabetes, and obesity (Anderson and Butcher 2006; Serdula et al. 1993; Whitaker et al. 1997; Wadden, Brownell, and Foster 2004; Watkins et al. 2003; Rosenberg et al. 2005; Whitaker 2004; Berkowitz et al. 2005; Gillman et al. 2003). In addition, the "electronic culture" options for entertainment and free time, including TV, video games, and the Internet, have proliferated. In 2005, more than 20 percent of high school students played video or computer games or used a computer for something other than school work for three or more hours on an average school day, and more than 35 percent of high school students watched TV for three or more hours on an average school day (CDC 2006).

School environments are a major influence on children's eating and activity habits, given the limited options children are given in a school setting. Nutrition standards for food available through school breakfast and lunch currently focus on meeting minimum standards and keeping costs low. In the past few decades, there has also been an influx in the availability of sodas, snack machines, and fast food on campuses and a reduction in physical education, recess, and recreation time (Institute of Medicine [IOM] 2006).

School environments are a major influence on children's eating and activity habits, given the limited options children are given in a school setting. Nutrition standards for food that is available through school breakfast and lunches currently focus on meeting minimum standards and keeping costs low.

The communities where children live also can either encourage or inhibit opportunities for physical activity. Through the "built environment," or the man-made aspects of communities, a number of trends have resulted in people being less active, including communities that foster driving rather than walking or biking, lack of public transit options, poor upkeep of sidewalk infrastructure, walking areas that are often unsafe or inconvenient, limited parks and recreation space, and poor upkeep and security in local parks (Dearry 2004).

Strategies for Combating Childhood Overweight

Over the past decade, experts have emphasized the need to develop obesity and overweight prevention and control strategies that focus on children. This approach is viewed as particularly significant because instilling in children the importance of healthy behaviors can help reduce their risk for obesity and related health issues throughout their lives.

A 2006 Cochrane review of twenty-two intervention programs aimed at children concluded that "the current evidence suggests that many diet and exercise interventions to prevent obesity in children are not effective in preventing weight gain, but can be effective in promoting a healthy diet and increased physical activity levels" (Summerbell et al. 2006). This review supports an argument for developing strategies that focus on promoting improved nutrition and physical activity rather than stressing weight loss as a primary approach. The following is a review of six different policy approaches to combating childhood obesity that focus on improving health as a primary objective.

1. Working with Families
and Improving Nutrition and Physical
Activity Opportunities at Home

Efforts to involve families in obesity-prevention efforts are viewed by many as an effective area for intervention activities. Programs that target improvements within home environments by reaching children via their parents or guardians "produce significant long-term results," according to a review, funded in part by the NIH, of a range of studies (Wadden, Brownell, and Foster 2004).

One example of an effective intervention strategy has involved working with mothers participating in the federally funded Women, Infants and Children (WIC) nutrition program to understand the benefits of providing healthier beverage options to children and encouraging more activity (McGarvey et al. 2004). An educational effort through a WIC clinic setting in Virginia in 2004 resulted in mothers providing more water to their children, rather than sugared beverages, and encouraging more active playtime (McGarvey et al. 2004). A program in Kentucky revealed that WIC mothers had the misconception that heavier children translated into healthier children. The program also found that WIC mothers introduced solid foods earlier than recommended (Baughcum et al. 1998). Targeted educational efforts resulted in mothers gaining an increased understanding of healthier feeding options for their children.

A number of studies have demonstrated a connection between the weight of parents, particularly mothers and children, suggesting strategies that address families as a unit may be particularly important, especially when children are young and "while parental influence is still strong and before obesity-promoting behaviors have become well ingrained" (McGarvey et al. 2004).

Other research has found that children whose mothers limited unhealthy food options at home had lower body-mass index (BMI) scores (Myles et al. 2003). And a 2005 review of literature on breastfeeding and obesity concluded that "breastfeeding is protective against obesity, although the precise magnitude of the association remains unclear. Increasing uptake of breastfeeding could form an important part of population strategies to prevent obesity" (Owen et al. 2005).

2. Reaching Preschool-Age Children
through Child Care

Some researchers have raised the concern that "little is known about the physical activity behavior of preschool-aged children or about the influence of preschool
attendance on physical activity" (Pate et al. 2004). Experts emphasize that "child
care represents an untapped rich source of strategies to help children acquire pos
itive health habits to prevent obesity" (Story, Kaphingst, and French 2006).

Currently, thirty-eight states and the District of Columbia have child care outdoor time requirements, eight states require at least one outdoor hour a day, and
five states (Delaware, Georgia, Illinois, Mississippi, and Tennessee) have additional nutrition, physical activity, and media use policies (Story, Kaphingst, and
French 2006).

Head Start, a federal–state program for the care of low-income three- and
four-year-olds, routinely measures the height and weight of children in the program. While it is unclear how this data is used, researchers suggest it could be a
rich area for future studies and interventions (Story, Kaphingst, and French
2006). Because participation in Head Start is based on socioeconomic status, children in the Head Start program are from low-income families and are therefore
at a greater risk of becoming overweight (Story, Kaphingst, and French 2006).

One example of a preschool curriculum focused on promoting health is the
"Color Me Healthy" program for four- and five-year-olds in North Carolina.
Color Me Healthy is a preschool curriculum program designed to teach children
ages four and five about nutrition and physical activity. It is currently in use in
nearly fifty counties in North Carolina, and teacher participants report that it is
generating positive results (Dunn et al. 2006). The curriculum includes lesson
plans for teachers; picture cards, posters, and music that promote healthy eating
and physical activity; newsletters to parents; and behavior incentives like hand
stamps.

3. Reaching Children through Schools
and in After-School Programs by Improving
Food and Physical Education
and Encouraging Physical Activity

School-based programs can yield positive results in preventing obesity, and a
number of studies call for "broader implementation of successful programs"
(Veugelers and Fitzgerald 2005). Children spend large portions of time at school,
and in before- and after-school programs, and they often consume two meals and
snacks in these settings.

The more than fourteen thousand school districts in the United States have
primary jurisdiction for setting school nutrition and physical activity policies.

States can establish policies or pass legislation that affect schools, but the locali-
ties typically have discretion in deciding if they will follow them. States may try
to create incentives for following policies, such as attaching compliance to state
funding. However, school districts may choose to ignore state policies.

Most schools participate in the school lunch, breakfast, and after-school programs in coordination with the U.S. Department of Agriculture (USDA) Food
and Nutrition Service (FNS). To qualify for federal subsidies to offer free or
reduced-cost meals to low-income children, schools must establish meal programs that comply with minimum nutrition standards. Under these standards,
the sale of "foods of minimal nutritional value" (e.g., candy, water ices, chewing
gum, and soft drinks) are restricted from being sold during meal times in cafeterias but are not restricted from being sold at any time outside of cafeterias
(Government Accountability Office [GAO] 2004; Brescoll, Kersh, and Brownell
2008 [this volume]). In recent years, sixteen states have taken legislative action to
require higher nutritional standards of school meals than "minimum" USDA
requirements (Trust for America's Health 2007).

Reports by the USDA, the GAO, and independent researchers have all found
nutrition in school lunches to be "substandard" (*The Food Institute Report* 2004;
Physicians Committee for Responsible Medicine 2004; Associated Press Online
2003; GAO 2004). In addition, the FNS, via new proposed regulations, advised
"school food personnel to be more careful about how they contract for the food that
will be served to children" (Center for Health and Health Care in Schools 2005).
In 2007, USDA requirements for school meals are expected to be updated to meet
the 2005 *Dietary Guidelines for Americans* (Trust for America's Health 2007).

Food is often available in schools through vending machines, school stores,
and á la carte lines in cafeterias. These foods, known as "competitive foods," are
not required to meet the USDA standards. Instead, standards are set by states or
local school systems (GAO 2004). Twenty-two states have taken legislative action
to set nutrition standards on foods sold outside of the school meal programs
(Trust for America's Health 2007). Twenty-six states have taken legislative action
to limit when and where foods that are not part of the school meal programs can
be sold during school hours (Trust for America's Health 2007).

Many schools receive revenue from the sale of competitive foods. Money from
food sales is often used to pay for special activities or items not covered by the
school's budget (GAO 2004). However, many schools do not consider the fact
that reduced sales within the regular school lunch programs due to "competitive"
food sales means the federal government allocates less money to the school lunch
programs in the future. Revenue generated from competitive foods, therefore,
often results in a reduction in funding for the school lunch program.

While every state has physical education requirements for students, these
requirements are often not enforced and often result in physical education programs of inadequate quality. Some states are considering ways to improve and
better implement their requirements. However, these requirements come without financial support, equating to an unfunded, and therefore burdensome, mandate placed on schools and school districts.

Many state education agencies argue that physical education policies are often not enforced because there are already too many other mandated curriculum requirements (Wisconsin Education Association Council 2004). Some education experts point out that the Elementary and Secondary Education Act (ESEA), known as the "No Child Left Behind Act," which emphasizes student achievement on standardized tests, is forcing school districts to divert limited resources away from programs that are not tested under ESEA, such as physical education and extracurricular sports (Wisconsin Education Association Council 2004). In addition, states often allow schools exemptions from physical education standards (Pyramid Communications 2003).

Some states are considering ways to improve and better implement their [physical education] requirements. However, these requirements come without financial support, equating to an unfunded, and therefore burdensome, mandate placed on schools and school districts.

Healthy People 2010 states that health education should include information about the consequences of unhealthy diets and inadequate physical activity. Health education seeks to teach students about maintaining good health, including proper nutrition and the value of physical activity, which are keys to controlling obesity. The CDC (1997) noted that health education can effectively promote students' health-related knowledge, attitudes, and behaviors. These education programs are intended to help students set a foundation for maintaining good nutritional habits and a physically active lifestyle.

Only two states—Colorado and Oklahoma—do not require schools to provide health education. However, in states that do require health education, few criteria have been set to ensure the quality of health education curricula or to establish a minimum credit requirement for graduating students (Trust for America's Health 2007).

A number of states have undertaken initiatives to screen students' BMI levels. The screenings are intended to help the states identify schools, school districts, and student populations that may need interventions to help reduce the prevalence of overweight. Results are typically mailed to parents as well. Twelve states have taken legislative action to support school efforts to test students' BMI levels as either part of health examinations or physical education activities (Trust for America's Health 2007). In 2003, California and Illinois enacted legislation requiring risk analysis and noninvasive screening of students for type 2 diabetes. In 2005, California also enacted a ballot initiative that encourages additional diabetes awareness and prevention efforts. Two other states, Pennsylvania and Texas, considered legislation to screen students for their potential at-risk status for type 2 diabetes, but the initiatives were not enacted.

Emerging school-based efforts have focused on improving the quality of food sold in schools, limiting sales of less nutritious foods, improving physical education and health education, and encouraging increased physical activity either within the school day or through extracurricular pursuits (see Graff 2008 [this volume]; Leviton 2008). Some communities have also invested in more comprehensive programs, such as a statewide initiative in Arkansas, and the Child and Adolescent Trial for Cardiovascular Health (CATCH) program involving ninety-six schools in four states.

Examples of Successes in School-Based Approaches

- The Child and Adolescent Trial for Cardiovascular Health (CATCH) elementary school program encompassing 3,714 students in ninety-six schools in four states focused on educating students, teachers, and staff and modifying school lunches and physical education (Luepker et al. 1996; Nader et al. 1999). The program showed positive results, with students consuming healthier diets and engaging in more physical activity. The findings suggest that a program that encompasses a school-based approach can yield improvements. Activity levels for students at the older age ranges of the study began to dissipate toward the end of the study, demonstrating an increased need to continue with middle and high school interventions.
- A 2001 study found that activity levels in students increased in school-based interventions involving supervision and access to recreational facilities (Sallis et al. 2001). Also, studies have shown that programs aimed at improving student participation in physical activity generally have positive results (Carrel et al. 2005). For example, one study of twenty-four high schools offering a Lifestyle Education and Activity Program (LEAP) resulted in increased activity among girls (Pate et al. 2005).

Arkansas: Breaking New Ground in Childhood Obesity Strategies

In 2003, Arkansas passed a comprehensive act to address childhood obesity. One component of the law required the annual measurement and confidential reporting of each student's BMI to his or her parents (Arkansas Center for Health Improvement 2005). During the 2004–2005 school year, 98 percent of public schools participated in the program. Thirty-eight percent of public school students were found to be overweight and at risk for obesity. The law also required every school district to create a school nutrition and physical activity advisory committee to develop policies and programs to address obesity.

Example of Action: The Alliance for a Healthier
Generation Works with Industry to Create Voluntary
Guidelines for Eliminating Sugary Drinks from Schools

In May 2006, the Alliance for a Healthier Generation, a partnership between the William J. Clinton Foundation and the American Heart Association, collaborated with the American Beverage Association and representatives of the three largest beverage distributors, Coca-Cola, PepsiCo, and Cadbury Schweppes, to combat the nation's childhood obesity epidemic by eliminating the sale of sugary drinks in schools. The initiative has the potential to help nearly 35 million students lead healthier lives by establishing guidelines in elementary, middle, and high schools across the country that would limit available beverages to the following (Clinton Foundation 2006):

Elementary Schools:

- Bottled water
- Up to 8-ounce servings of milk and 100-percent juice
- Low-fat and nonfat regular and flavored milk with up to 150 calories per 8 ounces
- 100-percent juice with no added sweeteners and up to 120 calories per 8 ounces

Middle School:

- Same as elementary school, except juice and milk may be sold in 10-ounce servings

High School:

- Bottled water
- No- or low-calorie beverages with up to 10 calories per 8 ounces
- Up to 12-ounce servings of milk, 100-percent juice, light juice, and sports drinks
- Low-fat and nonfat regular and flavored milk with up to 150 calories per 8 ounces
- 100-percent juice with no added sweeteners and up to 120 calories per 8 ounces
- Light juices and sports drinks with no more than 66 calories per 8 ounces
- At least 50 percent of beverages must be water or no- or low-calorie options

The above guidelines are to remain in effect before and after school hours when child care programs, clubs, arts, and athletic practices take place. The goal of the initiative is to implement these guidelines in 75 percent of schools by summer 2008 and in all schools by summer 2009. Success of implementation, however, is dependent upon the individual states, schools districts, and schools, as compliance with the guidelines is voluntary (from http://healthiergeneration.org/beveragekit/).

American Academy of Pediatrics' (2006) Physical Activity Guidelines

- *Infants and toddlers* should be "allowed to develop enjoyment of outdoor physical activity and unstructured exploration."
- *Preschool children (ages four to six)* should take part in "free play" and "be encouraged with an emphasis on fun, playfulness, exploration, and experimentation."
- *Elementary school children (ages six to nine)* should "improve their motor skills, visual tracking, and balance. Parents should continue to encourage free play. . . . Organized sports (soccer, baseball) may be initiated. . . ."

- *Middle school children (ages ten to twelve)* should "focus on enjoyment with family members and friends. . . .Emphasis on skill development and increasing focus on tactics and strategy as well. . . ."
- *Adolescents* should focus on activities that they and their friends enjoy, which is "crucial for long-term participation. Physical activities may include personal fitness preferences (e.g., dance, yoga, running), active transportation (walking, cycling), household chores, and competitive and non-competitive sports" (American Academy of Pediatrics 2006).

In addition to state initiatives, the CDC provides federal support to a number of school-based obesity initiatives. The agency has established a Coordinated School Health Program, which is a model for how to integrate a range of school and community efforts. These include physical education; health education; health services; nutrition services; counseling, psychology, and social services; encouraging healthier school environments; providing health promotion for school staff; and family and community involvement.

In addition, the CDC has created a School Health Index self-assessment and planning guide for schools; has developed a Physical Education Curriculum Analysis Tool in partnership with physical education experts across the country; and administers two surveys—School Health Policies and Programs Study and School Health Profiles—related to children's health in schools.

The CDC also awards Division of Adolescent and School Health (DASH) "cooperative agreement" funds to twenty-three states to support state and local efforts. The U.S. Department of Education is the lead agency for these cooperative agreements, which average $411,000, and works with state departments of health to strengthen school-based policies and programs that address obesity and chronic disease. The DASH grants support the planning and coordination of school-based programs that address all aspects of health in a school, including physical education and other physical activities, nutritional services, and health education; the implementation of the school health guidelines that address physical activity and healthy eating; statewide assessments of critical health behaviors that contribute to obesity and overweight in youth; local-level assessment of school health programs; the building of effective partnerships among state-level governmental and nongovernmental agencies in support of school health programs and policies; and the establishment of a state technical assistance and resource plan for school districts and schools.

4. Public Education Campaigns Aimed at Encouraging Better Nutrition and Activity

Acknowledging that marketing can be a strong vehicle for influencing attitudes and behavior, groups ranging from the Federal Trade Commission (FTC) to the IOM have issued reports encouraging the use of social marketing practices to promote healthier behaviors (e.g., increased physical activity) in children and youth (FTC 2006; IOM 2006).

Example of a Public Education Campaign Focused on "Tweens": VERB

To help address youth activity concerns and make use of marketing strategies, the CDC in 2001 created and funded a five-year, multiethnic, multimedia campaign called VERB for youth ages nine to thirteen to encourage more physical activity and increase awareness about the importance of exercise (Wong et al. 2004). In fiscal year 2006, VERB funding was zeroed out by Congress, eliminating the program.

A 2005 evaluation of the program found the following:

- Seventy-four percent of children knew about the campaign.
- Several subgroups of children—including perhaps those most at risk, "children from urban areas that were densely populated" and those whose activity was already quite low—demonstrated positive effects from the campaign, including "more median weekly sessions of free-time physical activity than did children who were unaware of VERB."
- As awareness of VERB increased, so did activity levels.
- Nine- and ten-year-olds who knew about the VERB campaign had 34 percent more activity sessions per week than those who did not know about the campaign (http://www.cdc.gov/youth campaign/research/outcome.htm).

5. Limiting the Marketing of Food to Children

Marketing food to children has been a controversial subject since the 1970s. In 1974, the food and marketing industries created a self-regulating Children's Advertising Review Unit (CARU) of the Council of Better Business Bureaus. A joint 2005 workshop and 2006 report by the FTC and the U.S. Department of Health and Human Services (HHS) on marketing food and beverages to children provided recommendations that continue to support CARU's self-policing strategy, stressing a hope that the food and marketing industries will offer more nutritious products with improved packaging to align with nutrition recommendations and to provide consumers with more detailed nutrition information (FTC 2006).

A 2006 IOM report also suggests that the food and beverage industries and restaurants should encourage healthier diets for children and youth through advertising and should work with the government, interest groups, and schools to improve marketing practices. The IOM report also suggests that government should use taxes, incentives, and subsidies to encourage better marketing practices among these industries, and that if self-regulation does not produce adequate change, legislation and regulation should be used. The report adds that a government agency should be funded and created to monitor and report on marketing practices. A number of companies have undertaken self-regulation efforts over the past year, including Kraft Co., Kellogg Co., and Walt Disney Co. In addition, in July 2007 a number of companies announced new self-restriction policies for marketing to children under age twelve, including Coca-Cola Co., McDonalds Corp., PepsiCo, General Mills Inc., Campbell Soup Co., Hershey Co., Unilever, Masterfoods USA, Kraft Foods Inc., and Cadbury Adams (Associated Press 2007). Decisions about voluntary restrictions vary on a company by company basis. For example, General Mills announced it will limit advertising of Trix cereal to children under age twelve but will not limit marketing of Cocoa Puffs, which has less than one gram of sugar per serving. As another example, PepsiCo, which owns Frito-Lay, Quaker Foods, Pepsi, and Gatorade, will only advertise two of its products to children under twelve, Baked Cheetos Cheese Flavored Snacks and Gatorade drinks (PepsiCo 2007).

6. Working with Doctors and Other Health Care Providers

Studies have shown that educating doctors about providing better counseling to patients about physical activity and nutrition has been an important factor in influencing changes in patient behavior (National Center for Chronic Disease Prevention and Health Promotion 1996). Children routinely have "well-care" examinations by doctors, providing a strong opportunity for evaluation and counseling related to nutrition and activity. Heightened attention from doctors and other health care providers may be an important strategy for helping at-risk and obese children better manage nutrition and activity.

The NIH recently provided a multiyear grant to several medical schools to create a nutrition curriculum and practice guidelines called the Nutrition Academic Award (National Heart, Lung, and Blood Institute 2006). The program's goal is to "encourage development or enhancement of medical school curricula to increase opportunities for students, house staff, faculty, and practicing physicians to learn nutrition principles and clinical practice skills with an emphasis on preventing cardiovascular diseases, obesity, diabetes, and other chronic diseases" (National Heart, Lung, and Blood Institute 2006).

Research featured in the 2006 *Future of Children* regarding childhood obesity suggested that "given the magnitude of the childhood obesity problem . . . pediatricians and other health care providers are going to have to step up and take a major role in the care and health of the obese child. Successfully treating obesity will require a major shift in pediatric care" (Caprio 2006, 210).

The American Academy of Pediatrics (2006) recommended that pediatricians ask parents a variety of questions to gauge children's physical activity, such as "the number of times per week their child plays outside for at least 30 minutes" and "the number of hours per day their child spends in front of a television, video game, or computer screen."

Experts Recommend School-Based and Family-Based Focus

Trust for America's Health's August 2006 report, *F as in Fat: How Obesity Policies Are Failing in America*, included a survey of state chronic disease directors

(CDDs) to find out which overweight and obesity prevention and reduction strategies experts believe are more important and should be prioritized.

CDDs are state-government-employed experts who focus on chronic disease prevention and public health promotion. They participate in each stage of health promotion, translating research into practice, developing programs at the local level, and evaluating the effectiveness of programs. They also use their experience to work for public policies that promote the health of their communities, state, and the nation.

In June 2006, the National Association of Chronic Disease Directors (NACCD) distributed information about the survey to CDDs via e-mail. The survey was administered through the Internet service Survey Monkey (www.survey monkey.com) and was available for a period of approximately two weeks. Twenty-six out of fifty CDDs responded to the survey.

Overall, the CDDs believe that there are no "quick fixes" to the obesity epidemic and that obesity prevention and reduction strategies require a holistic and long-term approach.

The CDDs were provided with a list of potential strategies for addressing the obesity crisis. They ranked four childhood obesity policies based on which ones they believed would have the greatest impact in reducing or controlling childhood obesity. On a scale of 1 to 4, with 1 representing the policy they felt would have the greatest impact, they ranked "school-based approaches, such as increasing physical education classes, more free recess/play time, or improving the nutritional content of foods sold in schools" as the top priority, with an average score of 2.33. They ranked "public education campaigns targeting parents and primary caregivers about the importance of healthy eating and physical activity for their children" second highest, with an average score of 2.41.

They ranked "improve built environment policies to create and improve recreational opportunities in schools and the community including accessibility of sidewalks, parks, and gymnasiums" third, with an average score of 2.55. CDDs were mixed about the strategy of "work[ing] with medical doctors and other health care professionals to make sure they are providing the necessary guidance about healthy eating and exercise at routine checkups, and [to] ensure that [this guidance is] reimbursed by third party payers," which they ranked fourth, with an average score of 2.82.

In a separate question, CDDs rated strategies to counter childhood obesity on a scale of 1 to 10, with 10 representing the strategy they felt would be most helpful in combating obesity in youth. They rated "parents should role model for and teach healthy eating to their children, as well as stress the importance of physical activity" at 9.11; "schools should increase the amount of physical education" at 8.67; "meal and vending contracts in schools should mandate healthier options with maximum nutritional value, rather than the current emphasis on minimum revenues" at 8.38; and "schools should improve the quality of physical education" at 8.29.

Conclusion: Walk the Talk

Short-term approaches to countering obesity have been repeatedly shown to fail over time. On the individual level, successful obesity intervention strategies incorporate dietary and physical activity changes into daily life on a permanent and ongoing basis. This requires a lifelong, comprehensive commitment to behavioral change. On the broader, public health level, efforts must focus on the long term as well. This requires the political will to provide enough funding to adequately support the development, implementation, and ongoing evaluation of large-scale obesity intervention studies (see Brescoll 2008).

Many segments of our society have an important role to play in antiobesity efforts. Individuals, families, communities, local governments, states, schools, employers, industry, and the federal government all have the opportunity, if not the direct responsibility, to recognize the costs and consequences of obesity—and the savings and benefits of health.

Many segments of our society have an important role to play in antiobesity efforts. Individuals, families, communities, local governments, states, schools, employers, industry, and the federal government all have the opportunity, if not the direct responsibility, to recognize the costs and consequences of obesity—and the savings and benefits of health.

Addressing such a pervasive social issue is challenging and may seem overwhelming. However, with the number of Americans—adults and children—facing obesity-related health problems, the problem is too important to ignore. Current efforts, however, are often limited in scope and resources.

A number of promising strategies to combat obesity based on recommendations from experts in the field are emerging, but much more needs to be done. Results from Trust for America's Health's CDD survey suggest that strategies must focus on supporting lifelong lifestyle changes and working with communities to help make it easier for people to make these changes in their lives. Public health experts must help policymakers to better identify specific, practical strategies that are both proven and cost-effective.

Additional research is needed to identify evidence-based interventions and best practices guidelines for programs. Results from current studies and Trust for America's Health's CDD survey call for additional resources for "translational" research that helps inform and improve long-term, community-based approaches.

However, while the need for translational research is critical, the nation cannot wait for the outcome of these studies to ramp up our efforts against obesity. The impact of obesity on the current population and the continuing rise in obesity rates, particularly among children, require the nation to take action now, based on the best evidence and practices that are currently known, and as more research is conducted.

References

American Academy of Pediatrics, Council on Sports Medicine and Fitness and Council on School Health. 2006. Active healthy living: Prevention of childhood obesity through increased physical activity. *Pediatrics* 117 (5): 1834-42.

Anderson, P. M., and Kristin F. Butcher. 2006. Childhood obesity: Trends and potential causes. *Childhood Obesity* 16 (1): 19-45.

Arkansas Center for Health Improvement. 2005. The 2005 Arkansas Assessment of Childhood and Adolescent Obesity, executive summary. http://www.achi.net/BMI_Info/Docs/2005/Results05/2005%20Executive%20Summary%20for%20the%20Web.pdf (accessed May 7, 2006).

Associated Press. 2007. Limiting junk food ads aimed at kids. http://www.azcentral.com/business/articles/0718biz-nokidads18-ON.html (accessed July 23, 2007).

Associated Press Online. 2003. Obstacles in way of health school lunch. December 7. [No longer available online]

Baughcum, A. E., K. A. Burklow, C. M. Deeks, S. W. Power, and R. C. Whitaker. 1998. Maternal feeding practices and childhood obesity. *Archives of Pediatrics & Adolescent Medicine* 152 (10): 1010-14.

Berkowitz, R. I., V. A. Stallings, G. Maislin, and A. J. Stunkard. 2005. Growth of children at high risk of obesity during the first 6 years of life: Implications for prevention. *American Journal of Clinical Nutrition* 81:140-46.

Birch, L. B. 2006. Child feeding practices and the etiology of obesity. *Obesity* 14:343-44.

Brescoll, Victoria L., Rogan Kersh, and Kelly D. Brownell. 2008. Assessing the feasibility and impact of federal childhood obesity policies. *Annals of the American Academy of Political and Social Science* 615: 173-89.

Burdette, H. L., and R. C. Whitaker. 2006. Maternal infant-feeding style and children's adiposity at 5 years of age. *Archives of Pediatrics & Adolescent Medicine* 160 (4): 513-20.

Caprio, S. 2006. Treating child obesity and associated medical conditions. *Childhood Obesity* 16 (1): 209-24.

Carrel, A. L., R. R. Clark, S. E. Peterson, B. A. Nemeth, J. Sullivan, and D. B. Allen. 2005. Improvement of fitness, body composition, and insulin sensitivity in overweight children in a school-based exercise program. *Archives of Pediatrics and Adolescent Medicine* 159:963-68.

Center for Health and Health Care in Schools. 2005. USDA cautions on school food contracts. http://www.healthinschools.org/ejournal/2005/jan1.htm (accessed May 6, 2006).

Clinton Foundation. 2006. Press release: Alliance for a Healthier Generation—Clinton Foundation and American Heart Association—and Industry leaders set healthy school beverage guidelines for U.S. schools. http://www.clintonfoundation.org/050306-nr-cf-hs-hk-usa-pr-healthy-school-beverage-guidelines-set-for-united-states-schools.htm (accessed May 3, 2006).

Cotterill, R. W., and A. W. Franklin. 1995. *The urban grocery store gap.* Storrs: Food Marketing Policy Center, University of Connecticut.

Datar, A., and R. Sturm. 2006. Childhood overweight and elementary school outcomes. *International Journal of Obesity* 30:1449–60.

Dearry, A. 2004. Editorial: Impacts of our built environment on public health. *Environmental Health Perspectives* 112 (1): A600-601.

Dietary Guidelines for Americans. 2005. U.S. Department of Health and Human Services, U.S. Department of Agriculture. http://www.health.gov/dietaryguidelines/dga2005/document/default.htm.

Dietz, W. H. 1998. Health consequences of obesity in youth: Childhood predictors of adult disease. *Pediatrics* 101 (3): 518-25.

Dunn, C., C. Thomas, D. Ward, K. Webber, C. Cullitan, and L. Pegram. 2006. Design and implementation of a nutrition and physical activity curriculum for child care settings. *Chronic Disease* 3 (2): A58.

Economic Research Service, U.S. Department of Agriculture. 1999. Rural poor's access to supermarkets and large grocery stores. *Family Economics and Nutrition Review* 12 (3): 90.

Federal Trade Commission. 2006. Perspectives of marketing, self-regulation, and childhood obesity: A report on a joint workshop of the Federal Trade Commission and the Department of Health and Human Services. http://www.ftc.gov/os/2006/05/PerspectivesOnMarketingSelf-Regulation&ChildhoodObesityFTCandHHSReportonJointWorkshop.pdf (accessed May 7, 2006).

Fisher, J. O., B. J. Rolls, and L. L. Birch. 2003. Children's bite size and intake of an entrée are greater with large portions than with age-appropriate or self-selected portions. *American Journal of Clinical Nutrition* 77:1164-70.

The Food Institute Report. 2004. *School lunch prices on the rise; efforts to offer healthier food continue.* Elmwood Park, NJ: The Food Institute.

Gillman, M. W., S. Rifas-Shiman, C. S. Berkey, A. E. Field, and G. A. Colditz. 2003. Maternal gestational diabetes, birth weight, and adolescent obesity. *Pediatrics* 111 (3): 221-26.

Government Accountability Office. 2004. School meal programs, competitive foods are available in many schools; actions taken to restrict them differ by state and locality. GAO Report-04-673. http://www.gao.gov/new.items/d04673.pdf (accessed July 14, 2004).

Graff, Samantha K. 2008. First Amendment implications of restricting food and beverage marketing in schools. *Annals of the American Academy of Political and Social Science* 615: 153-72.

Hardy, L. R., J. S. Harrell, and R. A. Bell. 2004. Overweight in children: Definitions, measurements, confounding factors, and health consequences. *Journal of Pediatric Nursing* 19: 376-84.

Institute of Medicine. 2006. *Food marketing to children and youth: Threat or opportunity?* Washington, DC: National Academies Press.

Johannsen, D. L., N. M. Johannsen, and B. L. Specker. 2006. Influence of parents' eating behaviors and child feeding practices on children's weight status. *Obesity* 14 (3): 431-39.

Leviton, Laura C. 2008. The school environment. *Annals of the American Academy of Political and Social Science* 615: 37-54.

Luepker, R. V., C. L. Perry, S. M. McKinlay, P. R. Nader, G. S. Parcel, E. J. Stone, L. S. Webber, J. P. Elder, H. A. Feldman, C. C. Johnson, et al. 1996. Outcomes of a field trial to improve children's dietary patterns and physical activity. The Child and Adolescent Trial for Cardiovascular Health, CATCH Collaborative Group. *Journal of the American Medical Association* 275 (10): 768-76.

McGarvey, E., A. Keller, M. Forrester, E. Williams, D. Seward, and D. E. Suttle. 2004. Feasibility and benefits of a parent-focused preschool child obesity intervention. *American Journal of Public Health* 94 (9): 1490–95.

Myles, F. S., S. Heshka, K. L. Keller, B. Sherry, P. E. Matz, A. Pietrobelli, and D. B. Allison. 2003. Maternal-child feeding patterns and child body weight. *Archives of Pediatrics & Adolescent Medicine* 157 (9): 926-32.

Nader, P. R., E. J. Stone, L. A. Lytle, C. L. Perry, S. K. Osganian, S. Kelder, L. S. Webber, J. P. Elder, D. Montgomery, H. A. Feldman, M. Wu, C. Johnson, G. S. Parcel, and R. V. Luepker. 1999. Three-year maintenance of improved diet and physical activity. The CATCH cohort. *Archives of Pediatrics and Adolescent Medicine* 153 (7): 695-704.

National Center for Chronic Disease Prevention and Health Promotion, U.S. Centers for Disease Control and Prevention. 1996. *Physical activity and health: A report of the Surgeon General.* http://www.cdc.gov/nccdphp/sgr/sgr.htm (accessed May 7, 2007).

National Health and Nutrition Examination Survey (NHANES), National Center for Health Statistics, U.S. Centers for Disease Control and Prevention. 2005-2006. Data sets and related documentation. http://www.cdc.gov/nchs/about/major/nhanes/datalink.htm (accessed May 20, 2006).

National Heart, Lung, and Blood Institute, National Institutes of Health. 2006. About the Nutrition Academic Award Program. http://www.nhlbi.nih.gov/funding/training/naa/about.htm (accessed May 8, 2006).

National Institutes of Diabetes and Digestive and Kidney Diseases (NIDDK), National Institutes of Health. 2005. Do you know the health risks of being overweight? Weight Control Network. http://win.niddk.nih.gov/publications/health_risks.htm (accessed June 6, 2005),

Nelson, J. C. K. Carpenter, and M. A. Chiasson. 2006. Diet, activity, and overweight among preschool-age children enrolled in the Special Supplemental Nutrition Program for Women, Infants, and Children (WIC). *Preventing Chronic Disease* 3 (2): 1-12.

Nielsen, S. J., and B. M. Popkin. 2003. Patterns and trends in food portion sizes, 1977-1998. *Journal of the American Medical Association* 289 (450): 3.

Owen, C. G., R. M. Martin, P. H. Whincup, G. D. Smith, and D. G. Cook. 2005. Effect of infant feeding on the risk of obesity across the life course: A quantitative review of published evidence. *Pediatrics* 115 (5): 1367-77.

Pate, R. R., K. A. Pfeiffer, S. G. Trost, P. Ziegler, and M. Dowda. 2004. Physical activity among children attending preschool. *Pediatrics* 114 (5): 1258-63.

Pate, R. R., D. S. Ward, R. P. Saunders, G. Felton, R. K. Dishman, and M. Dowda. 2005. Promotion of physical activity among high-school girls: A randomized controlled trial. *American Journal of Public Health* 95 (9): 1582-87.

PepsiCo. 2007. PepsiCo strengthens marketing practices to children. http://www.prnewswire.com/cgi-bin/stories.pl?ACCT=104&STORY=/www/story/07-18-2007/0004628074&EDATE= (accessed July 23, 2007).

Physicians Committee for Responsible Medicine. 2004. *2004 school lunch report card.* http://www.pcrm.org/health/reports/lunch2004_intro.html.

Potchuchuki, M. 2003. *Attracting grocery store retail investment to inner-city neighborhoods: Planning outside the box.* Detroit, MI: Wayne State University.

Prevention Institute for the Center for Health Improvement. 2003. Supermarket access in low-income communities. http://www.preventioninstitute.org/nutrition.html (accessed June 2006).

Putnam, J., J. Allshouse, and L. S. Kantor. 2002. US per capita food supply trends. *Food Review.* Washington, DC: U.S. Department of Agriculture.

Pyramid Communications. 2003. *Healthy schools for healthy kids.* The Robert Wood Johnson Foundation. http://www.rwjf.org/files/publications/other/HealthySchools.pdf (accessed May 7, 2006).

Rosenberg, T. J., S. Garbers, H. Lipkind, and M. A. Chiasson. 2005. Maternal obesity and diabetes as risk factors for adverse pregnancy outcomes: Differences among 4 racial/ethnic groups. *American Journal of Public Health* 95 (9): 1545-51.

Sallis, J. F., T. L. Conway, J. J. Prochaska, T. L. McKenzie, S. J. Marshall, and M. Brown. 2001. The association of school environments with youth physical activity. *American Journal of Public Health* 91 (4): 618-20.

Serdula, M. K., D. Ivery, R. J. Coates, D. S. Freedman, D. F. Williamson, and T. Byers. 1993. Do obese children become obese adults? A review of the literature. *Prevention Medicine* 22:167-77.

Stice, E., K. Presnell, and H. Shaw. 2005. Psychological and behavioral risk factors for obesity onset in adolescent girls: A prospective study. *Journal of Consulting and Clinical Psychology* 73 (2): 195-202.

Story, M., K. M. Kaphingst, and S. French. 2006. The role of child care settings in obesity prevention. *Childhood Obesity* 16 (1): 143-68.

Summerbell, C. D., E. Waters, L. D. Edmonds, S. Kelly, T. Brown, and K. J. Campbell. 2006. Interventions for preventing obesity in children. *The Cochrane Database of Systematic Reviews* 3. Hoboken, NJ: John Wiley. http://www.cochrane.org/reviews/en/ab001871.html (accessed June 7, 2006).

Trust for America's Health. 2006. *F as in fat: How obesity policies are failing in America.* Washington, DC: Trust for America's Health.

———. 2007. *F as in fat: How obesity policies are failing in America.* Washington, DC: Trust for America's Health.

U.S. Centers for Disease Control and Prevention (CDC). 1997. Guidelines for school and community programs to promote lifelong physical activity among young people. *Morbidity and Mortality Weekly Report* 46 (RR-6): 1-36.

———. 2006. Youth risk behavior surveillance—United States 2005. *MMWR Surveillance Summaries* 55 (SS-5): 1-108.

Veugelers, P. J., and A. L. Fitzgerald. 2005. Effectiveness of school programs in preventing childhood obesity: A multilevel comparison. *American Journal of Public Health* 95 (3): 432-35.

Wadden, T. A., K. D. Brownell, and G. D. Foster. 2004. Presentation on obesity: Responding to the global epidemic. *Journal of Consulting and Clinical Psychology* 70 (3): 510-25.

Watkins, M. L., S. A. Rasmussen, M. A. Honein, L. D. Botto, and C. A. Moore. 2003. Maternal obesity and risk for birth defects. *Pediatrics* 111 (5): 1152-58.

Whitaker, R. C. 2004. Predicting preschooler obesity at birth: The role of maternal obesity in early pregnancy. *Pediatrics* 114 (1): 29-36.

Whitaker R. C., J. A. Wright, M. S. Pepe, K. D. Seidel, and W. H. Dietz. 1997. Predicting obesity in young adulthood from childhood and parental obesity. *New England Journal of Medicine* 37 (13): 869–73.

Wisconsin Education Association Council. 2004. Physical education, extracurricular sports suffer under budget strains. http://www.weac.org/News/2003-04/jun04/phyed.htm (accessed May 7, 2006).

Wong, F., M. Huhman, C. Heitzler, L. Asbury, R. Bretthauer-Mueller, S. McCarthy, and P. Londe. 2004. VERB™—A social marketing campaign to increase physical activity among youth. http://www.cdc.gov/pcd/issues/2004/jul/04_0043.htm (accessed September 27, 2007).

Wrotniak, B. H., L. H. Epstein, R. A. Paluch, and J. N. Roemmich. 2004. Parent weight change as a predictor of child weight change in family-based behavioral obesity treatment. *Archives of Pediatric & Adolescent Medicine* 158 (4): 342-47.

SECTION FOUR

Comments

Keywords: childhood obesity; public policy; research

Mobilizing to Defeat the Childhood Obesity Epidemic

By
SENATOR TOM HARKIN

Currently, the United States is confronted with a public health crisis of the first order. Nearly 15 percent of American children and teenagers are obese. Most parents do not look at their seven-year-old child and see a candidate for heart disease, diabetes, or cancer later in life. However, a quarter of children between the ages of five and ten already show the early-warning signs of heart disease. It is of great concern when experts state that today's children could be the first generation in American history to have a shorter lifespan than their parent's generation. However, it is also of great concern to me that we do not have a clear understanding on the course to tackle and prevent childhood overweight and obesity. To address these challenges, I commend the authors in this special issue on childhood overweight in *The Annals of the American Academy of Political and Social Science*, who are examining the many contributing factors that can lead to overweight or obesity among children.

Children are facing an upward battle as several factors converge to increase their odds of becoming overweight or obese. The average child encounters junk-food vending machines at

Since first being elected to the U.S. Congress in 1974 and later to the U.S. Senate in 1984, Senator Tom Harkin (D-IA) has been a leader in the effort to improve health care for Iowans and all Americans. Along with Senator Arlen Specter (R-PA), he led the effort to double funding for the National Institutes of Health. He greatly increased funding for breast cancer research and launched a national breast and cervical cancer early detection program. He is principal cosponsor of the Stem Cell Research Enhancement Act, intended to lift the current restrictions on embryonic stem cell research. And in recent years, he has led the campaign to reorient the U.S. health care system toward wellness and disease prevention.

DOI: 10.1177/0002716207308840

school. Recess and physical education have been shortened or phased out of many schools; some elementary schools have been built without playgrounds. We allow our kids to vegetate in front of TV and computer screens five or more hours a day. Kids see tens of thousands of junk-food ads every year. Why should we be surprised when the final outcomes are twin epidemics of childhood obesity and diabetes?

Well, if the *problem* is us, then the *solution* can be us, too. We need to get junk food out of our schools and provide healthier options. We need to demand physical activity and physical education during the school day. We need corporate responsibility and we need to encourage media to advertise healthier foods. And finally, we need to mobilize entire communities to focus on better nutrition, increased physical activity, and a new culture of wellness.

I believe kids are eating more junk food for at least three reasons: One, because that is the food they were brought up to eat. Two, because it is available everywhere—including public schools. And three, because it is advertised and marketed ingeniously.

The Kaiser Family Foundation and the Institute of Medicine have examined food marketing to our kids. Current estimates find that the food industry spends more than $12 billion a year on marketing through television, movies, cell phones, and the Internet. Unfortunately only 2 percent of advertising is for fruits and vegetables; the majority of advertising focuses on snacks and candy that are high in fat, sugar, and sodium. I am cautiously optimistic about the new Council of Better Business Bureaus—Children's Food and Beverage Advertising Initiative (see http://www.cbbb.org/initiative/). I hope that the industry and media companies will honor their public pledges and shift their practices. I am also hopeful that the FCC Task Force on Media and Childhood Obesity that I cochair with Senator Sam Brownback (R-KS) will develop and implement real solutions that effectively deal with this public health problem.

Government; the entertainment, food, and advertising industries; schools; parents—we all have a responsibility to wake up and confront the childhood obesity epidemic. Denial is no longer an option.

In the Senate, I have been responding on multiple fronts, aiming to restrict junk food in schools, improve school lunch quality, expand physical education, build more sidewalks in communities, and address junk-food marketing to kids.

I believe that we need further research to develop a well-validated community assessment tool to measure the barriers in communities to youth participating in physical activity. My vision is to have every community in America focused on promoting health and preventing disease—instead of just dealing with the bad consequences of obesity, diabetes, and heart disease.

I also feel the U.S. Department of Agriculture needs to update its nutrition standards and apply them everywhere on school grounds, not just in the cafeteria. This would finally give us a tool to fight back against the junk-food invasion in our public schools.

In addition, we need incentives to help create more sidewalks and bike paths and to improve pedestrian and bicycle safety. We need to encourage federal, state, and regional agencies that receive federal transportation funding to incorporate pedestrian and bicycle safety measures when communities are built or modernized.

In the 2002 farm bill, I initiated the Fresh Fruit and Vegetable Program, which distributes fruits and vegetables, free of charge, to pupils in classrooms and elsewhere on school grounds. We began with one hundred schools in four states and one Indian reservation, and the program was a huge success. In 2004, the program was expanded to four more states and two more Indian reservations. My goal is to expand this program so that every state can participate.

Late in her life, Jackie Kennedy Onassis said, "If you bungle raising your children, I don't think whatever else you do well matters very much." The United States is a nation of unprecedented wealth and power. But I fear that, in so many respects, we are botching the raising of our children. We are cutting out opportunities for them to be physically active, serving unhealthy foods in schools, and advertising unhealthy foods on television, Web sites, and cell phones, to name a few. Very often, this is all being done to make money.

We must demand better from corporate America, from our schools, and from ourselves. Beyond re-creating America as a wellness society, we need to become a nation that cares passionately about the health and well-being of its children— a nation that will move mountains to defeat the twin epidemic of childhood obesity and diabetes.

Keywords: childhood overweight; childhood obesity; diabetes; public policy; media

As a nation, we must confront the epidemic increase in childhood obesity rates. As we seek innovative ways to protect the health and vitality of our young people, we usher in a new, and much-needed, era of cooperation between consumers, industry, health advocacy organizations, and media companies.

For several years, research has indicated that childhood obesity is on the verge of becoming an epidemic. In the last thirty years, the rate of overweight and obese children has risen to 16 percent, which is a 300 percent increase. The U.S. Surgeon General has identified being overweight and obese as one of the fastest growing causes of disease and death in America. Perhaps even more alarming, a recent study shows that, for the first time in modern history, the life expectancy of younger generations may decrease by as much as five years due to excessive weight.

In 2007, the Institute of Medicine (IOM) issued nutrition standards for foods in schools (see http://www.iom.edu/CMS/3788/30181/42502 .aspx). Congress directed the Centers for Disease Control, in partnership with the IOM,

Confronting Childhood Obesity

By
SENATOR SAM
BROWNBACK

Senator Sam Brownback (R-KS) has been a radio broadcaster, attorney, teacher, and administrator. He was elected to the House of Representatives in 1994. In 1996, he was elected to the U.S. Senate seat held by Bob Dole. In the U.S. Senate, he serves on the Appropriations, Judiciary, and Joint Economic Committees. He is the Ranking Member on the Joint Economic Committee, the Financial Services and General Government Appropriations Subcommittee, as well as the subcommittee responsible for the Constitution. He also cochairs the FCC Task Force on Media and Childhood Obesity with Senator Tom Harkin (D-IA), cochairs the Senate Cancer Coalition and the Human Rights Caucus, chairs the Senate Values Action Team, and is a founding member of the Senate Fiscal Watch Team.

DOI: 10.1177/0002716207308894

to review and generate recommendations outlining appropriate nutritional standards that could be used by schools when evaluating food services.

The study found that if competitive foods, such as name-brand snacks, are available for sale in a school, then fruits, vegetables, whole grains, and nonfat or low-fat milk and dairy products should also be made available. In addition, the IOM outlined that these products should also meet the 2005 Dietary Guidelines for Americans, which were designed to help children and adolescents develop healthful eating habits.

The negative health effects associated with obesity will not only affect our children's physical health but also their financial well-being. Currently, the cost of treating diabetes is $132 billion per year; we can only expect this figure to grow substantially as the number of cases of Type 2 diabetes rises. Already, an estimated 2 million children from ages twelve to nineteen have a prediabetic condition that is linked to obesity and inactivity.

Inactivity is another leading cause in the rise of childhood obesity. Children under the age of six spend almost two hours every day watching television, using computers, and playing video games. A recent Kaiser Family Foundation study found that children eight and older spend nearly six and a half hours a day consuming media. Our children live in a media-saturated environment. Every minute a child spends watching television, using the Internet, or playing video games is time in which he or she could instead exercise or practice other healthy habits.

As a father of five children, I understand the difficulty in limiting the time children spend with electronic media. However, we must encourage physical activity for the added health benefits that result from an active lifestyle. I firmly believe that if we are to end childhood obesity in this country, we must encourage our children to limit time spent on sedentary activities.

Limiting the amount of media our children consume would also limit the amount of food marketing to which our children are exposed. A recent study found that companies spend $15 billion per year on marketing and advertising to children under the age of twelve. This is twice the amount spent just ten years ago. Furthermore, the average child annually sees approximately forty thousand television ads; collectively children influence $500 billion in annual spending on advertised products, including food.

Clearly we must find ways to expose our children to healthier messages. That is why I joined Senator Tom Harkin (D-IA), Federal Communications Chairman Kevin Martin, and Federal Communications Commissioners Debbie Tate and Michael Copps to announce the formation of the FCC Task Force on Media and Childhood Obesity: Today and Tomorrow.

This voluntary task force has brought together individuals from the public and private sectors to address childhood obesity. In September 2007, the FCC Task Force issued a report to outline its proposal on how all sectors of our society—business, media, consumer, health organizations, and parents—can unite to end childhood obesity. I firmly believe that a voluntary solution is the best solution for this country.

Already we are seeing great strides from a number of companies that have voluntarily reduced the amounts of food products high in salt, fat, sugar, and calories marketed to our youth. Companies that participate in the Council of Better Business Bureaus (CBBB) Food and Beverage Advertising Initiative have already committed to voluntary restrictions on promoting products that do not meet certain nutrition guidelines to youth under twelve years old. This is a tremendous step forward in stemming the tide in the fight against childhood obesity.

I anticipate that like the CBBB initiative, the FCC Task Force will in fact build upon this great work and move industry, parents, and consumer and health advocacy organizations in a consolidated and cohesive effort in addressing the factors that contribute to childhood obesity.

Clearly, no single factor contributes to the growing obesity epidemic; likewise, no single "silver bullet" will end this very serious health issue. It will take our collective efforts to address this matter. Together, we can win the war against childhood obesity. Together, we can ensure the health and vitality of our nation. And together, we can make a lasting and positive difference in the life of every child in America.

Keywords: children; obesity; interventions; environment; social movement

What Can We Do to Control Childhood Obesity?

By
WILLIAM H. DIETZ
and
THOMAS N. ROBINSON

This issue of *The Annals* focuses on childhood obesity. Obesity now affects 18 percent of U.S. children and adolescents (Ogden et al. 2000). Among children and adolescents, as for adults, African American and Mexican American populations are disproportionately affected. Although only 25 percent of adult obesity begins in childhood, childhood-onset obesity that persists into adulthood is associated with more severe adult obesity than obesity that begins in adulthood (Freedman et al. 2001). Estimates from the Bogalusa Heart Study indicate that 50 percent of adults with a body mass index (BMI) greater than 40 (approximately one hundred pounds overweight) became obese before the age of eight (D. S. Freedman, unpublished data). Furthermore, the risk factors for adult disease are already present in childhood. For example, 60 percent of five- to ten-year-old children have at least one additional risk factor for cardiovascular disease, and 25 percent have two or more (Freedman et al. 1999). Because the diseases associated with obesity account for 25 percent of the increases in medical costs that have occurred since 1989 (Thorpe et al. 2004), the rapidly increasing prevalence of childhood obesity and its disproportionate impact on severe obesity in adulthood emphasize the need to develop appropriate preventive and therapeutic methods for children and adolescents.

The articles in this volume address the impact of a variety of environments on childhood obesity. Almost no environment exists that does not promote increased food intake or

NOTE: The findings and conclusions in this report are those of the authors and do not necessarily represent the views of the Centers for Disease Control and Prevention.

DOI: 10.1177/0002716207308898

ANNALS, *AAPSS*, 615, January 2008

inactivity. It follows from this observation that many creative opportunities exist to positively influence children's eating and activity behaviors in and across all of these environments. New policies for daycare centers, schools, and communities can be crafted and used to reconfigure environments to improve nutrition and increase physical activity. Like other examples of diseases linked to complex behaviors, it seems unlikely that the epidemic of obesity will respond to single interventions. One notable effort to apply multiple strategies simultaneously to improve nutrition and reduce inactivity is reflected in an amendment to the New York City Health Code that took effect in January 2007. The regulation, which applies to group day-care, reflects many of the most promising strategies for addressing childhood obesity (American Medical Association 2007), including allowing no television, video, or other screen viewing for children less than two years old; limiting viewing to sixty minutes per day of educational programs or programs that actively engage child movement for children older than two; requiring sixty minutes of physical activity daily; eliminating sugar-sweetened beverages; and providing low- or no-fat milk. No evaluation of the impact of this regulation is yet available.

Many creative opportunities exist to positively influence children's eating and activity behaviors in and across all of these environments.

As the reader of this issue of *The Annals* will quickly conclude, the many changes likely required in multiple environments to control childhood obesity

William H. Dietz, MD, PhD, is the director of the Division of Nutrition, Physical Activity, and Obesity at the Centers for Disease Control and Prevention (CDC). He is a member of the Institute of Medicine, a recipient of the Holroyd-Sherry award from the American Academy of Pediatrics (AAP) for his contributions to the field of children and the media, and the recipient of the 2006 Nutrition Research award from the AAP for outstanding research in pediatric nutrition. He has published more than 150 articles and is the editor of four books, including A Guide to Your Child's Nutrition.

Thomas N. Robinson, MD, MPH, is an associate professor of pediatrics and of medicine in the Division of General Pediatrics and the Stanford Prevention Research Center at Stanford University School of Medicine and director of the Center for Healthy Weight at Lucile Packard Children's Hospital at Stanford. He focuses on "solution-oriented" research, developing and evaluating health promotion and disease prevention interventions for children, adolescents, and their families. He is principal investigator on numerous National Institutes of Health (NIH)-funded prevention studies.

present an intimidating challenge. However, the multiple environments and causes also present a diverse set of opportunities for developing effective strategies. Like tobacco control, we believe that the necessary changes in nutrition, activity, and inactivity will likely require changes on the scale of a social movement. Based on experience with prior social movements, at least several interrelated goals must be achieved before the local changes currently under way in various settings converge to produce a unified national approach (McAdam and Scott 2005). These include the widespread perception of obesity as a threat, mobilization in response to that threat, and the connection of a variety of sectors around a common series of actions. Although obesity has received substantial attention from the media and is clearly perceived by physicians, public health practitioners, politicians, and foundations as a significant threat to health, it is uncertain whether parents and the general public perceive the threat at a level necessary to motivate a more broad-based social movement. Mobilizing the grassroots support necessary to elicit and sustain a social movement will almost certainly require a more widespread perception of obesity as a threat to families and children and greater positive beliefs about the benefits of changing the behaviors that promote obesity. Although single strategies may prevent or control obesity in a single setting or family, the experience with tobacco control suggests that multiple strategies employed in multiple settings will likely be required to achieve the population-wide changes in food intake and physical activity necessary to control the obesity epidemic. However, despite many individual efforts to change children's nutrition and physical activity in schools and communities around the country, these efforts have not yet morphed into a national interconnected network focused on common goals and strategies. Nonetheless, the intense interest in solutions to childhood obesity across multiple environments, reflected by this issue of *The Annals*, helps us move closer to the goal of a unified and coherent approach.

References

American Medical Association. 2007. *Expert committee releases recommendations to fight childhood and adolescent obesity.* http://www.ama-assn.org/ama/pub/category/17674.html.

Freedman, D. S., W. H. Dietz, S. R. Srinivasan, and G. S. Berenson. 1999. The relation of overweight to cardiovascular risk factors among children and adolescents: The Bogalusa Heart Study. *Pediatrics* 103: 1175–82.

Freedman, D. S., L. Kettel Khan, W. H. Dietz, S. R. Srinivasan, and G. S. Berenson. 2001. Relationship of childhood obesity to coronary heart disease risk factors in adulthood: The Bogalusa Heart Study. *Pediatrics* 108: 712–18.

McAdam, D., and W. R. Scott. 2005. Organizations and movements. In *Social movements and organization theory*, ed. G. F. Davis, D. McAdam, W. R. Scott, and M. N. Zald, 4–40. New York: Cambridge University Press.

Ogden, C. L., M. D. Carroll, L. R. Curtin, M. A. McDowell, C. J. Tabak, and K. M. Flegal. 2006. Prevalence of overweight and obesity in the United States, 1999–2004. *Journal of the American Medical Association* 295:1549–55.

Thorpe, K. E., C. S. Florence, D. H. Howard, and P. Joski. 2004. The impact of obesity on rising medical spending. *Health Affairs*, Jul–Dec, Suppl, Web Exclusives, W4–480–486.

SECTION FIVE

Quick Read Synopsis

QUICK READ SYNOPSIS

QUICK READ SYNOPSIS

Overweight and Obesity in America's Children: Causes, Consequences, Solutions

Special Editor: AMY B. JORDAN
The Annenberg Public Policy Center, University of Pennsylvania

Volume 615, January 2008

Prepared by Herb Fayer, Jerry Lee Foundation

DOI: 10.1177/0002716207311669

Childhood Overweight and the Relationship between Parent Behaviors, Parenting Style, and Family Functioning

Kyung Rhee, The Warren Alpert Medical School of Brown University

Background This article will explore the relationship between three levels of parental influence and its impact on dietary behaviors and the development of childhood overweight:
- specific parent feeding practices that are targeted toward the child with the intent to shape eating behaviors and intake;
- general parent behaviors that are not necessarily targeted at the child, such as food availability and parent modeling, but that also influence the development of child eating behaviors; and
- global influences like parenting style and family functioning that shape the socioemotional environment at home.

NOTE: Understanding the scope of parental influence may help to improve our efforts to prevent and treat childhood obesity.

Parent Behaviors Parents can shape their children's food preferences by exposing them to healthy foods at home and making them more easily accessible.
- Increasing the accessibility of fruits and vegetables can be helpful in increasing the consumption of these foods, particularly among children with low initial preferences for these foods.

- Helping parents increase availability and accessibility of targeted foods is important since it appears to increase the likelihood that children will eat these foods and can predict future consumption.
- Teaching parents to serve age-appropriate portions for children may be very beneficial and help children adjust their intake.

Modeling Parents can indirectly influence their children's eating habits by modeling good eating behaviors.
- The impact of modeling may also be enhanced by positive social responses that are tied to the food and eating environment.
- Unfortunately, modeling of negative behaviors can have an equally strong but opposite effect and has been associated with the development of emotional eating, snacking, and body dissatisfaction.
- Studies demonstrate that parents can indirectly shape child behaviors through modeling. Encouraging parents to adopt healthy behaviors themselves may aid in our efforts to curb childhood obesity.

Parenting Style Parenting style is the general pattern of parenting that provides the emotional background in which parent behaviors are expressed and interpreted by the child.
- It has been suggested that behavior delivered within the context of a more positive parenting style will have a different impact on the child than one delivered in a more negative parenting style.
- A positive parenting style, namely, the authoritative parenting style, is classified by high displays of sensitivity, emotional warmth, and involvement by the parent as well as high expectations and demands for maturity and self-control from the child.
  - This parenting style has been associated with positive childhood outcomes such as higher academic achievement, increased self-regulatory ability, more frequent use of adaptive strategies, fewer depressive symptoms, and fewer risk-taking behaviors.
- A critical dimension of parenting style is parental warmth and sensitivity toward the child. This dimension of maternal sensitivity is independently associated with a lower risk of child overweight by first grade.
  - Another study lends evidence to support the idea that the use of specific behavior modification strategies may be more effective when the child perceives greater involvement or warmth from the parent.

Family Functioning A broader dimension that may impact the ability of parents to control their child's weight is family functioning.
- While poor family functioning has been related to poorer adherence to treatment in families with cystic fibrosis and diabetes, its role in pediatric overweight management has not been thoroughly explored.
- Some studies suggest that families of obese children are more conflicted and less cohesive.
- Moens et al. (2007) found that parents with overweight children used more maladaptive control or management strategies regarding food than parents with nonoverweight children.

- Dysfunction in many aspects of family functioning, like managing daily routines, accomplishing tasks, fulfilling parenting roles that assist in pediatric weight control efforts, communicating with family members, and controlling child behaviors may contribute to the poor energy regulation capabilities of overweight children.
- Positive family interactions and order in the household may create an atmosphere that allows for greater acceptance by children of particular parent behaviors regarding overweight management

Conclusion   Parents not only help mold and shape specific behaviors in children but also influence their attitudes and beliefs about food and eating practices.

- Traditionally we have examined the impact of specific feeding practices on child intake and weight, but the socioemotional impact of parenting and the stability provided by effective family functioning can also play a role in the development of healthy eating behaviors.
- These larger parent-level influences interact with specific behaviors to modify their impact on childhood overweight. Understanding the impact of these more global parental influences and trying to intervene at this level may provide additional strategies to help curb childhood obesity.

NOTE: As we have seen, the impact of specific behaviors on childhood overweight must be considered within the context of the larger community and culture. It is with further understanding of these complex interactions that a more comprehensive and potentially more effective strategy can be implemented to help reduce the rates of overweight among our children.

Children's Healthy Weight and the School Environment

Laura C. Leviton, The Robert Wood Johnson Foundation

Background   This article outlines the promise and limitations of schools for preventing childhood obesity.

- While schools are unlikely to reverse the epidemic of childhood obesity by themselves, they are an important venue for prevention.
- Advocates have called for reforms to restore time spent on recess and physical education, to limit "competitive foods" (foods of little nutritional value that compete with the school breakfast and lunch), and to improve healthy offerings in the school cafeteria.
- The environmental factors in school seem readily apparent and somewhat easier to change than the many forces in communities that are contributing to the problem of childhood overweight.

School Issues There are limits to what schools can do about the obesity problem.

- Schools are often hard-pressed financially, forcing them to make choices about programs to save or cut, including physical education.

- Schools have been forced into a focus on academic achievement scores.
- School personnel often suffer from "innovation fatigue": they have seen many changes come and go.

Healthy Food

The food environments of schools are correlated with weight status—where school policies support frequent snacking and the availability of foods high in calories and fat, children's body mass index is greater.
- Two general forces affect the food environment:
  - whether the school food service follows the USDA dietary guidelines and
  - whether competitive foods are present.
- A big problem is that school districts come to rely on the revenues from competitive foods to support not only food service but also academic and extracurricular activities.

Obesity Prevention

The direct relationship between physical activity and obesity prevention is clear in the review of studies.
- Moderately intense physical activity for thirty to sixty minutes a day led to a reduction in percent body fat for overweight children and youth.
- No reduction in percent body fat for normal-weight children occurred in these studies. It is important to bear in mind that prevention means maintaining the weight of normal-weight children, so one might not expect to see a change in those with normal weight.
- Changing the school food environment—that is, the price, promotion, and availability of foods—has been found effective in changing children's choices of food during the school day.

Physical Activity

Enhanced physical education, which uses credentialed teachers, is effective in increasing children's physical activity.
- In a quasi-experiment, children receiving instruction from specialists or trained teachers were more physically active at the end of two years than were control students.
- Physical activity outside of school hours was unaffected.
- Children are generally more active at school when there is equipment such as basketball hoops, improvements in playgrounds, and supervision to organize active games.

Reducing TV Time

Television and video games may be implicated in the rise in childhood obesity, because too much time in these sedentary activities replaces physical activity and because many children snack while viewing television.

What Is Being Done?

As policy and environmental approaches are proposed and endorsed, we are seeing a familiar pattern: local initiatives are taking the lead, followed by state and federal actions.
- At the federal level, resources have been provided for some time for training and technical assistance.
- National voluntary efforts combat childhood obesity through changes in school programs and environment.
- State legislatures and departments of education have been active in the past few years in passing new laws and regulations.
- At the district level change has been slow.

QRS

Conclusion   The school environment can contribute to an overall energy balance in children's lives.
- At a minimum, schools can reverse decades of policies and environmental changes that have helped'to produce the obesity epidemic.
- Moving beyond the school walls, coordinated efforts include farm-to-school programs, safe routes that permit children to walk to school, use of the school facility by community organizations for active after school time, and a host of other efforts.
- The available evidence is that implementation is the key, and implementation is a long, hard road for any school program.

Childhood Overweight and the Built Environment: Making Technology Part of the Solution rather than Part of the Problem

Amy Hillier, University of Pennsylvania

Background   The changing nature of how children engage with their environment is one factor in the dramatic increase in childhood overweight.
- Children are engaging much less with the world outside their homes in terms of physical activity and much more in terms of eating.
- Technological innovations have contributed to these changes.
- The media expose them to highly coordinated advertising campaigns, many of which target children with junk food and sweets.
- This article reviews many innovations in combating childhood obesity, including the use of geospatial technologies, electronic food and travel diaries, digital audio players, Web sites, and cell phones.

NOTE: "Built environment" describes everything that children encounter when they step outside their door in their immediate neighborhood area.

Advertising   Children have their greatest exposure to advertising through broadcast and cable television. Much of what they see advertised is food.
- Fast-food restaurants regularly partner with movies aimed at children and advertise special promotions on TV.
- The movie industry also does promotions for fast-food restaurants.
- Outdoor advertising has become increasingly creative in how it uses technology to target groups such as children.
- Increasingly sophisticated computer, television, and audio options keep children sedentary during much of their free time while exposing them to coordinated advertising campaigns disproportionately promoting unhealthy foods.

Research Ops   All of the technological improvements in the past ten years provide limitless opportunities for researchers to advance the understanding of how children interact with the built environment and how to intervene to reduce childhood overweight.

- Geospatial technologies including geographic information systems (GIS) and global positioning systems (GPS) are increasingly used by researchers to model the built environment.
- Research studies have used GIS to measure walkability and accessibility.
- Researchers have used GPS to monitor park and trail usage and accelerometers to measure physical activity levels.

Eating and Travel Behavior

Technology is moving ahead to measure eating and travel behavior.
- The National Cancer Institute is developing a Web-based instrument called Automated Self-Administered 24-Hour Recall to assess eating behavior.
- The author hopes to develop Food and Environment Diaries for Urban Places (FED-UP), a video game–like food and travel diary that students would complete online using a map interface.
  - This program would use cell phones and GPS devices.

Improving the Built Environment

Policy makers, software companies, and government officials have found ways to use technology to reshape the built environment.
- For example, GIS and spatial modeling are being used to design healthier and more livable communities consistent with the research findings about walkability and mixed land use.
- At least two computer games have been developed to encourage healthy eating.
- A number of new technologically based games hold promise for reengaging children in physical activity and outdoors.

Solutions

So how do we find solutions for the misuse of media and technology in the fight against childhood overweight?
- Part of the answer involves a conceptualization of childhood overweight that makes children active participants in solutions.
  - We must meet children where they are, and that means understanding why they are so interested in Wii, DDR, MySpace, YouTube, cell phones, text messaging, and other technologies that distinguish their childhoods dramatically from previous generations.
- The companies that create the most successful video games, cell phones, and Web sites must be viewed as potential allies in the fight against childhood overweight.
  - It is unlikely that researchers and health advocates can develop and distribute new technologies like these on a large scale without the help of the entertainment industries.

NOTE: Ultimately, we need to help children make better choices over their life course, creating what King et al. (2002) described as "choice-enabling" environments. This means that all children need to have access to healthy foods and recreation; then we can focus on helping them to make good choices. They must see evidence that their choices can make a difference for themselves and for society, that childhood overweight is a problem, and that the problem is not intractable.

Q
R
S

Childhood Obesity Prevention: Successful Community-Based Efforts

Laure DeMattia, assistant clinical professor at the
Medical College of Wisconsin; and Shannon Lee Denney,
University of Wisconsin–Milwaukee

Background

The rates of childhood obesity have tripled since the 1960s, with more than 33.3 percent of children now at risk for obesity.

- The resulting excess weight puts children at risk for complicating diseases that are likely to persist into adulthood.
- As these overweight and obese children age, their health will continue to deteriorate and will further burden our health care system.
- While it may seem inequitable for the nation to incur the cost of prevention for what is largely considered an individual's problem, the taxpayers' current cost is astonishing at more than $117 billion per year.
- We need short-term, intermediate, and long-term evaluation to have a sustained improvement of the childhood obesity epidemic.
  - There is a greater chance of success in addressing the childhood obesity epidemic if public, private, and voluntary organizations would combine and share respective resources to create a coordinated and sustained effort.
  - One recommendation—industry, communities, and schools build partnerships with government, academia, and foundations.

Ecological Model

The Ecological Model of Childhood Overweight focuses specifically on characteristics that could affect an individual child's weight status in relation to the multiple environments in which that child is embedded.

- The first system is the individual child's genetic environment.
  - Children have different rates of growth and energy requirements, which vary by sex and age.
  - Additionally, if a child has two overweight parents in comparison to a child who does not have an overweight parent, a slight increase in dietary intake of the genetically susceptible child may show a larger increase in weight gain compared to the child with no familial obesity.
- The next system that influences a child's weight status is the family environment.
  - Neighborhood safety can influence the physical activity levels of children.
  - Living in neighborhoods without a grocery store is associated with reduced access to fresh fruits and vegetables. Increasing intake of fruits and vegetables is one way to displace energy-dense, low-nutrient foods that contribute to childhood obesity.

- American families are eating more outside their homes than any period before in history.
- According to the Growing Up Today Study, the length and exclusivity of breastfeeding is associated with reduced risk of childhood obesity.
- The Ecological Model forces us to take into account the larger community in which the child lives.
  - Studies often cite barriers to adopting healthy behaviors, such as lack of accessibility of recreational opportunities, decreased access to healthy food options, and lack of time to implement physical activity.
  - Community efforts outside of legislation are occurring at the local grassroots and academic levels.
  - Mixed use of land may help reduce obesity. Urban sprawl increases the probability of chronic disease by providing fewer opportunities for physical activity and appealing to less active people who are drawn to car-friendly areas.
  - Schools are an ideal location for education and for intervention against inactivity and poor nutritional intake.

Federal Policies   Federal policies that will help support individual behavior changes are as follows:

- Develop tax incentives for schools.
- Improve accessibility to grocery stores and farmers markets by making the sale of healthy options more lucrative.
- Introduce regulation by the Food and Drug Administration requiring that all chain restaurants place clear calorie information at point of sale.
- Promote breastfeeding and protect a mother's ability to do so at work.
- Mandate physical activity as part of the curriculum for all students.

Starting Point   Evolving research has shown that fetal malnutrition and maternal prepregnancy obesity are placing children at a lifelong risk of obesity.

- Prenatal counseling is where we need to start.
- Following up in the postnatal time period will potentially help parents learn about appropriate portion size and food choice.
- Targeting lower-income and overweight mothers for weight loss classes can improve the food choices of their young children.

Conclusion   Small victories to reverse childhood obesity are being realized.

- While small victories are occurring, we see a future where this generation of children may not outlive their parents.
- Research shows that early intervention and prevention are more effective and less costly than treatment of adolescent or adult obesity.
- Increasing our national investment of research dollars, policy change, program funding, and health care benefits aimed at the prevention and early intervention of childhood obesity will change the environment to support individuals' behaviors that reduce their risk of obesity.

The Effects of Food Marketing
on Children's Preferences: Testing the Moderating
Roles of Age and Gender

Ariel Chernin, Center on Media and Child Health,
Harvard University

QRS

Summary

This study examined the influence of food marketing on children's preferences and tested whether age and gender moderated the effects of ad exposure.
- There is strong evidence that commercials shape children's food preferences and short-term eating habits and increase the number of purchase requests children direct to parents.
- Results indicated that exposure to food commercials increased children's preferences for the advertised products.
- Age did not moderate this effect; younger and older children were equally persuaded by the commercials.
- Boys were more influenced by the commercials than girls.

Age

Age has been proposed as a moderator of advertising effects, with the frequent assumption that younger children are more susceptible to advertising than older children.
- Little conclusive evidence supports the assertion that younger children are more vulnerable to advertisers' messages than older children.
- Most studies have been conducted with samples that cover very narrow age ranges. Therefore, the moderating effect of age has been largely inferred from comparisons between different studies conducted with separate populations of children.
- This is problematic because differences in study design, stimuli, and measures limit one's ability to make valid inferences.
- Livingstone and Helsper (2004) tentatively concluded that older children and teenagers are more influenced by food advertising than younger children.

Discussion

This study examined the influence of commercials on children.
- Exposure to commercials significantly increased children's preferences for the advertised products.
- The products appealed equally to younger and older children, and there was no evidence of an interaction between ad exposure and age on product preference.
- Future research should examine the relationship between children's emotional responses to advertising and their preferences for advertised products, as well as the relative contributions of affective and cognitive variables in explaining persuasion outcomes.
- While age did not moderate the effects of ad exposure, there was a significant interaction between exposure to the ads and gender.

Limitations

Several limitations of the present research should be noted.
- The study was conducted with a convenience sample of children, which potentially limits the generalizability of the findings.
- Children identified their preferred cereals and drinks from images and did not actually consume the products.
- It is potentially problematic that not all of the drink options were available in stores at the time the study was conducted.
- It should be noted that the regression model explained only a small amount of variance in product preference. The model likely omitted variables that could have contributed additional explanatory power.

Conclusion

While efforts to restrict advertising to young children are well-intentioned, it has yet to be conclusively demonstrated that younger children are inherently more persuadable than older children.
- In fact, given that older children have more control over their diets than younger children, perhaps older children's responses to food marketing should be of greater concern.
- Media literacy education is a possible avenue for intervention that can be tailored to children of different ages.

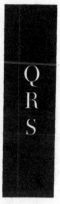

Children, Television Viewing, and Weight Status: Summary and Recommendations from an Expert Panel Meeting

Amy B. Jordan, University of Pennsylvania; and Thomas N. Robinson, Stanford University

Background

Research has indicated a wide range of factors believed to contribute to obesity among children, but of growing concern is the potential contribution made by children's media use.
- Children spend more time in TV viewing than any other home activity.
- In April 2006, an expert panel was convened to address the topic of children, television, and weight status and to do the following:
  - examine the evidence for and mechanisms underlying the television viewing/childhood weight connection,
  - identify the most promising public health strategies to diminish the negative effects of television viewing and other screen media behaviors on childhood obesity based on current knowledge and expert opinion, and
  - develop a research agenda to diminish the negative effects of television viewing and other screen media behaviors.

Causal Mechanisms

There are four hypothesized mechanisms through which television viewing may lead to childhood overweight:
- lower resting energy expenditure,
- displacement of physical activity,

- food advertising leading to greater energy intake, and
- eating while viewing leading to greater energy intake.

Interventions   The expert panel identified a number of strategies.
- Eliminate TV from children's bedrooms.
- Encourage mindful viewing by monitoring screen media watched, budgeting TV time, fostering media literacy, and making program choices for children.
- Turn off the TV while eating.
- Use school-based curricula to reduce children's screen time.
- Provide training for health care professionals to counsel on reducing children's media use.

Research   A goal of the meeting was to develop a research agenda that will best inform
Agenda   strategies to diminish the negative effects of television viewing and other screen media behaviors on childhood obesity.
- Feasibility and pilot studies are needed to assess screen media reduction strategies and interventions to reduce weight gain and/or obesity.
- Randomized controlled trials are needed to be able to infer causality and estimate effect sizes with a high degree of confidence.
  - Efficacy studies identify and explore mechanisms leading to reduced screen time and/or reduced weight gain or obesity.
  - Efficacy trials identify individual or group characteristics that define who responds more or less to various interventions.
- Another priority research area identified by the panel is developing better measures of screen media use and/or exposure.

Funding   The panel recognized that their recommendations will depend on the availability of funding.
- Research funding is particularly needed for early-stage feasibility and pilot studies and efficacy and effectiveness studies.
- Empirical evidence offers the best chances of answering questions of relevance to parents, health professionals, schools, public health professionals, and agencies and public policy makers.

Calories for Sale: Food Marketing to Children in the Twenty-First Century

Susan Linn, Harvard Medical School; and Courtney L. Novosat,
Campaign for Commercial-Free Childhood

Background   Children are targets for a maelstrom of marketing for all sorts of products, enabled by sophisticated technology and minimal government regulation.
- A significant proportion of marketing that targets children is for energy-dense, low-nutrient food.

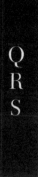

- Digital technology allows marketers to find more direct, personalized gateways to reach young audiences that sidestep parental authority and bank as much on the unknowing parent as the gullible child.
- The authors argue that parents can no longer keep pace either with innovations in advertising or increased spending, suggesting the need for tighter government regulations on food marketing to children.
- The unprecedented escalation of childhood obesity mirrors the equally unprecedented escalation of largely unregulated marketing to children.

NOTE: In 1984 the FCC "rescinded all restrictions on the amount of commercial content" in favor of a self-regulatory policy still in effect today.

Corporate Marketing

Corporations want to expose their brand in as many different places as possible, or almost anywhere children turn in the course of their day.
- Brand licensing is particularly prevalent on television and is used to fund programs aimed at children, even on public television.
- Product placement is technically prohibited by law in children's television programming but is rampant in the prime-time programs that are children's favorites—also in films and video games.
- Contests or sweepstakes targeting children are frequently partnered with films or foods along with other promotions and tie-ins.
- Marketing to a captive audience in schools is especially effective.
- Ninety-four percent of high schools, 84 percent of middle schools, and 58 percent of elementary schools allowed the sale of soda or other soft drinks on their premises.
- Advertising frequently appears on school property including corporate names and logos on educational materials and programs.
- Fund-raising involves fast-food, candy, and junk-food sponsors.

Technology

The vast array of new technologies makes it possible for companies to target children without parental knowledge or consent.
- The Internet is rife with marketing opportunities via such sites as Facebook, MySpace, and Yahoo.
- Video game example—in 2006, Burger King released three video games for multiple platforms featuring its King character.
- Cell phone example—Frito-Lay created an integrated marketing approach to promote Black Pepper Jack Doritos using text messaging, billboards, and the Internet alongside TV and radio spots.

Family Stress

The sheer volume of marketing targeted at children is stressful for families.
- Corporations often undermine parental authority by encouraging children to nag. They inundate children with images that tend to portray adults as incompetent, mean, or absent.

Regulation

There is a call for increased regulation of food marketing to children. The current administration, however, is philosophically opposed to regulation.
- We need significant grassroots pressure from advocacy groups.
- Warnings or idle threats are insufficient; only an "on the books" policy will quell the onslaught of food marketing to kids.

Q
R
S

Conclusion

The rise of childhood obesity mirrors the unprecedented increase of food marketing aimed at children.
- Companies bypass parents and target children directly in myriad ways.
- While food companies and the marketing industry tout self-regulation, the rise in childhood obesity suggests that self-regulation has failed.
- From a public health perspective, what makes the most sense is to prohibit marketing brands of food to children altogether.
- We should also question the wisdom of depending on the food and media industries to promote healthy eating to children.

Suggestions

The following are suggestions for changes in policy that would limit the amount of child-targeted junk-food marketing:
- Congress should restore to the Federal Trade Commission its full capacity to regulate marketing to children.
- The marketing and sale of brands associated with unhealthy food products in schools should be prohibited, including corporate-sponsored teaching materials.
- Corporate tax deductions for advertising and marketing junk food to children could be eliminated.
- Product placement of food brands in all media could be discouraged.
- Food companies should be prohibited from using advertising techniques that exploit children's developmental vulnerabilities.
- Licensed media characters to market food products to young children should be prohibited.
- We should support a truly commercial-free Public Broadcasting System that would provide programming for children free of any marketing, including brand licensing.

First Amendment Implications of Restricting Food and Beverage Marketing in Schools

Samantha K Graff, Public Health Law & Policy

Background

By allowing junk-food and soda companies to saturate the school atmosphere with their products and messages, schools may be helping to fuel the American childhood obesity epidemic.
- A growing movement urges public school districts to limit nonnutritious food and beverage marketing on campus.
- A school may be inhibited not only by monetary and political pressures but also by legal questions relating to the First Amendment.
- This article seeks to demystify how the First Amendment bears upon efforts to restrict food and beverage marketing in public schools.
- The article distinguishes between two First Amendment standards of review that a court could apply to a school district advertising policy—a

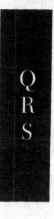

forum analysis and the commercial speech test—and argues that a forum analysis is the appropriate approach.
- The article identifies three types of advertising policies that should survive judicial review under a forum analysis.

Advertising Regulations

Under the Supreme Court's commercial speech doctrine, courts treat government restrictions on advertising as a First Amendment speech issue.

Options to Avoid First Amendment Scrutiny

The public schools could combat the rampant promotion of unhealthy food and drinks on their campuses in at least two ways without invoking First Amendment scrutiny.
- They could restrict the sale of certain categories of products without restricting advertising for such products.
- They could draft individual contracts with vendors that do not permit certain sales and advertising practices.

Possible First Amendment Legal Standards

From a First Amendment perspective, a policy limiting advertising of nonnutritious foods and beverages in public schools has two attributes: it involves a content-based government regulation on public property of advertising.
- As a result, if the policy is challenged in court, one of two First Amendment standards of review could apply: a forum analysis (focusing on the location of the speech regulation) or the commercial speech test (focusing on the type of speech being regulated).
- A forum analysis is a more lenient standard of review than the commercial speech test. It would require a school district policy to limit nonnutritious food and beverage advertising on campus to be "reasonable" and "viewpoint-neutral."

A Forum Analysis Should Apply

Plain logic, Supreme Court precedent, and Ninth Circuit precedent provide three sources of support for the conclusion that a forum analysis is the appropriate standard of review for a school district policy limiting advertising of nonnutritious foods and beverages on campus.

Conceptualizing a Policy to Survive a Forum Analysis

A school district policy limiting junk food and soda marketing has a good chance of surviving a forum analysis (i.e., of being "reasonable" and "viewpoint-neutral") if it bans:
- all advertising on campus,
- all food and beverage advertising on campus, and
- advertising on campus for those foods and drinks that are not allowed to be sold on campus.

However, a school district policy is unlikely to pass a forum analysis if it forbids advertising on campus for a category of food and drink products while simultaneously allowing the sale on campus of those same products.

Conclusion

Q R S

Marketing goods and services, including junk food and soda, to public school students results in a collision between two classic American ideals.

- On one hand, our society nurtures a belief that a public school should be a protected environment in which students learn wholesome information and skills in preparation for democratic citizenship.
- On the other hand, we believe in the free market, accepting that access to new groups of consumers, including our nation's youth, bolsters the strength of our economy.

A well-developed body of constitutional law suggests that while the First Amendment keeps a tight rein on government entities that want to restrict advertising intended for adult consumers, it gives public school districts significant leeway to curb advertising directed at their student bodies.

Assessing the Feasibility and Impact of Federal Childhood Obesity Policies

Victoria L. Brescoll, Yale University; Rogan Kersh, New York University; and Kelly D. Brownell, Yale University

Background

This article surveys national experts in nutrition and health policy on the public health impact and the political feasibility of fifty-one federal policy options for addressing childhood obesity.

- The aim of this article is to explore which childhood obesity policies are most likely to create optimal defaults for healthy eating and physical activity in children.
- Policies that were viewed as politically infeasible but having a great impact on childhood obesity emphasized outright bans on certain activities.
- In contrast, education and information dissemination policies were viewed as having the potential to receive a favorable hearing from national policy makers but little potential public health impact.
- A central need for the field is to develop the means to make high-impact policies more politically feasible.

Unhealthy Eating

In the United States, large portions, high consumption of soft drinks and high-calorie fast foods, low costs for high-calorie foods and higher costs for fruits and vegetables, limited access to healthy foods for the poor, and massive marketing campaigns targeting children are linked to poor diet, high risk for excess weight gain, and in some cases diseases such as diabetes.

- More than 17 percent of American children and adolescents are overweight or obese, with certain subgroups, such as African American youth, having even higher prevalence rates.
- This has led to increased incidences of hypertension, diabetes, and even heart attacks among obese children.

- Research has shown that the school food environment and food-related policies are associated with children's weight; snack foods, desserts, pastries, candy, and soft drinks are available in most schools.

Policy Study   One problem facing policy makers and other opinion leaders is that there is little guidance about which policy proposals would have the greatest public health impact and which would be the most politically feasible.

- Given the gravity of the problem and the potential cost of implementing these policies, it is crucial to know two basic things about these policies:
  - Their political feasibility—will they receive a favorable hearing from policy makers?
  - Their potential public health impact—what is the likelihood that they will help reduce and/or prevent childhood obesity?

The Data   Examining the policy study data qualitatively reveals five major themes.

- Policies viewed as being politically infeasible but having a great impact on obesity emphasized outright bans on certain activities.
- Nutrition labeling on menus in schools (including school vending machines and providing parents with nutritional information about school lunches) were seen as moderately feasible but low-impact relative to other policies.
- Policies in which the federal government would impose mandates on schools were generally seen as politically infeasible.
- Education and information dissemination policies, such as increasing federal funding for nutrition education, teaching healthy meal preparation and cooking skills to children, and providing nutritional information to parents about school lunches might receive a favorable policy hearing but might have little public impact.
- Increased funding for research was seen by both nutrition and policy experts as being impactful and politically feasible.

NOTE: Both nutrition and policy experts emphasized that to effectively combat childhood obesity, a wide array of these policies needs to be enacted. They also repeatedly mentioned the need to involve parents in childhood obesity policies, although this was not included in the list of policies that they evaluated. In addition, they mentioned the need to reform school lunches and expand the free fruit and vegetable program.

Conclusion   This study is a first step in outlining areas of childhood obesity legislation that seem politically plausible and genuinely significant if implemented.

- Future research should expand on this study by paring down the number of policies and performing structured interviews with a subset of nutrition and policy experts.
- It remains troubling that a commitment toward a problem as serious as childhood obesity can change so rapidly with the political winds.
- We need a dynamic approach, one in which public health and policy experts work specifically to increase the political feasibility of high-impact policies.

- The above will involve changing public opinion, creating a stronger scientific foundation for policies, and examining novel legal and legislative approaches.
- Passing impactful legislation now, such as that which has been identified in this article, can prevent profound public health problems as the next generation of American citizens develops and matures.

Generation O: Addressing Childhood Overweight before It's Too Late

Laura M. Segal and Emily A. Gadola, Trust for America's Health

Background

Because of the serious health consequences of childhood obesity, there is an urgent need to make practical decisions now to address the problem, based on common sense, the best prevailing research, and the advice of experts.
- This starts with addressing the contributing factors behind the real culprits—poor nutrition and inadequate physical activity.
- We need to develop overweight prevention and control strategies focused on instilling in children the importance of healthy behaviors.
- This article reviews policy recommendations and intervention strategies for addressing childhood overweight.

NOTE: The fight against obesity and physical inactivity must include well-funded, long-term approaches; a research agenda that emphasizes longitudinal studies; and a fresh look at what constitutes "success" and how it is measured.

School

School environments are a major influence on children's eating and activity habits, given the limited options children are given in a school setting.
- Nutrition standards of school breakfast and lunches wrongly focus on meeting minimum standards and keeping costs low.
- There has also been an influx in the availability of sodas, snack machines, and fast food on campuses and a reduction in the amount of physical education, recess, and recreation time.

NOTE: School-based efforts have focused on improving the quality of food sold in schools, limiting sales of less nutritious foods, improving physical education and health education, and encouraging increased physical activity.

Communities

The communities where children live also can either encourage or inhibit opportunities for physical activity.
- A number of trends have resulted in people being less active, including communities that foster driving rather than walking or biking, lack of public transit options, poor upkeep of sidewalk infrastructure, walking areas that are often unsafe or inconvenient, and so on.

Families   Efforts to involve families in obesity-prevention efforts are viewed by many
                  as an effective area for intervention activities.
                  • Parents need to understand the benefits of providing healthier beverage
                    options to children and encouraging more activity.
                  • A number of studies have demonstrated a connection between the weight
                    of parents, particularly mothers, and children.

Head Start   Head Start could be a rich area for future studies and interventions.

Healthy   Healthy People 2010 states that health education should include information
People 2010   about the consequences of unhealthy diets and inadequate physical activity.

Government   In addition to state initiatives, the CDC provides federal support to a num-
                  ber of school-based obesity initiatives.
                  • The agency has established a Coordinated School Health Program—a
                    model for how to integrate a range of school and community efforts.
                  • The CDC also awards Division of Adolescent and School Health (DASH)
                    "cooperative agreement" funds to twenty-three states to support state and
                    local efforts. The DASH grants support the planning and coordination of
                    school-based programs that address all aspects of health in a school.

Public   Groups ranging from the Federal Trade Commission (FTC) to the Institute
Education   of Medicine (IOM) have issued reports encouraging the use of social mar-
                  keting practices to promote healthier behaviors (e.g., increased physical
                  activity) in children and youth.
                  • In addition, the food and beverage industries and restaurants should
                    encourage healthier diets for children and youth through advertising.
                  • Government should use taxes, incentives, and subsidies to encourage better
                    marketing practices among the above industries.
                  • Also, educating doctors about providing better counseling to patients
                    about physical activity and nutrition has been an important factor in influ-
                    encing patient behavior change.
                  • Parents should role model for and teach healthy eating to their children,
                    as well as stress the importance of physical activity.

Conclusion   Short-term approaches to countering obesity have been repeatedly shown to
                  fail over time.
                  • On the individual level, successful obesity intervention strategies incorpo-
                    rate dietary and physical activity changes into daily life on a permanent
                    and ongoing basis.
                  • We need the political will to provide enough funding to adequately sup-
                    port the development, implementation, and ongoing evaluation of large-
                    scale obesity intervention studies.
                  • Individuals, families, communities, local governments, states, schools,
                    employers, industry, and the federal government all have the opportunity
                    to recognize the costs and consequences of obesity.
                  • Results from Trust for American's Health's Chronic Disease Directors
                    (CDD) survey suggest that strategies must focus on supporting lifelong
                    lifestyle changes.
                  • Public health experts must help policy makers to better identify specific,
                    practical strategies that are both proven and cost-effective.

The Content You Want, the Convenience You Need.

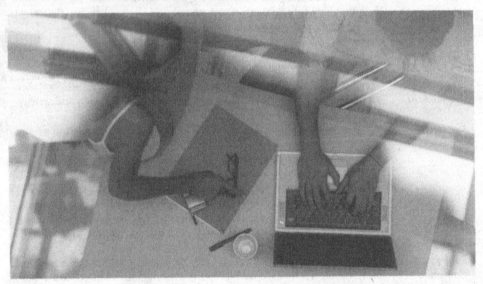

SAGE Journals Online
Online Journal Delivery Platform

SAGE Journals Online hosts SAGE's prestigious and highly cited journals and represents one of the largest lists in the social sciences as well as an extensive STM offering. The platform allows subscribing institutions to access individual SAGE journal titles and provides users with dramatically enhanced features and functionality, including flexible searching and browsing capabilities, customizable alerting services, and advanced, toll-free inter-journal reference linking.

Librarian-friendly features include
- Familiar HighWire subscription and administration tools
- Perpetual access to purchased content
- Temporary backfile access to 1999 (where available)
- Enhanced subscription options for most titles
- COUNTER-compliant reports
- User-friendly usage statistics
- Open-URL compliant
- Pay-per-view options

⑤SAGE Publications
www.sagepublications.com

⑤SAGE JOURNALS *Online*

Printed in the United States
By Bookmasters